Helicobacter Pylori Infection: Pathophysiology, Epidemiology and Management

Helicobacter Pylori Infection: Pathophysiology, Epidemiology and Management

Edited by Jordan Phillips

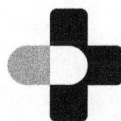

AMERICAN
MEDICAL PUBLISHERS
www.americanmedicalpublishers.com

American Medical Publishers,
41 Flatbush Avenue,
1st Floor, New York,
NY 11217, USA

Visit us on the World Wide Web at:
www.americanmedicalpublishers.com

ISBN: 978-1-63927-143-6

Cataloging-in-Publication Data

Helicobacter pylori infection : pathophysiology, epidemiology and management / edited by Jordan Phillips.
    p. cm.
Includes bibliographical references and index.
ISBN 978-1-63927-143-6
1. Helicobacter pylori infections. 2. Helicobacter pylori infections--Pathophysiology.
3. Helicobacter pylori infections--Epidemiology. 4. Helicobacter pylori
infections--Treatment. 5. Gastroenterology. I. Phillips, Jordan.
RC840.H38 H45 2022
616.330 14--dc23

Table of Contents

Preface

It is often said that books are a boon to mankind. They document every progress and pass on the knowledge from one generation to the other. They play a crucial role in our lives. Thus I was both excited and nervous while editing this book. I was pleased by the thought of being able to make a mark but I was also nervous to do it right because the future of students depends upon it. Hence, I took a few months to research further into the discipline, revise my knowledge and also explore some more aspects. Post this process, I begun with the editing of this book.

Helicobacter pylori refers to a microaerophilic bacterium that is usually found in stomach. It is generally in the shape of a helix. Its shape is developed from penetrating the mucoid lining of the stomach. It is infectious and can cause chronic gastritis, gastric ulcers and duodenal ulcers. Helicobacter pylori infection does not have major visible symptoms except minor abdominal pains and nausea. Helicobacter pylori is also associated with a wide range of diseases such as atherosclerosis, alzheimer's disease, multiple sclerosis, coronary artery disease, periodontitis, parkinson's disease, Guillain–Barré syndrome, rosacea, psoriasis, chronic urticaria, etc. It is diagnosed using invasive and non-invasive methods. Invasive means include histological examination with endoscopic biopsy and rapid urease test. Non-invasive methods involve stool antigen tests, carbon urea breath test, etc. This book unfolds the unexplored aspects related to the epidemiology and management of helicobacter pylori infection. It also provides significant information on helicobacter pylori to help develop a good understanding of its treatment. The book is appropriate for students seeking detailed information in this area as well as for experts.

I thank my publisher with all my heart for considering me worthy of this unparalleled opportunity and for showing unwavering faith in my skills. I would also like to thank the editorial team who worked closely with me at every step and contributed immensely towards the successful completion of this book. Last but not the least, I wish to thank my friends and colleagues for their support.

Editor

Helicobacter pylori infection and circulating ghrelin levels

Chidi V Nweneka[1][*][†], Andrew M Prentice[1,2][†]

Abstract

Background: The nature of the association between ghrelin, an orexigenic hormone produced mainly in the stomach, and *Helicobacter pylori (H pylori)*, a bacterium that colonises the stomach, is still controversial. We examined available evidence to determine whether an association exists between the two; and if one exists, in what direction.

Methods: We reviewed original English language studies on humans reporting circulating ghrelin levels in *H pylori* infected and un-infected participants; and circulating ghrelin levels before and after *H pylori* eradication. Meta-analyses were conducted for eligible studies by combining study specific estimates using the inverse variance method with weighted average for continuous outcomes in a random effects model.

Results: Seventeen out of 27 papers that reported ghrelin levels in *H pylori* positive and negative subjects found lower circulating ghrelin levels in *H pylori* positive subjects; while 10 found no difference. A meta-analysis of 19 studies with a total of 1801 participants showed a significantly higher circulating ghrelin concentration in *H pylori* negative participants than in *H pylori* positive participants (Effect estimate (95%CI) = -0.48 (-0.60, -0.36)). However, eradicating *H pylori* did not have any significant effect on circulating ghrelin levels (Effect estimate (95% CI) = 0.08 (-0.33, 0.16); Test for overall effect: Z = 0.67 (P = 0.5)).

Conclusions: We conclude that circulating ghrelin levels are lower in *H pylori* infected people compared to those not infected; but the relationship between circulating ghrelin and eradication of *H pylori* is more complex.

Background

The relationship between ghrelin, a 28-amino acid peptide secreted primarily by the oxyntic cells of the stomach [1] and involved in body mass regulation, and *Helicobacter pylori (H pylori)*, a bacterium that colonises the stomach, has remained controversial. The first report suggesting an association between the two was that by Nwokolo et al [2] who examined the effect of *H pylori* eradication on plasma ghrelin levels in 12 healthy adult male and female subjects. They reported that eradicating *H pylori* from the subjects was associated with an increase in plasma ghrelin levels. At about the same time, Gockel et al [3] reported that *H pylori* had no effect on plasma ghrelin levels in a study of 39 age- and BMI-matched *H pylori* positive and negative women. Subsequently a number of other papers, including animal studies, have explored this relationship [4-7]. A number of review articles have also appeared exploring this relationship [8,9]; but none of these has been conducted systematically.

Considering the putative role of ghrelin in body mass regulation, understanding this association could help in maximizing its benefits, and also provide further insight into the physiology of appetite and body mass regulation. The objective of this review is to examine available evidence to determine whether or not a relationship exists between ghrelin and *H pylori* infection; and where one exist, to investigate the direction of the association. Specifically, this review sets out to answer three questions: 1) Is *H pylori* infection associated with circulating ghrelin levels? 2) what is the effect of eradicating *H pylori* infection on circulating ghrelin levels?; and 3) what is the effect of *H pylori* infection on ghrelin producing cells in the stomach?

---

* Correspondence: cnweneka@mrc.gm
† Contributed equally
[1]Nutrition Programme, Medical Research Council Laboratories, The Gambia, P.O. Box 273, Banjul, The Gambia

Methods

Literature search strategy and data extraction

A comprehensive search of the scientific literature (Medline (OVID), OvidMedline (R) 1950 - October Week 2 plus In-process & Non-indexed citations, Embase (1980 to 2010 week 41), and ISI Web of Knowledge) was conducted using the search terms "ghrelin AND *helicobacter pylori*". The search was repeated several times. The last search was conducted on October 29, 2010. Further searches were conducted using Google scholar; while the bibliography of original and review articles were searched for studies with ghrelin and *helicobacter pylori* in their titles. Duplicate searches were first removed; thereafter, the abstracts of retrieved articles were reviewed for relevance prior to accessing the full paper. Only English-language primary studies on humans were included provided that the authors assessed at least one of the following: 1) compared circulating ghrelin concentration in *H pylori* positive and negative subjects; 2) compared the effect of eradicating *H pylori* on circulating ghrelin levels; or 3) compared gastric ghrelin in *H pylori* positive and negative subjects or changes in gastric ghrelin after *H pylori* eradication. Letters in response to published articles, commentaries, and editorials were excluded. Conference abstracts that had not been published as full papers were included where the full abstracts could be retrieved, provided that such conference abstract contained enough information for either the qualitative or the quantitative synthesis. However, where a conference abstract has been published as a full paper, the full paper was retrieved and the conference proceeding excluded.

Efforts were made to contact authors of conference abstracts whose full paper publications could not be traced to inquire if the paper had been published as a full paper and if not, to get further details about the study. Efforts were also made to contact authors of papers where some relevant information was missing to request for the missing information or for further clarifications. We contacted 18 authors [2,6,10-25]; but only nine authors [2,14, 18,21-26] responded and provided the needed information. We were unable to contact one author [27].

We also attempted to group the papers reviewed by study teams in other to assess the spread of the papers reviewed. In deciding whether different papers were published by the same research groups, similarity in authorship was examined. Where at least one author contributed to different publications, those publications were deemed to have emanated from the same research group.

Outcomes evaluated

Outcomes evaluated included: differences in circulating ghrelin levels between *H pylori* positive and negative subjects; changes in circulating ghrelin concentration after *H pylori* eradication; differences in ghrelin mRNA between *H pylori* positive and negative subjects; changes in ghrelin mRNA after *H pylori* eradication; differences in ghrelin immunoreactive cells between *H pylori* positive and negative subjects; changes in ghrelin immunoreactive cells after cure; correlation between ghrelin immunoreactive cells with severity of *H pylori* infection; correlation between gastric and plasma ghrelin; correlation between ghrelin mRNA and plasma ghrelin; and correlation between cells and plasma ghrelin.

Data synthesis

The data extracted were classified into three classes: 1) data comparing circulating ghrelin concentration in *H pylori* positive and negative subjects; 2) data comparing the circulating ghrelin concentration before and after *H pylori* eradication; and 3) data assessing any of the gastric ghrelin parameters. Each of these classes was supposed to answer a specific question (Table 1). The variables were re-coded in forms that would make analysis easier (Table 2). Table 3 lists the papers excluded from the review and the reasons for their exclusion.

Statistical analysis

Simple proportions were used to determine the frequency of occurrence of each categorical variable considered; and association between different variables assessed using Fisher's exact chi^2 test. Continuous variables like sample size and duration of follow-up was initially summarized using medians and inter-quartile ranges and later categorized as shown in Table 2. Multiple logistic regression analysis was used to assess confounding. The descriptive analysis was conducted using Stata version 8 (StataCorp LP, College Station, Texas, USA).

Meta-analysis

We conducted meta-analyses of summary statistics from individual studies that compared circulating ghrelin levels between *H pylori* positive and *H pylori* negative subjects; and for studies that compared circulating ghrelin levels before and after eradication of *H pylori*. For each study, the mean circulating ghrelin concentrations and standard deviations (sd) for the different comparison groups were used to generate standardized mean differences (SMDs) and 95% confidence intervals (95% CI) since different studies used different units to measure ghrelin concentration, and some studies measured plasma ghrelin while others measured serum ghrelin. For studies that reported standard errors of mean, standard deviation was derived using the formula provided in the Cochrane Handbook of clinical reviews: SD = SEM × √N (http://www3.interscience.wiley.com/homepages/106568753/handbook.pdf). Studies that reported only medians and 95% CI or interquartile ranges

Table 1 Research questions explored by the review

Research question	Explanatory data
Is *H pylori* infection associated with circulating ghrelin levels?	Data comparing circulating ghrelin concentration in *H pylori* positive and negative subjects
What is the effect of eradicating *H pylori* on circulating ghrelin levels?	Data comparing the circulating ghrelin concentration before and after *H pylori* eradication
What is the effect of *H pylori* infection on ghrelin expression in the stomach?	Data assessing any of the gastric ghrelin parameters

(IQR) [2,6] were not included in the meta-analysis. Table 4 lists studies excluded from the meta-analysis and the reasons for their exclusion.

Study specific estimates were combined using the inverse variance method with weighted average for continuous outcomes in a random effects model. Heterogeneity was assessed using the chi-squared method and the I^2 method described by Higgins et al [28,29]. For studies that reported different sub-groups separately [30-32] those sub-groups were included as separate papers in the meta-analysis. Chuang et al, [30] reported ghrelin levels for males and females separately. While the data for males did not increase the heterogeneity of the studies, inclusion of the data for females introduced significant heterogeneity to the analysis. All the papers that resulted in significant heterogeneity of the studies in the meta-analysis were removed from the meta-analysis. A separate meta-analysis conducted for this sub-group of excluded studies revealed a significant heterogeneity (P=0.0001; I^2 = 86%) and the effect size was very small and not significant (SMD -0.13 [-0.33, 0.06], Test for overall effect: Z = 1.36 (P = 0.17)). These papers were therefore completely excluded from the meta-analysis and described in a narrative. Sensitivity analysis was conducted to assess the contribution of each study to the pooled estimate by excluding individual studies one at a time and recalculating the pooled SMD estimates for the remaining studies. Funnel plots were used initially to assess publication bias and later confirmed using Begg's and Egger's tests. The meta-analyses were conducted using Review Manager Version 5 (RevMan 5; http://www.cc-ims.net/revman/download), while the Begg's and Egger's tests were conducted using Stata version 8 after downloading the installation files for the tests from the internet.

Results
Search results
The literature search yielded 1361 papers (404 from databases and 957 from Google Scholar) plus one unpublished paper. After removing duplicate articles, reviews, commentaries and letters (written in response to published articles), 166 papers (including one conference abstract and one unpublished paper) were left. These were further screened using titles and abstract to assess for eligibility, resulting in the exclusion of 106 articles (Figure 1). The full texts of the remaining 60 articles (excluding the conference abstract) were

Table 2 Dictionary of variables used in the review

Variable	Coding scheme
Study Team	A, B, C etc
Design	Cohort, Cross-sectional, Case control, Experimental
Healthy	Healthy only, Sick only, Both
Region	Asia, Africa, Europe, North America, South America
Gender	Male only, Female only, Both
Age	Children only, Adults only, Both
Number of methods used to assess *H pylori*	One method; two or more methods
Type of ghrelin assay used	Commercial RIA, in-house RIA, Commercial ELISA, Commercial EIA
Sample storage	-70°C and below; above -70°C
Sample type	Serum; Plasma
Weight	Normal, Low, Various, High
Difference in circulating ghrelin concentration between *H pylori* + & - subjects	Lower, no difference, higher
Changes in circulating ghrelin after cure	Increased, decreased, no change
Duration of follow-up	4 weeks & below; Above 4 weeks
Sample size	Two categorizations were done: 1) 50 & below, 51-200, 201 and above; 2) Above 20, Below 20

Table 3 Papers excluded from the review

	Reason for exclusion
Suzuki et al, 2006 [54]	Did not report ghrelin levels in *H pylori* positive & *H pylori* negative patients
Nunes et al, 2006 [27]	Not sufficient information in abstract and authors could not be contacted for further clarifications
Campana et al, 2007 [56]	All subjects were *H pylori* negative
Isomoto et al, 2005 [52]	Compared only *H pylori* strains
Checchi et al, 2007 [10]	Did not compare serum ghrelin levels in *H pylori* positive & *H pylori* negative subjects
Wu et al, 2005 [57]	Did not assess ghrelin
Shinomiya et al, 2005 [58]	Did not compare the difference in ghrelin between *H pylori* positive & *H pylori* negative subjects
Suzuki et al, 2005 [59]	Did not assess ghrelin
Sundbom et al, 2007 [60]	Did not assess *H pylori*
Huang et al, 2007 [61]	Did not assess *H pylori*
Nishizawa et al, 2006 [62]	Did not assess *H pylori*
Ando et al, 2006 [63]	Did not assess ghrelin
Kempa et al, 2007 [64]	All subjects were *H pylori* negative
Ates et al, 2008 [65]	Did not assess *H pylori*
Wang et al, 2006 [66]	Did not assess ghrelin
Doki et al, 2006 [67]	Did not assess *H pylori*
Gao et al, 2008 [68]	Excluded people with *H pylori*
Cherian et al, 2009 [69]	Did not assess ghrelin
Kebapcilar et al, 2009 [70]	Did not assess ghrelin
Dutta et al, 2009 [71]	Did not assess ghrelin
Gen et al, 2010 [72]	Did not assess ghrelin
Taniaka-Shintani et al, 2005 [1]	Examined only ghrelin immunoreactive cells

retrieved. Twenty-two papers were subsequently dropped from the review (Table 3), and another 11 from the meta-analysis (Table 4).

Is *H pylori* infection associated with circulating ghrelin levels?

Table 5 is an evidence table of studies that compared circulating ghrelin levels in *H pylori* positive and *H pylori* negative individuals. Twenty-six studies compared circulating ghrelin levels between *H pylori* positive and negative subjects. The analysis of one of the studies [30] was stratified by gender, yielding different results; this study was therefore entered into the evidence table as two separate papers with each gender representing one paper, bringing the total number of papers reviewed to 27. One paper [22] was not included in the evidence table because the grouping of the subjects studied did not permit a straight forward

Table 4 Papers excluded from the meta-analysis

Nwokolo et al, 2003 [2]	Reported median values & 95% CI; also measured integrated ghrelin levels rather than the discrete measurement that other authors used. The authors stated that the median values were used because the sample size was small and the data were skewed
Mendez-Sanchez et al, 2007 [49]	Studied ghrelin immuno-reactive cells, did not provide data on plasma ghrelin levels
Salles et al, 2006 [19]	Ghrelin values not provided. Only P-values
Gao et al, 2009 [15]	Ghrelin values not provided
Choe et al, 2007 [6]	Median & IQR provided. Further clarifications not provided by the authors
Czesnikiewicz-Guzik et al, 2005 [12]	Insufficient information for meta-analysis
Czesnikiewicz-Guzik et al, 2007 [13]	Insufficient information for meta-analysis
Masaoka et al [51]	This was a case study with only one subject
Stec-Michalska et al, 2009 [24]	Measured only gastric ghrelin
Liew et al, 2006 [47]	Assessed only gastric ghrelin
Konturek et al, 2006 [17]	The numbers of *H pylori* positive and negative participants were not provided and the authors did not respond to requests for further information.

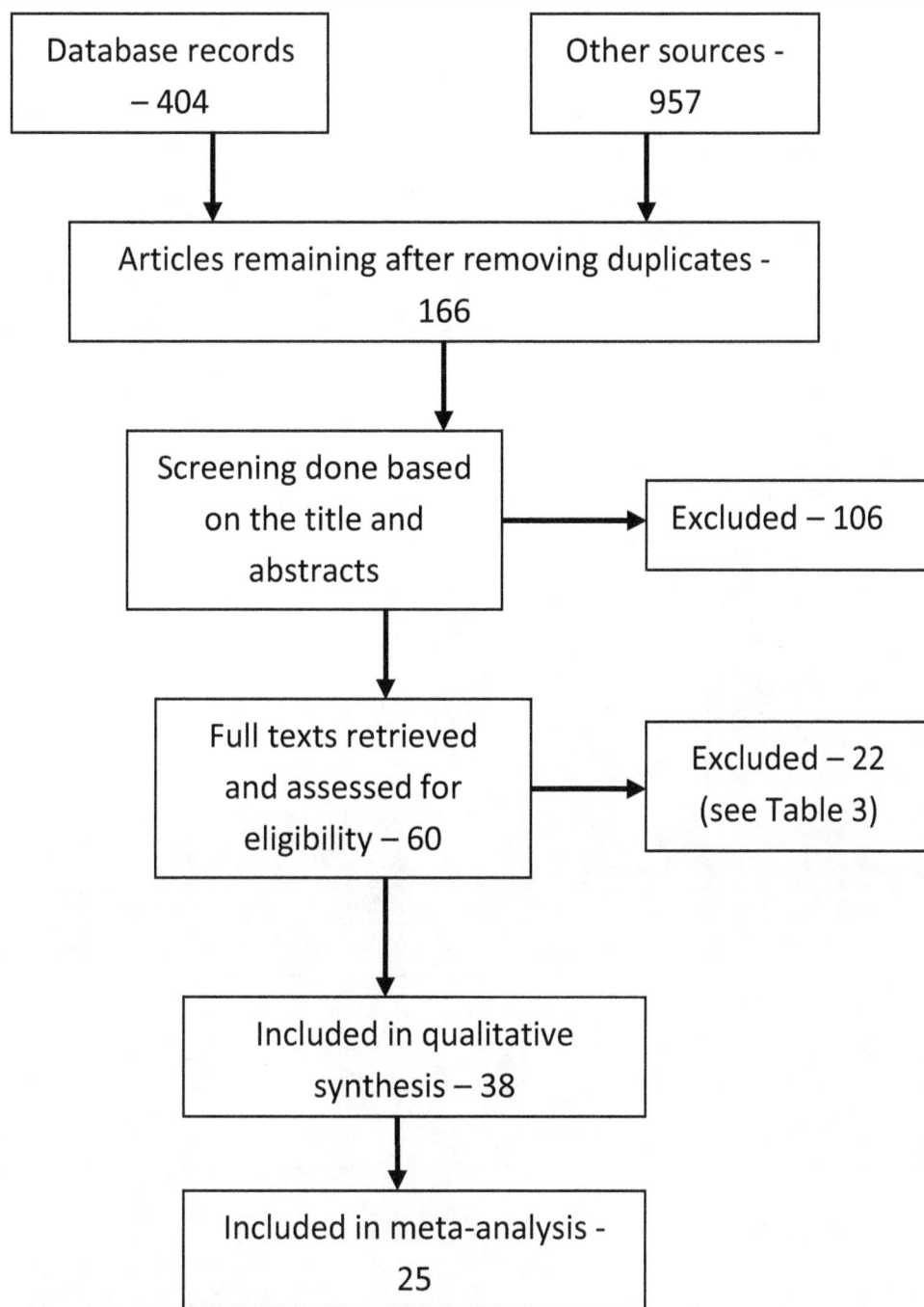

Figure 1 PRISMA flow chart showing information flow in the selection of papers for the review.

comparison of the *H pylori* positive and *H pylori* negative subjects. The paper was therefore reviewed in a separate narrative. Table 6 summarises the characteristics of the studies included in the evidence table. Most of the studies (77%) investigated both males and females, 85% studied only adults and 52% studied sick subjects mainly subjects with gastrointestinal symptoms (64.7%) and Cancer (17.65%). Thirteen (48.2%) of the studies [15,21,30,33-41] were conducted in Asia; 11 (40.7%) [3,11,12,17,19,26,31, 32,42-44] in Europe and three (11.1%) [14,18,45] in North America. Twenty-two percent of the studies reviewed were contributed by one research group alone, while Japan contributed 30% of the papers. More than two-thirds of the studies used radioimmunoassay to measure serum or plasma ghrelin, 55.6% assessed *H pylori* using two or more methods,

Table 5 Evidence table of studies that compared circulating ghrelin levels in Hp+ and Hp- individuals

Reference & Country	Study Team	Design	Healthy	Gender	Age	Method of H pylori assessment	Ghrelin assay kit	Overnight fast	Sample storage	Sample type	Weight	Sample size	Ghrelin levels in Hp+ vs Hp-
Kawashima et al, 2009; Japan [38]	A	Cohort	Both	Both	Adults	Serology	Commercial EIA	Yes	-80	Plasma	Normal	220	Lower
Plonka et al, 2006; Poland [32]	B	Cohort	Healthy	Both	Both	Modified UBT plus ELISA	Commercial RIA	Yes	-80	Serum		538	Lower
Isomoto et al, 2005; Japan [36]	C	Cohort	Sick	Both	Adults	RUT, histology (Giemsa stain)	In-house RIA	Yes	-80	Plasma	Normal	81	Lower
Roper et al, 2008; USA [18]	D	Cross-sectional	Healthy	Men	Adults	serology, histology & RUT or positive culture	Commercial EIA	Yes	-20	Serum	Normal	256	No Difference
Pacifico et al, 2008; Italy [26]	E	Cohort	Both	Both	Children	Culture of gastric specimen or histology + RUT	Commercial RIA	Yes	-70	Serum	Normal	85	No Difference
Gokcel, 2003; Turkey [3]	F	Case control	Sick	Women	Adults	Not stated	Commercial EIA	Yes	Not stated	Plasma	Normal	39	No Difference
Plonka et al, 2006; Poland [43]	B	Case control	Healthy	Both	Children	Serology and UBT	Commercial RIA	Yes	-80	Serum	Various	287	Lower
Shiotani et al, 2005; Japan [21]	G	Case control	Healthy	Both	Adults	Detection of HP IgG ab in the urine	Commercial ELISA	Yes	Not stated	Serum	Various	132	Lower
Osawa et al, 2005; Japan [40]	C	Case control	Sick	Men	Adults	Culture & histology	In-house RIA	Yes	-30	Plasma	Normal	160	Lower
Chuang et al*, 2009; Taiwan [30]	H	Cross-sectional	Sick	Men	Adults	Not described	Commercial RIA	Yes	-72	Plasma	low to normal	145	Lower
Chuang et al*, 2009; Taiwan [30]	H	Cross-sectional	Sick	Women	Adults	Not described	Commercial RIA	Yes	-72	Plasma	low to normal	196	No Difference
Alonso et al, 2007; Spain [42]	P	Cross-sectional	Sick	Both	Adults	UBT, histology (Giemsa stain)	Commercial RIA	Yes	-80	Plasma	Normal	15	Lower
Salles et al, 2006; France [19]	I	Cross-sectional	Sick	Both	Adults	UBT, serology, culture, histology & PCR	Commercial RIA	Yes	-80	Plasma	low to normal	62	Lower
Jun et al, 2007; Korea [37]	J	Cross-sectional	Sick	Both	Adults	RUT, histology (Giemsa stain)	Commercial RIA	Yes	-70	Plasma	Normal	63	No Difference
D'Onghia et al, 2007; Italy [31]	K	Case control	Both	Both	Adults	ELISA	RIA	Yes	-20	Serum	Various	79	Lower
Gao et al, 2009; China [15]	L	Case control	Healthy	Both	Adults	Serology & UBT.	Commercial RIA	Yes	-80	Plasma	Normal	100	Lower
Isomoto et al, 2005; Japan [35]	C	Cross-sectional	Sick	Both	Adults	Anti-IgG antibody, 13C-UBT, or RUT	In-house RIA	Yes	-80	Plasma	Normal	89	Lower
Isomoto et al, 2005; Japan [41]	C	Cross-sectional	Sick	Both	Adults	Serology, UBT or RUT	In-house RIA	Yes	-80	Plasma	Normal	249	Lower
An et al, 2007; Korea [33]	Q	Cohort	Sick	Both	Adults	Not stated	Commercial ELISA	Yes	-70	Plasma	Normal	41	No difference
Nishi et al, 2005; Japan [39]	C	Cross-sectional	Both	Both	Adults	Serology & UBT	In-house RIA	Yes	-80	Plasma	Normal	74	Lower
Czesnikiewicz-Guzik et al, 2005; Poland [12]	B	Cross-sectional	Healthy	Women	Adults	UBT	Not stated	Not stated	Not stated	Serum	Not Stated	100	Lower

Table 5 Evidence table of studies that compared circulating ghrelin levels in Hp+ and Hp- individuals *(Continued)*

Konturek et al, 2006; Poland [17]	B	Cross-sectional	Healthy	Both	Both	UBT & serology	Human RIA	Yes	-80	Serum	Not Stated	180	Lower
Cindoruk et al, 2007; Turkey [11]	M	Cohort	Sick	Both	Adults	Either histology or UBT	RIA	Yes	-80	Plasma	Normal	50	No Difference
Isomoto et al, 2004; Japan [34]	C	Cohort	Sick	Both	Adults	Serology	Commercial RIA	Yes	-80	Plasma	Normal	68	Lower
de Martel, 2007; USA [14]	N	Case control	Sick	Both	Adults	In-house ELISA	Commercial ELISA	Yes	-80	Serum	Various	110	No Difference
Shak et al, 2008, USA [45]	R	Cohort	Healthy	Both	Adults	Serology	Commercial EIA	Yes	-20	Plasma	Obese	24	No difference
Uzzan et al, 2007 [44]	S	Cohort	Healthy	Both	Adults	Histology	Commercial RIA	Yes	Not stated	Serum	Obese	13	No difference

* These are from the same paper reporting the same study but were separated because the analysis was stratified by gender and the results for males and females were completely different; hence the decision to separate them.

Table 6 Summary of the characteristics of the studies reviewed in Table 5

Characteristic		n	n %
Study Design	Case control	7	25.93
	Cohort	9	33.33
	Cross-sectional	11	40.74
Gender studied	Both	21	77.78
	Men	3	11.11
	Women	3	11.11
Region	Asia	13	48.15
	Europe	11	40.74
	North America	3	11.11
Health status	Both	4	14.81
	Healthy	9	33.33
	Sick	14	51.85
Age Group	Adults	23	85.19
	Both	2	7.41
	Children	2	7.41
Type of Sickness	Cancer	3	17.65
	GI symptoms	11	64.71
	Others†	3	17.64
HP assessment methods used	Not Described	5	18.52
	One	7	25.93
	Two or more	15	55.56
Assay Type	Commercial EIA	4	14.81
	Commercial ELISA	3	11.11
	Commercial RIA	14	51.85
	In-house RIA	5	18.52
	Not stated	1	3.7
Sample Size	50 and below	6	22.22
	51-200	16	59.26
	201 and above	5	18.52
Sample Storage	-70C and above	19	70.37
	Below -70C	4	14.81
	Not Described	4	14.81
Sample type	Plasma	17	62.96
	Serum	10	37.04
BMI of participants	Normal	15	57.69
	Not Stated	2	7.69
	Obese	2	7.69
	Various	4	15.38
	low to normal	3	11.54

†Others include Crohn's disease (1), diabetes mellitus (1) and multiple conditions (1).

and in all the studies except one, samples were collected after overnight fast. All comparisons were based on the pre-meal ghrelin levels. In most of the studies (70.4%), the samples were stored at a temperature of -70°C or below until analysed; ghrelin was measure in plasma samples in 63% of the studies, while the participants were of normal weight in 58% of the studies. The sample sizes for the different studies ranged from 13 to 538 (median: 89; IQR: 62, 180).

Overall, 17 studies (63%) reported that circulating ghrelin concentrations were lower in *H pylori* positive subjects. Ten studies from Asia (76.9%) and seven from Europe (63.6%) found that circulating ghrelin levels in *H pylori* positive subjects were lower compared to *H pylori* negative subjects. The rest of the studies, including the three from the USA did not find any difference between *H pylori* positive and negative subjects. There was a weak association between the region of the world where the study was conducted and the finding of a lower circulating ghrelin level in *H pylori* positive subjects compared to *H pylori* negative subjects (Fisher's exact test = 0.07). This completely disappeared after controlling for gender, age, health status, type of sample used, storage conditions, BMI, and the sample size.

Zub-Pokrowiecka et al [22] investigated ghrelin changes in the plasma and gastric mucosa among participants with various gastric diseases. Their subjects were divided into four groups - Group 1 had gastric cancer and concomitant *H pylori* infection; group 2 had antral gastritis, duodenal ulcer and *H pylori* infection; group 3 had atrophic gastritis of the fundus and corpus of the stomach but no *H pylori* infection; while group 4 had no gastric lesions and no *H pylori* infection. These researchers reported that the fasting plasma ghrelin concentrations varied among the different groups as follows (in descending order): group 2, group 4, group 1 and group 3.

Meta-analysis

Twenty-one of the 26 studies reviewed in this section qualified for inclusion in the meta-analysis. Of these 21 studies, three studies provided ghrelin values for the different categories of subjects studied. Chuang et al [30] presented their results by gender; D'Onghia et al [31] presented their results according to whether the subjects were healthy controls or had colo-rectal cancer; and Plonka et al [32] presented their results for adults and children separately. Because each of these features could affect the circulating ghrelin concentration, the different categories were entered into the meta-analysis as separate papers bringing the total number of papers included to 24 with a total of 2244 participants. Table 4 lists studies excluded from the meta-analysis. Four papers were subsequently removed from the final analysis because they added significant heterogeneity to the analysis

(Figure 2). The analysis showed that circulating ghrelin concentration was significantly lower in *H pylori* positive participants than in *H pylori* negative participants (Effect estimate (95%CI) = -0.48 [-0.60, -0.36]). Figure 2 is a forest plot of SMDs of circulating ghrelin concentration between *H pylori* positive and *H pylori* negative subjects. There was no significant heterogeneity among the studies (Heterogeneity: Chi² = 24.21, df = 19 (P = 0.19); I² = 22%). Examination of the funnel plot (Figure 3) suggests some publication bias but the Egger and Begg's tests indicated no publication bias (Begg's test: z = 1.20 (continuity corrected), P = 0.23 (continuity corrected); Egger's bias coefficient = -59.99, P = 0.116). A sensitivity analysis indicated that all the studies included in the meta-analysis contributed approximately equally to the pooled estimate (Table 7). Three of the studies dropped from the meta-analysis did not find any difference in the circulating ghrelin levels between *H pylori* positive and *H pylori* negative subjects [14,26,30]. However, Plonka et al [32] found a significantly lower circulating ghrelin levels among a group of *H pylori* positive Polish shepherds compared to their *H pylori* negative controls. Adding these four papers (excluded because of heterogeneity)

only slightly increased the effect estimate (-0.42 [-0.57, -0.27]) but still showed that *H pylori* infection was associated with a lower circulating ghrelin concentration.

What is the effect of eradicating *H pylori* on circulating ghrelin levels?

Table 8 presents an evidence table of the studies that reported the effect of eradicating *H pylori* on circulating ghrelin levels. Thirteen papers were reviewed 12 of which were cohort studies and one RCT. Five of the 13 studies were conducted in Japan; 3 in Korea (both in Asia) and four in Europe. The only study from Africa was an unpublished paper by our team. Table 9 is a summary of the characteristics of the studies in Table 8.

In 11 studies, the subjects fasted overnight, and for 3 hours (between 6am and 9am) in one study, before being bled. Osawa et al [46] did not indicate whether their subjects were fasted or not. The sample sizes varied from 3 to 134; median value was 16 (IQR: 9, 43). The duration of follow-up varied from 4 weeks to 52 weeks (median follow-up time: 4.5 weeks; IQR: 4 weeks, 12 weeks). Jang et al [16] were not clear on the duration of follow-up of their subjects.

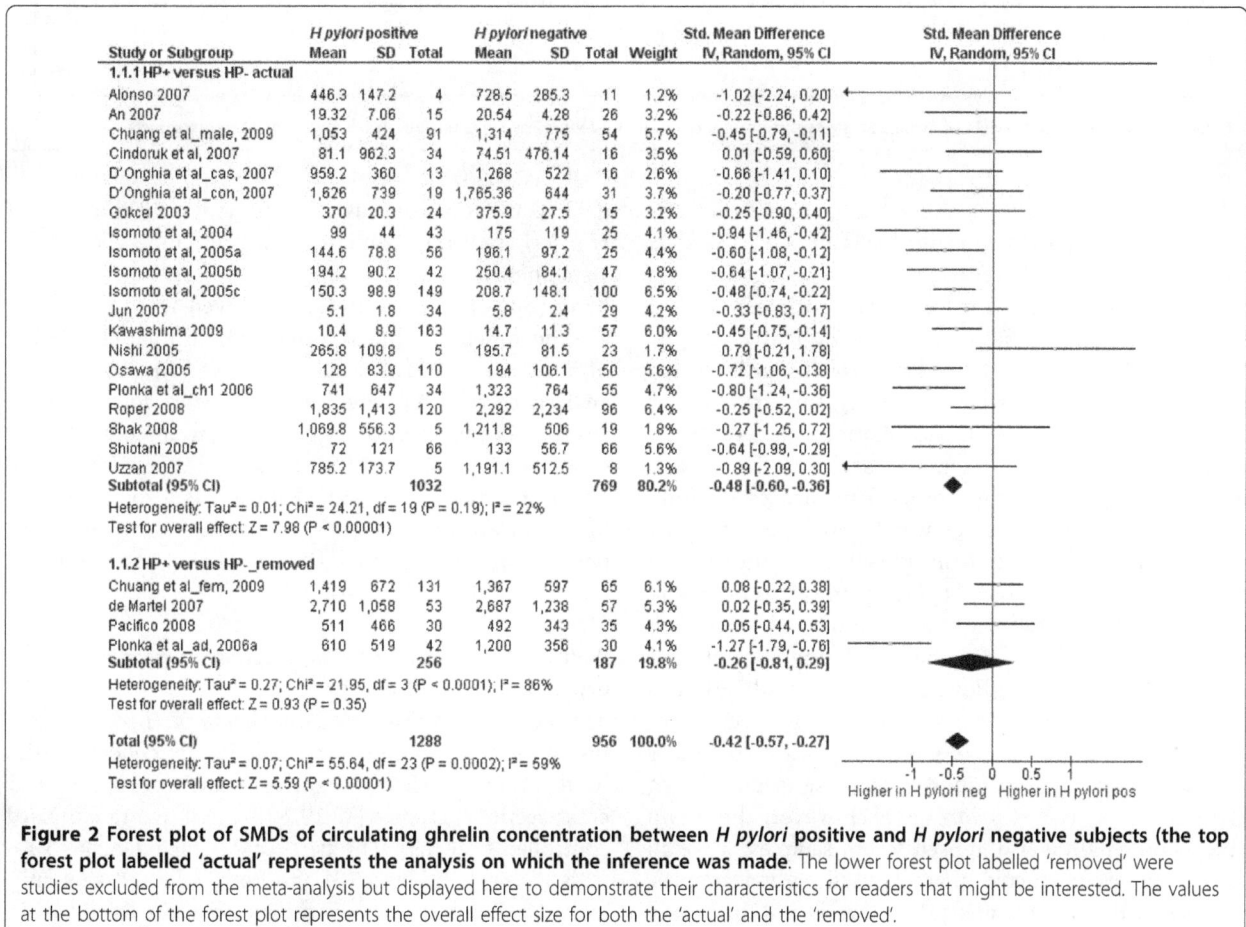

Study or Subgroup	H pylori positive Mean	SD	Total	H pylori negative Mean	SD	Total	Weight	Std. Mean Difference IV, Random, 95% CI	Std. Mean Difference IV, Random, 95% CI
1.1.1 HP+ versus HP- actual									
Alonso 2007	446.3	147.2	4	728.5	285.3	11	1.2%	-1.02 [-2.24, 0.20]	
An 2007	19.32	7.06	15	20.54	4.28	26	3.2%	-0.22 [-0.86, 0.42]	
Chuang et al_male, 2009	1,053	424	91	1,314	775	54	5.7%	-0.45 [-0.79, -0.11]	
Cindoruk et al, 2007	81.1	962.3	34	74.51	476.14	16	3.5%	0.01 [-0.59, 0.60]	
D'Onghia et al_cas, 2007	959.2	360	13	1,268	522	16	2.6%	-0.66 [-1.41, 0.10]	
D'Onghia et al_con, 2007	1,626	739	19	1,765.36	644	31	3.7%	-0.20 [-0.77, 0.37]	
Gokcel 2003	370	20.3	24	375.9	27.5	15	3.2%	-0.25 [-0.90, 0.40]	
Isomoto et al, 2004	99	44	43	175	119	25	4.1%	-0.94 [-1.46, -0.42]	
Isomoto et al, 2005a	144.6	78.8	56	196.1	97.2	25	4.4%	-0.60 [-1.08, -0.12]	
Isomoto et al, 2005b	194.2	90.2	42	250.4	84.1	47	4.8%	-0.64 [-1.07, -0.21]	
Isomoto et al, 2005c	150.3	98.9	149	208.7	148.1	100	6.5%	-0.48 [-0.74, -0.22]	
Jun 2007	5.1	1.8	34	5.8	2.4	29	4.2%	-0.33 [-0.83, 0.17]	
Kawashima 2009	10.4	8.9	163	14.7	11.3	57	6.0%	-0.45 [-0.75, -0.14]	
Nishi 2005	265.8	109.8	5	195.7	81.5	23	1.7%	0.79 [-0.21, 1.78]	
Osawa 2005	128	83.9	110	194	106.1	50	5.6%	-0.72 [-1.06, -0.38]	
Plonka et al_ch1 2006	741	647	34	1,323	764	55	4.7%	-0.80 [-1.24, -0.36]	
Roper 2008	1,835	1,413	120	2,292	2,234	96	6.4%	-0.25 [-0.52, 0.02]	
Shak 2008	1,069.8	556.3	5	1,211.8	506	19	1.8%	-0.27 [-1.25, 0.72]	
Shiotani 2005	72	121	66	133	56.7	66	5.6%	-0.64 [-0.99, -0.29]	
Uzzan 2007	785.2	173.7	5	1,191.1	512.5	8	1.3%	-0.89 [-2.09, 0.30]	
Subtotal (95% CI)			1032			769	80.2%	-0.48 [-0.60, -0.36]	
Heterogeneity: Tau² = 0.01; Chi² = 24.21, df = 19 (P = 0.19); I² = 22%									
Test for overall effect: Z = 7.98 (P < 0.00001)									
1.1.2 HP+ versus HP-_removed									
Chuang et al_fem, 2009	1,419	672	131	1,367	597	65	6.1%	0.08 [-0.22, 0.38]	
de Martel 2007	2,710	1,058	53	2,687	1,238	57	5.3%	0.02 [-0.35, 0.39]	
Pacifico 2008	511	466	30	492	343	35	4.3%	0.05 [-0.44, 0.53]	
Plonka et al_ad, 2006a	610	519	42	1,200	356	30	4.1%	-1.27 [-1.79, -0.76]	
Subtotal (95% CI)			256			187	19.8%	-0.26 [-0.81, 0.29]	
Heterogeneity: Tau² = 0.27; Chi² = 21.95, df = 3 (P < 0.0001); I² = 86%									
Test for overall effect: Z = 0.93 (P = 0.35)									
Total (95% CI)			1288			956	100.0%	-0.42 [-0.57, -0.27]	
Heterogeneity: Tau² = 0.07; Chi² = 55.64, df = 23 (P = 0.0002); I² = 59%									
Test for overall effect: Z = 5.59 (P < 0.00001)									

-1   -0.5   0   0.5   1
Higher in H pylori neg   Higher in H pylori pos

Figure 2 Forest plot of SMDs of circulating ghrelin concentration between *H pylori* positive and *H pylori* negative subjects (the top forest plot labelled 'actual' represents the analysis on which the inference was made. The lower forest plot labelled 'removed' were studies excluded from the meta-analysis but displayed here to demonstrate their characteristics for readers that might be interested. The values at the bottom of the forest plot represents the overall effect size for both the 'actual' and the 'removed'.

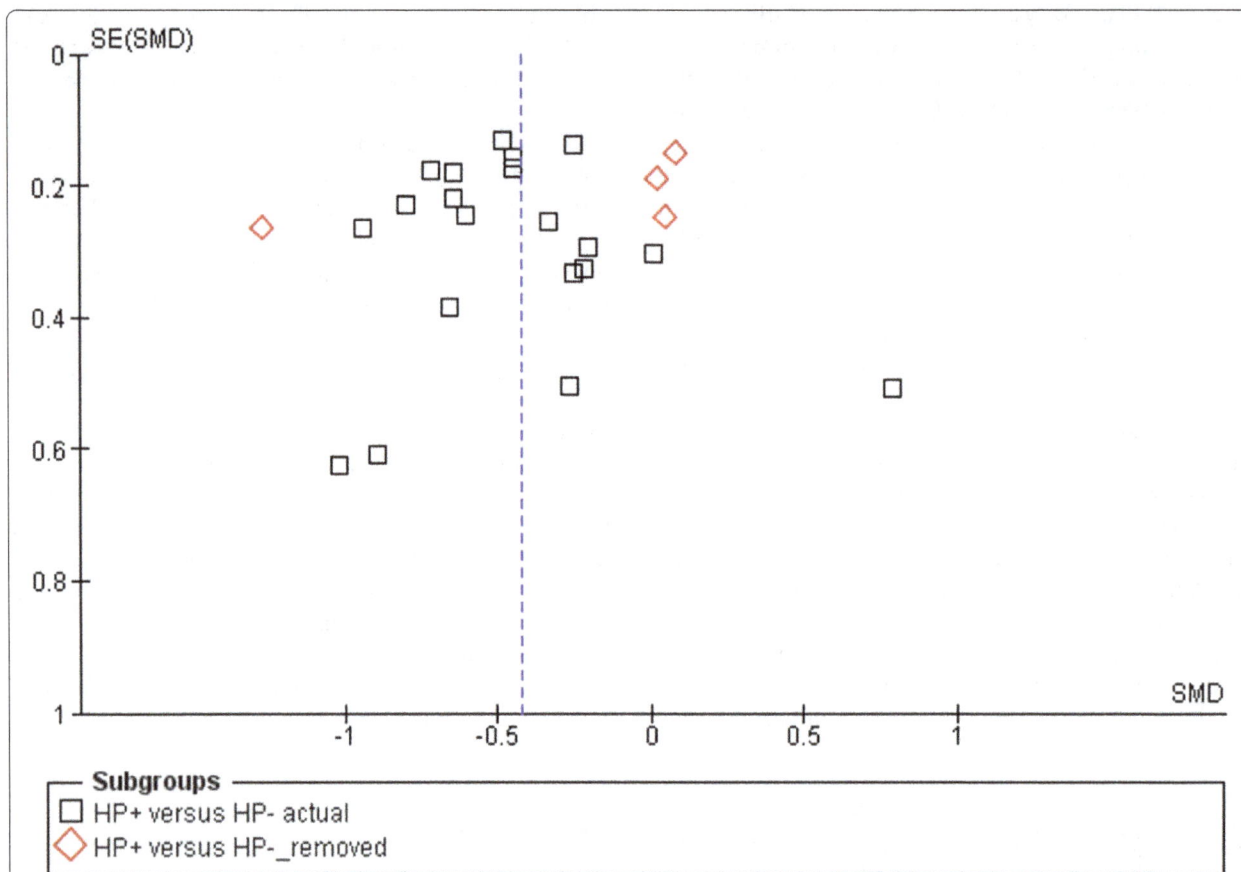

Figure 3 Funnel plot of SMDs of circulating ghrelin concentration between *H pylori* positive and *H pylori* negative subjects.

In seven studies (53.9%) there was no significant difference in circulating ghrelin levels pre- and post *H pylori* eradication. Three studies (23.1%) reported an increase above the pre-eradication level while 3 (23.1%) reported a decrease below the pre-eradication levels. Cross tabulation of the following variables with change in circulating ghrelin levels following cure of *H pylori* infection did not show any association: the age of the participants, the type of sample used, duration of follow-up, sample size, weight of participants, temperature at which the blood samples were stored, the assay kit used to measure circulating ghrelin, the number of methods used to assess *H pylori*, gender, country and the region where the study was conducted. Although not statistically significant, the circulating ghrelin concentration decreased following *H pylori* eradication in the two studies that measured ghrelin using serum samples (Fisher's exact test 0.08). Similarly, the two studies conducted on children found a decrease in circulating ghrelin levels after *H pylori* cure. However, these two studies on children also utilised serum samples; while all the 11 studies conducted in adults used plasma samples. From this descriptive analysis, there is not sufficient

data to make a conclusive statement on the effect of *H pylori* eradication on circulating ghrelin levels.

Meta-analysis

Nine (out of the 13 studies reviewed in this section) were included in a meta-analysis with a total population of 592. The excluded studies are listed in Table 4. The analysis showed that eradicating *H pylori* does not have any significant effect on circulating ghrelin levels (Effect estimate (95% CI) = -0.08 [-0.33, 0.16]; Test for overall effect: Z = 0.67 (P = 0.5)). Figure 4 is a forest plot of SMDs of circulating ghrelin concentration pre- and post-eradication of *H pylori*. The funnel plot indicated publication bias (Figure 5).

What is the effect of *H pylori* infection on ghrelin expression in the stomach?

Thirteen studies examined the effects of *H pylori* infection on gastric ghrelin. This includes six cohort studies [6,36,44,46-48], 2 case-control studies [40,49], four cross-sectional studies [18,19,24,37] and one randomised controlled trial [23]. The participants included sick subjects (7), well subjects (3) and both well and sick subjects (2). Eight studies were conducted in Asia, two in

Table 7 Sensitivity analysis of studies included in the meta-analysis

Studies excluded	SMD (95%CI)	Test for overall effect
Alonso et al, 2007	-0.47 [-0.59, -0.35]	Z = 7.80 (P < 0.00001)
An et al, 2007	-0.49 [-0.61, -0.37]	Z = 7.88 (P < 0.00001)
Chuang et al_male, 2009	-0.48 [-0.61, -0.35]	Z = 7.39 (P < 0.00001)
Cindoruk et al, 2007	-0.49 [-0.61, -0.38]	Z = 8.48 (P < 0.00001)
D'Onghia et al_case, 2007	-0.47 [-0.60, -0.35]	Z = 7.64 (P < 0.00001)
D'Onghia et al_control, 2007	-0.49 [-0.61, -0.37]	Z = 7.95 (P < 0.00001)
Gokcel et al, 2003	-0.49 [-0.61, -0.36]	Z = 7.84 (P < 0.00001)
Isomoto et al, 2004	-0.46 [-0.57, -0.35]	Z = 7.96 (P < 0.00001)
Isomoto et al, 2005a	-0.47 [-0.60, -0.35]	Z = 7.47 (P < 0.00001)
Isomoto et al, 2005b	-0.47 [-0.59, -0.34]	Z = 7.43 (P < 0.00001)
Isomoto et al, 2005c	-0.48 [-0.61, -0.35]	Z = 7.14 (P < 0.00001)
Jun et al, 2007	-0.49 [-0.61, -0.36]	Z = 7.72 (P < 0.00001)
Kawashima et al, 2009	-0.48 [-0.61, -0.35]	Z = 7.32 (P < 0.00001)
Nishi et al, 2005	-0.49 [-0.59, -0.39]	Z = 9.72 (P < 0.00001)
Osawa et al, 2005	-0.46 [-0.58, -0.34]	Z = 7.45 (P < 0.00001)
Plonka et al_ch1 2006	-0.46 [-0.58, -0.34]	Z = 7.65 (P < 0.00001)
Roper et al, 2008	-0.51 [-0.63, -0.39]	Z = 8.37 (P < 0.00001)
Shak et al, 2008	-0.48 [-0.60, -0.36]	Z = 7.79 (P < 0.00001)
Shiotani et al, 2005	-0.46 [-0.59, -0.34]	Z = 7.33 (P < 0.00001)
Uzzan et al, 2007	-0.47 [-0.59, -0.35]	Z = 7.76 (P < 0.00001)

France, one each in Poland, Brazil and USA. Ten studies recruited both males and females, and three recruited males only. All the sick participants had gastrointestinal symptoms. Different methods were used to assess *H pylori* infection either alone or in combination: histology (11 studies), culture (3), rapid urease assay (5), serology (3), urea breath test (2) and PCR (4). Ten of the 13 studies were conducted on normal weight subjects, two on obese subjects and one on subjects of different body weights. Due to the different gastric ghrelin parameters assessed, a meta-analysis was not possible.

Five studies assessed gastric ghrelin contents: one found it to be lower in *H pylori* positive subjects [36], three [6,18,44] found no significant difference between *H pylori* positive and negative participants, and one [24] found increased levels in *H pylori* positive participants. Isomoto et al [36] compared gastric ghrelin peptide contents in the endoscopic biopsies from the corpus of 56 *H pylori* positive and 25 *H pylori* negative subjects using radio-immunoassay. They reported significantly lower gastric ghrelin content in the *H pylori* positive subjects than the *H pylori* negative subjects. Roper et al [18] studied 216 adult males of normal BMI presenting for routine endoscopy consisting of 120 *H pylori* positive and 96 *H pylori* negative subjects. Although they did not find any significant difference in the gastric ghrelin levels between *H pylori* positive and *H pylori* negative subjects, they reported a very wide variation in the concentration of ghrelin in the gastric juice (from <80 to

776,000 pg/ml) with the *H pylori* positive subjects having higher gastric juice ghrelin levels than the *H pylori* negative subjects. Choe et al [6] did not find any significant difference in the gastric ghrelin levels between *H pylori* positive and *H pylori* negative subjects using biopsied tissues.

Four studies examined the expression of ghrelin mRNA in gastric mucosa [19,36,37,40]. Three studies found ghrelin mRNA expression to be lower in *H pylori* positive subjects than in *H pylori* negative subjects, while Jun et al [37] found no difference. Five studies assessed the quantity of ghrelin immunoreactive cells in the gastric mucosa [36,40,47-49]; all of which found that *H pylori* positive subjects had fewer ghrelin-producing cells than in uninfected subjects. However, in the study by Isomoto et al [36], this difference did not achieve statistical significance.

Five studies compared the various gastric ghrelin parameters before and after *H pylori* eradication [6,23,36, 46,48]. Choe et al [6] did not find any significant difference in the ghrelin concentration in the antrum, corpus and fundus pre- and post- *H pylori* eradication. Lee et al [23] reported a randomized controlled trial on *H pylori* positive volunteers without peptic ulcer or any other gastrointestinal symptoms in which the treatment group received triple *H pylori* eradication regimen while the control group did not receive any treatment. These authors reported a significant increase in gastric ghrelin mRNA expression following eradication compared to

Table 8 Evidence table of studies that examined changes in circulating ghrelin levels following *H pylori* eradication

Reference & Country	Study Team	Design	Healthy	Gender	Age category	HP assess	Ghrelin assay Kit	Sample storage	Sample type	Weight	Sample size	Circulating Ghrelin levels after cure	Follow-up (wks)
Nwokolo et al, 2003; UK [2]	A	Cohort	Healthy	Both	Adults	Serology and UBT	Commercial RIA	-20	Plasma	Various	10	Increased	6
Jang et al, 2008; Korea [16]	B	Cohort	Sick	Both	Adults	RUT plus histology & confirmed by UBT	Commercial RIA	-70	Plasma	Normal	16	Increased	Not stated
Osawa et al, 2006; Japan [46]	C	Cohort	Healthy	Men	Adults	Bacterial culture & histology	In-house RIA	Not stated	Plasma	Normal	134	Decreased	12
Czesnikiewicz-Guzik et al, 2007; Poland [13]	D	Cohort	Sick	Women	Adults	UBT; culture of saliva & supragingival dental plaques + serology	Commercial RIA	-80	Plasma	Not stated	49	Increased	4
Lee et al, 2010; Korea [23]	B	RCT	Healthy	Both	Adults	RUT, histology (Giemsa stain)	ELISA	-70	Plasma	Normal	9	No difference	5
Choe et al, 2007, Korea [6]	E	Cohort	Sick	Both	Adults	histology & PCR	Commercial ELISA	-70	Plasma	Normal	8	No difference	4
Pacifico et al, 2008; Italy [26]	F	Cohort	Both	Both	Children	Culture of gastric specimen or histology + RUT	RIA	-70	Serum	Normal	22	Decreased	52
Nweneka, et al, unpublished; Gambia	G	Cohort	Sick	Both	Children	UBT	Commercial RIA	-70	Serum	Low	3	Decreased	4
Isomoto et al, 2005 [36]; Japan	C	Cohort	Sick	Both	Adults	RUT, histology (Giemsa stain)	In-house RIA	-80	Plasma	Normal	43	No difference	4
Isomoto et al, 2005; Japan[35]	C	Cohort	Sick	Both	Adults	RUT, histology (Giemsa stain)	In-house RIA	-80	Plasma	Normal	10	No difference	4
Kawashima et al, 2009; Japan [38]	H	Cohort	Both	Both	Adults	Serology	Commercial EIA	-80	Plasma	Normal	49	Increased	23
Cindoruk et al, 2007; Turkey [11]	I	Cohort	Sick	Both	Adults	Either histology or UBT	RIA	-80	Plasma	Normal	23	No difference	12
Isomoto et al, 2004; Japan [34]	C	Cohort	Sick	Both	Adults	Serology	Commercial RIA	-80	Plasma	Normal	9	No difference	4

Table 9 Summary of the characteristics of the studies reviewed in Table 8

Characteristic		n	%
Study Design	Cohort	12	92.31
	RCT	1	7.69
Gender studied	Both	11	84.62
	Men	1	7.69
	Women	1	7.69
Region	Africa	1	7.69
	Asia	8	61.54
	Europe	4	30.77
Health status	Both	2	15.38
	Healthy	3	23.08
	Sick	8	61.54
Age Group	Adults	11	84.62
	Children	2	15.38
Type of Sickness	GI Symptoms	9	90
	PEM	1	10
HP assessment methods used	One	3	23.08
	Two or more	10	76.92
Assay Type	ELISA	2	15.38
	Commercial RIA	8	61.54
	In-house RIA	3	23.08
Sample Size	Above 20	6	46.15
	Below 20	7	53.85
Sample Storage	-70°C and below	11	84.62
	Above -70°C	1	7.69
	Not described	1	7.69
Sample type	Plasma	11	84.62
	Serum	2	15.38
BMI of participants	Normal	10	76.92
	Others	3	23.07
Duration of follow-up	4 weeks & below	6	46.15
	Above 4 weeks	6	46.15
	Not recorded	1	7.69
Change in ghrelin after cure	Decreased	3	23.08
	Increased	3	23.08
	No difference	7	53.85

the control group. Osawa et al [46] also reported an increase in ghrelin mRNA expression following *H pylori* cure. Although Isomoto et al [36] found a tendency towards increase in ghrelin mRNA expression following cure of *H pylori*, this increase was not significant. Tatsuguchi et al [48], on the other hand, found an increase in ghrelin immunoreactive cells following *H pylori* eradication in 50 patients with either peptic ulcer disease or gastritis, while in 11 patients who did not respond to eradication therapy, there was no difference in the number of ghrelin immunoreactive cells pre-and post-eradication therapy.

Three studies [36,47,49] found a negative correlation between ghrelin producing cells in the gastrum and the severity of *H pylori* infection. Gastric ghrelin content and gastric ghrelin mRNA expression were both positively correlated with plasma ghrelin concentration [36,46].

Discussion

The potential role of ghrelin in body mass regulation makes understanding its interactions with *Helicobacter pylori*, a highly prevalent gastrointestinal infection, important. To address this issue, we asked three questions: how does *H pylori* infection affect circulating ghrelin levels; how does eradicating *H pylori* affect circulating ghrelin; and how does *H pylori* infection affect gastric ghrelin and ghrelin producing cells.

The results of our analysis has conclusively shown that circulating ghrelin levels are significantly higher in *H pylori* negative people than in those infected with *H pylori* (P = 0.00001). Our results also suggest that eradicating *H pylori* does not have any significant effect on circulating ghrelin. Although there was no significant heterogeneity between the group of studies that compared circulating ghrelin concentrations before and after *H pylori* eradication, this result should be interpreted with the following caveats in mind: 1) three of the studies [34-36] included in the meta-analysis came from the same research group; and together accounted for 29% of the effect size; 2) the paper by Osawa et al [46] which reported higher ghrelin levels before *H pylori* eradication compared to the levels after eradication on its own contributed 26.2% of the effect; and 3) the sample sizes of most of the other studies were relatively small. Interestingly, all the smaller studies, except one, found higher circulating ghrelin levels post-eradication. Even among the subjects studied by Osawa et al [46], plasma ghrelin increased in 50 patients and decreased in 84 patients, although the overall effect was a decrease post-eradication. They were however, able to show that pre-eradication elevation of ghrelin was associated with a

Study or Subgroup	Pre-eradication			Post-eradication			Weight	Std. Mean Difference IV, Random, 95% CI
	Mean	SD	Total	Mean	SD	Total		
Cindoruk et al, 2007	78.34	486.5	23	88.67	533.3	23	11.9%	-0.02 [-0.60, 0.56]
Isomoto et al, 2004	142	33	9	166	113	9	5.9%	-0.27 [-1.20, 0.65]
Isomoto et al, 2005a	136.1	72.3	43	155.5	93.6	43	16.9%	-0.23 [-0.65, 0.19]
Isomoto et al, 2005b	176.5	79.5	10	191.3	120.4	10	6.5%	-0.14 [-1.02, 0.74]
Jang et al, 2008	30.12	40.92	16	40.75	167.93	16	9.3%	-0.08 [-0.78, 0.61]
Kawashima 2009	10.3	10.5	49	13.1	7	49	18.0%	-0.31 [-0.71, 0.09]
Lee 2010	18.64	5.08	9	21.27	3.58	9	5.7%	-0.57 [-1.52, 0.38]
Nweneka, et al, 2004	3,056	522	3	868	312	3	0.3%	4.07 [-0.17, 8.31]
Osawa 2006	120	72.9	134	103	61.4	134	25.5%	0.25 [0.01, 0.49]
Total (95% CI)			**296**			**296**	**100.0%**	**-0.08 [-0.33, 0.16]**

Heterogeneity: Tau² = 0.05; Chi² = 13.10, df = 8 (P = 0.11); I² = 39%
Test for overall effect: Z = 0.67 (P = 0.50)

Higher post-eradication   Higher pre-eradication

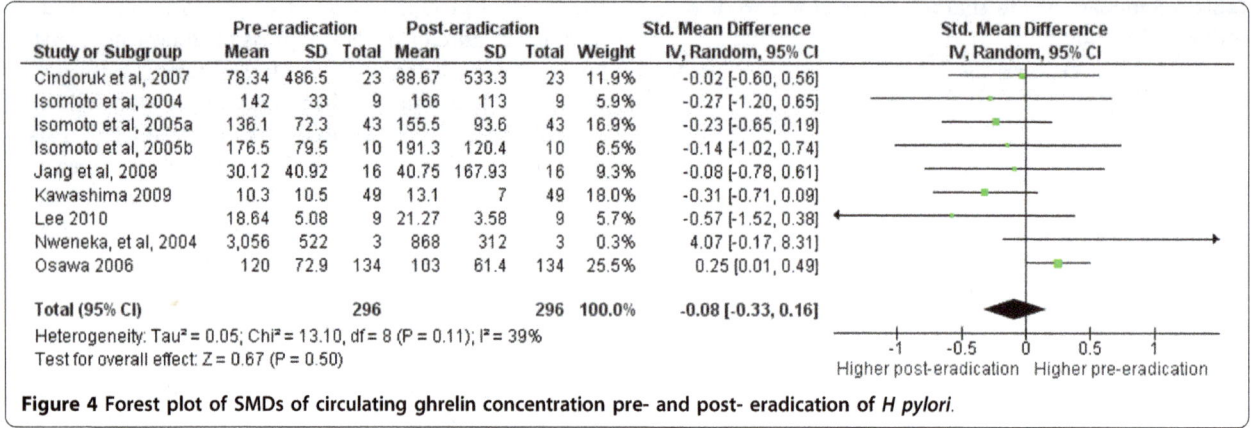

Figure 4 Forest plot of SMDs of circulating ghrelin concentration pre- and post- eradication of *H pylori*.

fall in ghrelin post-eradication. In our unpublished data, we also found that elevated ghrelin concentration pre-eradication was associated with a fall post-eradication. These two observations suggest that in addition to other factors, the pre-eradication ghrelin level determines the direction of response of ghrelin post-eradication.

The heterogeneity of the studies examining the effect of *H pylori* on gastric ghrelin expression as well as the small number of studies that examined different aspects of this relationship did not allow a meta-analysis to be performed. However, the descriptive data suggests that available evidence is still discrepant; although the weight of evidence seems to favour lower ghrelin mRNA and ghrelin immunoreactive cells in association with *H pylori* infection [19,36,40,47-49]. The ultimate effect of *H pylori* on gastric ghrelin appears to be dependent on the duration of infection and the extent of *H pylori*-induced damage to the gastric mucosa. At least three

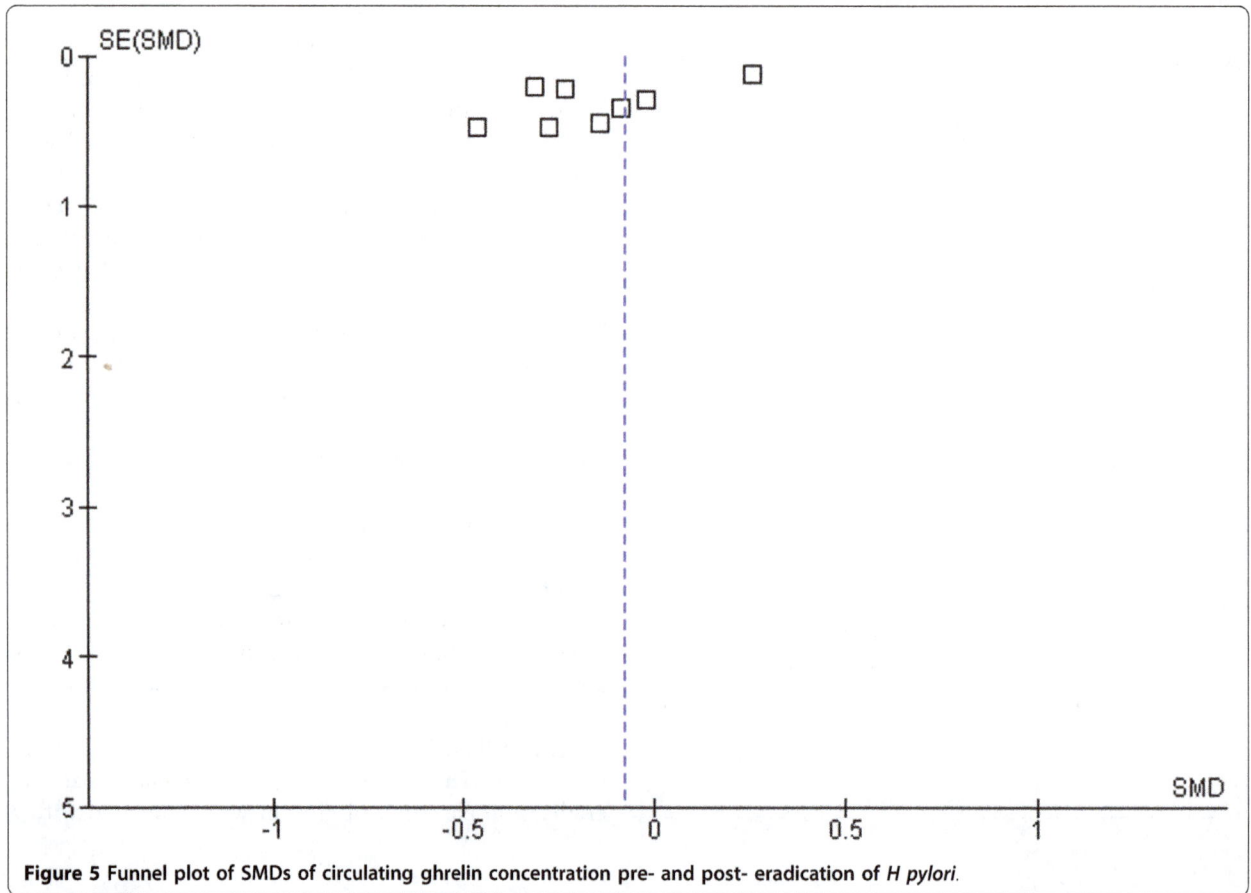

Figure 5 Funnel plot of SMDs of circulating ghrelin concentration pre- and post- eradication of *H pylori*.

studies found a negative correlation between number of ghrelin producing cells and the severity of *H pylori* infection [36,47,49].

The close anatomical proximity between the site of *H pylori* infection and the site of ghrelin production might result in the loss of ghrelin producing cells as part of the *H pylori* associated gastritis, causing reduced ghrelin production. However, such effect will not be restricted to *H pylori* infection and could occur in any other condition associated with gastritis. For example, Checchi et al [10] studied 233 patients with autoimmune gastritis (indicated by elevated parietal cell antibody (PCA)) and 211 control subjects, and found that mean serum ghrelin levels in PCA positive patients were significantly lower than in PCA negative patients, similar to the results found in *H pylori* infection by some studies. This decrease remained significant even after excluding patients with *H pylori* infection, suggesting that the *H pylori* infection was not necessarily responsible for the reduction in serum ghrelin. Again, the region of the stomach biopsied could also affect the results. Jang et al [16] reported that after ulcer healing and *H pylori* eradication, there was a significant increase in the levels of ghrelin mRNA. But while corpus ghrelin mRNA increased after cure and *H pylori* eradication, anthral ghrelin mRNA decreased, suggesting a differential response by the ghrelin producing cells in the different regions of the stomach. In healthy *H pylori* infected subjects however, Lee et al [23] found a significant increase in fundic ghrelin mRNA after eradication of *H pylori* (P = 0.0002) but no change in the anthral ghrelin mRNA (P = 0.5), suggesting a more complex relationship between gastric ghrelin production and *H pylori* infection. Teasing out this relationship will require more rigorous investigation.

If *H pylori* infection is associated with a lower circulating ghrelin, it is biologically plausible that its eradication will be associated with an increase in circulating ghrelin. But if *H pylori* reduces circulating ghrelin by destroying ghrelin producing cells, then the effect of eradicating it on circulating ghrelin would depend on the duration of infection, the amount of damage to ghrelin-producing cells, and the time it takes for these cells to regenerate. Indeed several studies have found a negative correlation between the number of ghrelin producing cells and the severity of gastritis [36,47,49]. And in one study, there was no change in ghrelin levels post-eradication after 4 weeks of follow-up, but the level progressively increased with follow-up, achieving, in some subjects, significant increase after 6 months of follow-up [36]. In contrast, mice infected with *H pylori* for 6-8 months had higher ghrelin levels compared to time-matched controls, which normalised

two months post-eradication [50]. However, Masaoka et al [51] did not find any change in circulating ghrelin levels 2 years after successful eradication of *H pylori* in an adult man.

The discrepancy in the response to *H pylori* eradication could also be related to the strain of *H pylori*. Isomoto et al [52] found that strain diversity in *H pylori* was associated with plasma and gastric ghrelin levels in humans. Patients with type I strain (which express the virulence factors cytotoxin-associated gene product (CagA) and Vacuolating cytotoxin A (VacA)) have lower circulating ghrelin levels than those with the less virulent type II strain which does not express the virulence factors. This finding also argues for a possible racial difference in the association between circulating ghrelin levels and *H pylori* infection: in regions where type I strain is dominant, one would expect to see reduced circulating ghrelin levels. While such speculation is attractive, it might not be entirely correct [53]. In this review, the effect of region and country of study on the relationship between *H pylori* and ghrelin was very weak, and appears to be confounded by several other factors.

The underlying clinical condition of the subject might also be affecting the results. Suzuki et al [54] studied plasma ghrelin in patients with peptic ulcer disease. They found that plasma ghrelin levels were significantly higher in patients with duodenal ulcer as well as those with gastric ulcer compared to those with chronic gastritis. Among the subjects that were *H pylori* positive, plasma ghrelin was significantly higher in patients with duodenal or gastric ulcer than in those with non-ulcer chronic gastritis. After treatment for the ulcer (with healing), no significant change was found in the plasma ghrelin levels (i.e. pre-and post eradication levels were similar). Most of the studies reviewed here recruited subjects with varying degrees and types of gastrointestinal pathology. If each of these gastrointestinal diseases affects ghrelin production differently as suggested by Suzuki et al [54], then the discrepancies noted in this review are to be expected. Compensation from other sources of ghrelin production might also explain the various inconsistencies highlighted in this review. For example, Suzuki et al [55] infected Mongolian gerbils with *H pylori* and assessed the plasma and gastric ghrelin levels at 17 and 23 weeks after the infection. They found a significant decrease in gastric ghrelin in the *H pylori* positive gerbils compared to the controls, but also found a significant increase in plasma ghrelin levels in the *H pylori* positive group. This same group also found increased plasma ghrelin and decreased gastric ghrelin levels in IL-1R1 knockout mice [4] suggesting that other sources of ghrelin might have contributed to the increased plasma ghrelin.

Limitations and implications for research and practice

The major limitation of this review is the use of only English language papers, which raises the possibility of some publication bias. Another limitation in conducting this review is that all except one of the papers were observational studies, most of which did not primarily set out to assess the relationship between ghrelin and *H pylori*; but assessed both parameters in relation to other objectives. Well designed randomised clinical trials are needed to verify the conclusions made by this review. Also, many of the studies included participants with diverse disease conditions whose impacts on ghrelin secretion have not been investigated before. The best approach to solve the riddle of the relationship between ghrelin and helicobacter pylori might be to study otherwise healthy participants with asymptomatic *H pylori* infection.

Conclusions

From available evidence, circulating ghrelin concentration is lower in people infected with *H pylori* compared to those not infected with the bacterium. However, a more complex relationship exists between circulating ghrelin levels and eradication of *H pylori*. This relationship may be modulated by the strain of infecting *H pylori*, the duration of follow-up, the extent of *H pylori*-induced gastritis and other underlying pathology. More studies are needed to further elucidate the impact of *H pylori* eradication on circulating ghrelin concentration.

Acknowledgements
The authors wish to acknowledge all the authors that responded to our inquiries particularly those that provided us with their raw data sets.

Author details
[1]Nutrition Programme, Medical Research Council Laboratories, The Gambia, P.O. Box 273, Banjul, The Gambia. [2]MRC International Nutrition Group, London School of Hygiene & Tropical Medicine, Keppel Street, London, UK.

Authors' contributions
CVN conceived the paper, conducted the literature search, initial analysis and took lead in the writing. AMP critically reviewed the analysis, and the initial drafts, and participated in writing subsequent drafts. Both authors read and approved the final manuscript.

Competing interests
The authors declare that they have no competing interests. Funding for this study was provided by the UK Medical Research Council.

References
1. Taniaka-Shintani M, Watanabe M: Distribution of ghrelin-immunoreactive cells in human gastric mucosa: comparison with that of parietal cells. *Journal of gastroenterology* 2005, 40(4):345-349.
2. Nwokolo CU, Freshwater DA, O'Hare P, Randeva HS: Plasma ghrelin following cure of Helicobacter pylori. *Gut* 2003, 52(5):637-640.
3. Gokcel A, Gumurdulu Y, Kayaselcuk F, Serin E, Ozer B, Ozsahin AK, Guvener N: Helicobacter pylori has no effect on plasma ghrelin levels. *European Journal of Endocrinology* 2003, 148(4):423-426.
4. Abiko Y, Suzuki H, Masaoka T, Nomura S, Kurabayashi K, Hosoda H, Kangawa K, Hibi T: Enhanced plasma ghrelin levels in Helicobacter pylori-colonized, interleukin-1-receptor type 1-homozygous knockout (IL-1R1-/-) mice. *World J Gastroenterol* 2005, 11(27):4148-4153.
5. Anania C, Pacifico L, Castronovo A, Neaga M, Ferrara E, Schiavo E, Bonamico M, Chiesa C: Long-term effects of Helicobacter pylori eradication on the levels of circulating ghrelin and leptin concentrations and on body composition in prepubertal children. *Helicobacter* 2007, 12(4):393-393.
6. Choe YH, Lee JH, Lee HJ, Paik KH, Jin DK, Song SY, Lee JH: Ghrelin Levels in Gastric Mucosa before and after Eradication of Helicobacter pylori. *Gut Liver* 2007, 1(2):132-137.
7. Choi JY, Hahm KB: [Ghrelin; influences on Helicobacter pylori-associated gastric diseases]. *Korean J Gastroenterol* 2006, 48(2):75-81.
8. Osawa H: Ghrelin and Helicobacter pylori infection. *World J Gastroenterol* 2008, 14(41):6327-6333.
9. Weigt J, Malfertheiner P: Influence of Helicobacter pylori on gastric regulation of food intake. *Curr Opin Clin Nutr Metab Care* 2009, 12(5):522-525.
10. Checchi S, Montanaro A, Pasqui L, Ciuoli C, Cevenini G, Sestini F, Fioravanti C, Pacini F: Serum ghrelin as a marker of atrophic body gastritis in patients with parietal cell antibodies. *Journal of Clinical Endocrinology & Metabolism* 2007, 92(11):4346-4351.
11. Cindoruk M, Yetkin I, Deger SM, Karakan T, Kan E, Unal S: Influence of H pylori on plasma ghrelin in patients without atrophic gastritis. *World Journal of Gastroenterology* 2007, 13(10):1595-1598.
12. Czesnikiewicz-Guzik M, Bielanski W, Guzik TJ, Loster B, Konturek SJ: Helicobacter pylori in the oral cavity and its implications for gastric infection, periodontal health, immunology and dyspepsia. *J Physiol Pharmacol* 2005, 56(Suppl 6):77-89.
13. Czesnikiewicz-Guzik M, Loster B, Bielanski W, Guzik TJ, Konturek PC, Zapala J, Konturek SJ: Implications of oral Helicobacter pylori for the outcome of its gastric eradication therapy. *Journal of Clinical Gastroenterology* 2007, 41(2):145-151.
14. de Martel C, Haggerty TD, Corley DA, Vogelman JH, Orentreich N, Parsonnet J: Serum ghrelin levels and risk of subsequent adenocarcinoma of the esophagus. *American Journal of Gastroenterology* 2007, 102(6):1166-1172.
15. Gao X, Kuang H, Liu X, Duan P, Yang Y, Ma Z: Circulating ghrelin/obestatin ratio in subjects with Helicobacter pylori infection. *Nutrition* 2009, 25(5):506-511.
16. Jang EJ, Park SW, Park JS, Park SJ, Hahm KB, Paik SY, Sin MK, Lee ES, Oh SW, Park CY, et al: The influence of the eradication of Helicobacter pylori on gastric ghrelin, appetite, and body mass index in patients with peptic ulcer disease. *Journal of gastroenterology and hepatology* 2008, 23(Suppl 2): S278-285.
17. Konturek PC, Czesnikiewicz-Guzik M, Bielanski W, Konturek SJ: Involvement of Helicobacter pylori infection in neuro-hormonal control of food intake. *Journal of Physiology & Pharmacology* 2006, 57(Suppl 5):67-81.
18. Roper J, Francois F, Shue PL, Mourad MS, Pei Z, Olivares de Perez AZ, Perez-Perez GI, Tseng CH, Blaser MJ: Leptin and ghrelin in relation to Helicobacter pylori status in adult males. *Journal of Clinical Endocrinology & Metabolism* 2008, 93(6):2350-2357.
19. Salles N, Menard A, Georges A, Salzmann M, de Ledinghen V, de Mascarel A, Emeriau JP, Lamouliatte H, Megraud F: Effects of Helicobacter pylori infection on gut appetite peptide (leptin, ghrelin) expression in elderly inpatients. *Journals of Gerontology Series A-Biological Sciences & Medical Sciences* 2006, 61(11):1144-1150.
20. Shindo T, Futagami S, Hiratsuka T, Horie A, Hamamoto T, Ueki N, Kusunoki M, Miyake K, Gudis K, Tsukui T, et al: Comparison of Gastric Emptying and Plasma Ghrelin Levels in Patients with Functional Dyspepsia and Non-Erosive Reflux Disease. *Digestion* 2009, 79(2):65-72.
21. Shiotani A, Miyanishi T, Uedo N, Iishi H: Helicobacter pylori infection is associated with reduced circulating ghrelin levels independent of body mass index. *Helicobacter* 2005, 10(5):373-378.
22. Zub-Pokrowiecka A, Rembiasz K, Konturek SJ, Budzynski A, Konturek PC, Budzynski P: Ghrelin in diseases of the gastric mucosa associated with Helicobacter pylori infection. *Med Sci Monit* 2010, 16(10):CR493-500.
23. Lee ES, Yoon YS, Park CY, Kim HS, Um TH, Baik HW, Jang EJ, Lee S, Park HS, Oh SW: Eradication of Helicobacter pylori increases ghrelin mRNA

expression in the gastric mucosa. *Journal of Korean Medical Science* 2010, **25**(2):265-271.

24. Stec-Michalska K, Malicki S, Michalski B, Peczek L, Wisniewska-Jarosinska M, Nawrot B: Gastric ghrelin in relation to gender, stomach topography and Helicobacter pylori in dyspeptic patients. *World Journal of Gastroenterology* 2009, **15**(43):5409-5417.

25. Suzuki H, Masaoka T, Hosoda H, Nomura S, Ohara T, Kangawa K, Ishii H, Hibi T: Plasma ghrelin concentration correlates with the levels of serum pepsinogen I and pepsinogen I/II ratio - A possible novel and non-invasive marker for gastric atrophy. *Hepato-Gastroenterology* 2004, **51**(59):1249-1254.

26. Pacifico L, Anania C, Osborn JF, Ferrara E, Schiavo E, Bonamico M, Chiesa C: Long-term effects of Helicobacter pylori eradication on circulating ghrelin and leptin concentrations and body composition in prepubertal children. *European Journal of Endocrinology* 2008, **158**(3):323-332.

27. Nunes FA, Alves JS, Diniz MTC, Barbosa AJA: Helicobacter pylori infection and density of gastric ghrelin-producing cells in obese and Nonobese patients. *Helicobacter* 2006, **11**(4):368-368.

28. Higgins JP, Thompson SG, Deeks JJ, Altman DG: Measuring inconsistency in meta-analyses. *BMJ* 2003, **327**(7414):557-560.

29. Higgins JP, Thompson SG: Quantifying heterogeneity in a meta-analysis. *Stat Med* 2002, **21**(11):1539-1558.

30. Chuang CH, Sheu BS, Yang HB, Lee SC, Kao AW, Cheng HC, Chang WL, Yao WJ: Gender difference of circulating ghrelin and leptin concentrations in chronic Helicobacter pylori infection. *Helicobacter* 2009, **14**(1):54-60.

31. D'Onghia V, Leoncini R, Carli R, Santoro A, Giglioni S, Sorbellini F, Marzocca G, Bernini A, Campagna S, Marinello E, *et al*: Circulating gastrin and ghrelin levels in patients with colorectal cancer: correlation with tumour stage, Helicobacter pylori infection and BMI. *Biomedicine & Pharmacotherapy* 2007, **61**(2-3):137-141.

32. Plonka M, Konturek PC, Bielanski W, Pawlik T, Brzozowski T, Konturek SJ: Relationship between ghrelin and Helicobacter pylori infection in Polish adult shepherds and their children. *Alimentary Pharmacology & Therapeutics* 2006, **24**:160-168.

33. Cindoruk M, Yetkin I, Deger SM, Karakan T, Kan E, Unal S: Influence of H pylori on plasma ghrelin in patients without atrophic gastritis. *World J Gastroenterol* 2007, **13**(10):1595-1598.

34. Isomoto H, Nakazato M, Ueno H, Date Y, Nishi Y, Mukae H, Mizuta Y, Ohtsuru A, Yamashita S, Kohno S: Low plasma ghrelin levels in patients with Helicobacter pylori-associated gastritis. *American Journal of Medicine* 2004, **117**(6):429-432.

35. Isomoto H, Ueno H, Nishi Y, Wen CY, Nakazato M, Kohno S: Impact of Helicobacter pylori infection on ghrelin and various neuroendocrine hormones in plasma. *World Journal of Gastroenterology* 2005, **11**(11):1644-1648.

36. Isomoto H, Ueno H, Saenko VA, Mondal MS, Nishi Y, Kawano N, Ohnita K, Mizuta Y, Ohtsuru A, Yamashita S, *et al*: Impact of Helicobacter pylori infection on gastric and plasma ghrelin dynamics in humans. *American Journal of Gastroenterology* 2005, **100**(8):1711-1720.

37. Jun DW, Lee OY, Lee YY, Choi HS, Kim TH, Yoon BC: Correlation between gastrointestinal symptoms and gastric leptin and ghrelin expression in patients with gastritis. *Digestive Diseases & Sciences* 2007, **52**(10):2866-2872.

38. Kawashima J, Ohno S, Sakurada T, Takabayashi H, Kudo M, Ro S, Kato S, Yakabi K: Circulating acylated ghrelin level decreases in accordance with the extent of atrophic gastritis. *Journal of Gastroenterology* 2009, **44**(10):1046-1054.

39. Suzuki H, Nishizawa T, Tsuchimoto K, Hibi T: [Helicobacter pylori infected gastric mucosa–inflammation, atrophy and carcinogenesis]. *Nippon Saikingaku Zasshi* 2005, **60**(3):453-457.

40. Osawa H, Nakazato M, Date Y, Kita H, Ohnishi H, Ueno H, Shiiya T, Satoh K, Ishino Y, Sugano K: Impaired production of gastric ghrelin in chronic gastritis associated with Helicobacter pylori. *Journal of Clinical Endocrinology & Metabolism* 2005, **90**(1):10-16.

41. Isomoto H, Nishi Y, Ohnita K, Mizuta Y, Kohno S, Ueno H, Nakazato M: The Relationship between Plasma and Gastric Ghrelin Levels and Strain Diversity in Helicobacter pylori Virulence. *Am J Gastroenterol* 2005, **100**(6):1425-1427.

42. Alonso N, Granada ML, Salinas I, Reverter JL, Flores L, Ojanguren I, Martinez-Caceres EM, Sanmarti A: Plasma ghrelin concentrations in type 1 diabetic patients with autoimmune atrophic gastritis. *European Journal of Endocrinology* 2007, **157**(6):763-769.

43. Plonka M, Bielanski W, Konturek SJ, Targosz A, Sliwowski Z, Dobrzanska M, Kaminska A, Sito E, Konturek PC, Brzozowski T: Helicobacter pylori infection and serum gastrin, ghrelin and leptin in children of Polish shepherds. *Digestive & Liver Disease* 2006, **38**(2):91-97.

44. Uzzan B, Catheline JM, Lagorce C, Bon C, Cohen R, Perret GY, Benamouzig R: Expression of ghrelin in fundus is increased after gastric banding in morbidly obese patients. *Obesity Surgery* 2007, **17**(9):1159-1164.

45. Shak JR, Roper J, Perez-Perez GI, Tseng CH, Francois F, Gamagaris Z, Patterson C, Weinshel E, Fielding GA, Ren C, *et al*: The effect of laparoscopic gastric banding surgery on plasma levels of appetite-control, insulinotropic, and digestive hormones. *Obesity Surgery* 2008, **18**(9):1089-1096.

46. Osawa H, Kita H, Ohnishi H, Nakazato M, Date Y, Bowlus CL, Ishino Y, Watanabe E, Shiiya T, Ueno H, *et al*: Changes in plasma ghrelin levels, gastric ghrelin production, and body weight after Helicobacter pylori cure. *Journal of Gastroenterology* 2006, **41**(10):954-961.

47. Liew PL, Lee WJ, Lee YC, Chen WY: Gastric ghrelin expression associated with Helicobacter pylori infection and chronic gastritis in obese patients. *Obes Surg* 2006, **16**(5):612-619.

48. Tatsuguchi A, Miyake K, Gudis K, Futagami S, Tsukui T, Wada K, Kishida T, Fukuda Y, Sugisaki Y, Sakamoto C: Effect of Helicobacter pylori infection on ghrelin expression in human gastric mucosa. *Am J Gastroenterol* 2004, **99**(11):2121-2127.

49. Mendez-Sanchez N, Pichardo-Bahena R, Vasquez-Fernandez F, Lezama-Mora JI, Leon-Canales AL, Barredo-Prieto B, Gonzalez-Avila D, Ponciano-Rodriguez G, Uribe M: Effect of Helicobacter pylori infection on gastric ghrelin expression and body weight. *Revista de Gastroenterologia de Mexico* 2007, **72**(4):359-364.

50. Bercik P, Verdu EF, Foster JA, Lu J, Scharringa A, Kean I, Wang L, Blennerhassett P, Collins SM: Role of gut-brain axis in persistent abnormal feeding behavior in mice following eradication of Helicobacter pylori infection. *American Journal of Physiology - Regulatory Integrative & Comparative Physiology* 2009, **296**(3):R587-594.

51. Masaoka T, Suzuki H, Imaeda H, Hosoda H, Ohara T, Morishita T, Ishii H, Kangawa K, Hibi T: Long-term strict monitoring of plasma ghrelin and other serological markers of gastric diseases after Helicobacter pylori eradication. *Hepato-Gastroenterology* 2005, **52**(61):1-4.

52. Isomoto H, Nishi Y, Ohnita K, Mizuta Y, Kohno S, Ueno H, Nakazato M: The Relationship between Plasma and Gastric Ghrelin Levels and Strain Diversity in Helicobacter pylori Virulence. *American Journal of Gastroenterology* 2005, **100**(6):1425-1427.

53. Hussein NR, Mohammadi M, Talebkhan Y, Doraghi M, Letley DP, Muhammad MK, Argent RH, Atherton JC: Differences in virulence markers between Helicobacter pylori strains from Iraq and those from Iran: potential importance of regional differences in H. pylori-associated disease. *Journal of clinical microbiology* 2008, **46**(5):1774-1779.

54. Suzuki H, Masaoka T, Nomoto Y, Hosoda H, Mori M, Nishizawa T, Minegishi Y, Kangawa K, Hibi T: Increased levels of plasma ghrelin in peptic ulcer disease. *Alimentary pharmacology & therapeutics* 2006, **24**:120-126.

55. Suzuki H, Masaoka T, Hosoda H, Ota T, Minegishi Y, Nomura S, Kangawa K, Ishii H: Helicobacter pylori infection modifies gastric and plasma ghrelin dynamics in Mongolian gerbils. *Gut* 2004, **53**(2):187-194.

56. Campana D, Nori F, Pagotto U, De Iasio R, Morselli-Labate AM, Pasquali R, Corinaldesi R, Tomassetti P: Plasma acylated ghrelin levels are higher in patients with chronic atrophic gastritis. *Clin Endocrinol (Oxf)* 2007, **67**(5):761-766.

57. Wu MS, Lee WJ, Wang HH, Huang SP, Lin JT: A case-control study of association of Helicobacter pylori infection with morbid obesity in Taiwan. *Archives of Internal Medicine* 2005, **165**(13):1552-1555.

58. Shinomiya T, Fukunaga M, Akamizu T, Irako T, Yokode M, Kangawa K, Nakai Y, Nakai Y: Plasma acylated ghrelin levels correlate with subjective symptoms of functional dyspepsia in female patients. *Scandinavian Journal of Gastroenterology* 2005, **40**(6):648-653.

59. Suzuki H, Masaoka T, Sakai G, Ishii H, Hibi T: Improvement of gastrointestinal quality of life scores in cases of Helicobacter pylori-positive functional dyspepsia after successful eradication therapy. *Journal of gastroenterology and hepatology* 2005, **20**(11):1652-1660.

60. Sundbom M, Holdstock C, Engstrom E, Karlsson FA: **Early changes in ghrelin following Roux-en-Y gastric bypass: Influence of vagal nerve functionality?** *Obesity Surgery* 2007, **17(3)**:304-310.

61. Huang Q, Fan YZ, Ge BJ, Zhu Q, Tu ZY: **Circulating ghrelin in patients with gastric or colorectal cancer.** *Digestive diseases and sciences* 2007, **52(3)**:803-809.

62. Nishizawa T, Suzuki H, Nomoto Y, Masaoka T, Hosoda H, Mori M, Ohara T, Morishita T, Kangawa K, Hibi T: **Enhanced plasma ghrelin levels in patients with functional dyspepsia.** *Alimentary Pharmacology & Therapeutics* 2006, **24**:104-110.

63. Ando T, Minami M, Ishiguro K, Maeda O, Watanabe O, Mizuno T, Fujita T, Takahashi H, Noshiro M, Goto H: **Changes in biochemical parameters related to atherosclerosis after Helicobacter pylori eradication.** *Alimentary Pharmacology & Therapeutics* 2006, **24**:58-64.

64. Kempa A, Krzyzanowska-Swiniarska B, Miazgowski T, Pilarska K: **Not insulin but insulin sensivity, leptin, and cortisol are major factors regulating serum acylated ghrelin level in healthy women.** *Journal of Endocrinological Investigation* 2007, **30**:659-665.

65. Ates Y, Degertekin B, Erdil A, Yaman H, Dagalp K: **Serum ghrelin levels in inflammatory bowel disease with relation to disease activity and nutritional status.** *Digestive diseases and sciences* 2008, **53(8)**:2215-2221.

66. Wang HH, Lee WJ, Liew PL, Yang CS, Liang RJ, Wang W, Lin JT, Wu MS: **The influence of Helicobacter pylori infection and corpus gastritis on the postoperative outcomes of laparoscopic vertical banded gastroplasty.** *Obesity Surgery* 2006, **16(3)**:297-307.

67. Doki Y, Takachi K, Ishikawa O, Miyashiro I, Sasaki Y, Ohigashi H, Nakajima H, Hosoda H, Kangawa K, Sasakuma F, *et al*: **Ghrelin reduction after esophageal substitution and its correlation to postoperative body weight loss in esophageal cancer patients.** *Surgery* 2006, **139(6)**:797-805.

68. Gao XY, Kuang HY, Liu XM, Ma ZB, Nie HJ, Guo H: **Plasma obestatin levels in men with chronic atrophic gastritis.** *Peptides* 2008, **29(10)**:1749-1754.

69. Cherian S, Forbes D, Sanfilippo F, Cook A, Burgner D: **Helicobacter pylori, helminth infections and growth: a cross-sectional study in a high prevalence population.** *Acta Paediatrica* 2009, **98(5)**:860-864.

70. Kebapcilar L, Sari I, Renkal AH, Alacacioglu A, Yuksel A, Ilhan E, Alkan B, Yuksel D, Kozaci DL, Gunay N: **The Influence of Helicobacter pylori Eradication on Leptin, Soluble CD40 Ligand, Oxidative Stress and Body Composition in Patients with Peptic Ulcer Disease.** *Internal Medicine* 2009, **48(24)**:2055-2059.

71. Dutta SK, Arora M, Kireet A, Bashandy H, Gandsas A: **Upper Gastrointestinal Symptoms and Associated Disorders in Morbidly Obese Patients: A Prospective Study.** *Digestive Diseases and Sciences* 2009, **54(6)**:1243-1246.

72. Gen R, Demir M, Ataseven H: **Effect of Helicobacter pylori Eradication on Insulin Resistance, Serum Lipids and Low-Grade Inflammation.** *Southern Medical Journal* 2010, **103(3)**:190-196.

Accuracy of endoscopic diagnosis of *Helicobacter pylori* infection according to level of endoscopic experience and the effect of training

Kazuhiro Watanabe[1†], Naoyoshi Nagata[1*†], Takuro Shimbo[2†], Ryo Nakashima[1†], Etsuko Furuhata[1†], Toshiyuki Sakurai[1†], Naoki Akazawa[1†], Chizu Yokoi[1†], Masao Kobayakawa[1†], Junichi Akiyama[1†], Masashi Mizokami[3†] and Naomi Uemura[4†]

Abstract

Background: Accurate prediction of *Helicobacter pylori* infection status on endoscopic images can contribute to early detection of gastric cancer, especially in Asia. We identified the diagnostic yield of endoscopy for *H. pylori* infection at various endoscopist career levels and the effect of two years of training on diagnostic yield.

Methods: A total of 77 consecutive patients who underwent endoscopy were analyzed. *H. pylori* infection status was determined by histology, serology, and the urea breast test and categorized as *H. pylori*-uninfected, -infected, or -eradicated. Distinctive endoscopic findings were judged by six physicians at different career levels: beginner (<500 endoscopies), intermediate (1500–5000), and advanced (>5000). Diagnostic yield and inter- and intra-observer agreement on *H. pylori* infection status were evaluated. Values were compared between the two beginners after two years of training. The kappa (K) statistic was used to calculate agreement.

Results: For all physicians, the diagnostic yield was 88.9% for *H. pylori*-uninfected, 62.1% for *H. pylori*-infected, and 55.8% for *H. pylori*-eradicated. Intra-observer agreement for *H. pylori* infection status was good (K > 0.6) for all physicians, while inter-observer agreement was lower (K = 0.46) for beginners than for intermediate and advanced (K > 0.6). For all physicians, good inter-observer agreement in endoscopic findings was seen for atrophic change (K = 0.69), regular arrangement of collecting venules (K = 0.63), and hemorrhage (K = 0.62). For beginners, the diagnostic yield of *H. pylori*-infected/eradicated status and inter-observer agreement of endoscopic findings were improved after two years of training.

Conclusions: The diagnostic yield of endoscopic diagnosis was high for *H. pylori*-uninfected cases, but was low for *H. pylori*-eradicated cases. In beginners, daily training on endoscopic findings improved the low diagnostic yield.

Keywords: Helicobacter pylori, Endoscopic training, Diagnostic yield, Endoscopic career level, Inter-observer agreement, Intra-observer agreement

Background

Since the discovery of *Helicobacter pylori* in 1982 [1], the association between *H. pylori* infection and gastric cancer has been well established [2]. Moreover, recent studies have shown that eradication of *H. pylori* prevents development of metachronous gastric cancer [3,4]. However, gastric cancer can occur in not only *H. pylori*-infected patients, but also *H. pylori*-eradicated patients. Therefore, it is extremely important to determine *H. pylori* infection status (uninfected, infected, or eradicated) by regular screening endoscopy.

Among patients with *H. pylori*-infected gastric mucosa, atrophic change is considered to be a risk of gastric cancer [2]. In Asia, especially in Japan, severe atrophic gastritis is more common than in the West [5,6], and it is considered highly detectable on endoscopy in these regions [5]. Therefore, endoscopic visualization of *H. pylori* infection

* Correspondence: nnagata_ncgm@yahoo.co.jp
†Equal contributors
[1]Department of Gastroenterology and Hepatology, National Center for Global Health and Medicine, 1-21-1 Toyama, Shinjuku-ku, Tokyo 162-8655, Japan

of the gastric mucosa is useful for the early detection of gastric cancer, and education of beginner endoscopists on this paradigm is becoming an important clinical issue. However, the value of endoscopic diagnosis of *H. pylori* infection status remains unclear [7-11].

In this paper, we identify the accuracy and reproducibility of endoscopic diagnosis of *H. pylori*-uninfected, -infected, and -eradicated status. Moreover, we compare scores of endoscopists with various levels of experience, and we identify the effect of two years of training on beginner endoscopists.

Methods
Subjects
A total of 148 consecutive dyspeptic patients who had undergone upper gastrointestinal endoscopy and who were diagnosed strictly for *H. pylori* infection at the National Center for Global Health and Medicine (NCGM) between December 2008 and April 2009 were selected from an endoscopic electronic database. Exclusion criteria included the use of non-steroidal anti-inflammatory drugs (NSAIDs), anti-thrombogenic drugs, and proton pump inhibitor and patients with a history of gastric surgery, hemorrhagic disease, liver cirrhosis, end-stage renal disease requiring dialysis, severe heart failure with any symptoms, and early or advanced gastric cancer, because these conditions can affect the mucosal appearance of the stomach [12-15]. After exclusion, 77 patients were selected for analysis.

Written informed consent was obtained from all participants in accordance with the Declaration of Helsinki and its subsequent revision. The study protocol was approved by the Ethics Committee of the NCGM (approval No. 811).

Gold standard for diagnosis of H. pylori infection status
H. pylori infection was evaluated by the presence of serum immunoglobulin G antibody against *H. pylori* (HM-CAP, Enteric Products, Westbury, NY), a ^{13}C urea breath test (UBT; with a cut-off value of 2.5‰; Ubit, Otsuka Pharmaceuticals, Tokyo, Japan), and histological examination with toluidine blue staining. For histological evaluation, three endoscopic biopsy specimens were taken from the greater curvature of the upper gastric body, angulus, and antrum.

Subjects with a history of *H. pylori* eradication who were confirmed negative by histologic examination of gastric biopsy specimens and a negative ^{13}C-UBT were defined as eradicated patients. Subjects without a history of *H. pylori* eradication who were confirmed negative based on the results of all three methods were defined as uninfected patients. The remaining subjects in whom neither status was confirmed were defined as infected patients.

Endoscopic assessment of H. pylori infection status
All endoscopies were performed by well-trained endoscopists using a high resolution videoendoscope (GIF-260H, Olympus Medical Systems, Tokyo, Japan) with a pre-endoscopic oral solution containing dimethylpolysiloxane (Balgin Antifoaming Oral Solution 2%, Kaigen Co., Ltd., Osaka, Japan).

We routinely record about 50–60 images at fixed sites of the esophagus, stomach, and duodenum in all cases and save them to the electronic endoscopic database (Solemio ENDO, Olympus Medical Systems). We selected six photos of specific sites of the antrum, angulus, lesser and greater curvature of the lower body, greater curvature of the upper body, and cardia of the stomach (Figure 1) from the electronic endoscopic database in each case, and endoscopic findings were then evaluated.

The following 11 distinctive endoscopic findings related to *H. pylori* infection status (uninfected, infected, and eradicated) were used for analysis: regular arrangement of collecting venules (RAC) [16], atrophic change [17,18], rugal hyperplasia [19], edema [20], spotty erythema [20], linear erythema [20], hemorrhage [20], exudate [20], fundic gland polyp [21], xanthoma [22], and motteled patchy erythema (MPE) [23]. Before judging, we held several seminars to obtain a consensus on the relation between *H. pylori* infection status and distinctive endoscopic findings [16-23] using typical images selected from the electronic endoscopic database. We then judged *H. pylori* infection status and categorized it as *H. pylori*-uninfected, *H. pylori*-infected, or *H. pylori*-eradicated on the basis of endoscopic findings. Endoscopic images were assessed by six endoscopists who were grouped according to endoscopic experience as follows: two beginner (<500 upper endoscopies), two intermediate (1500–5000 upper endoscopies), and two advanced (>5000 upper endoscopies). All six endoscopists were blinded to the clinical information of examined cases.

Training for endoscopic assessment of H. pylori infection status
Training of beginners was conducted in a systematical manner over two years of daily clinical practice and entailed the following: 1) recording the presence or absence of the 11 distinctive endoscopic findings into the electronic endoscopic database for all patients; 2) recording the prediction of *H. pylori* infection status on the basis of endoscopic findings. Two years after initial diagnosis, diagnosis of *H. pylori* infection status and endoscopic findings were reassessed in the same manner for all cases.

Statistical analysis
Diagnostic yield was calculated as a positive predictive value using the results of the endoscopic evaluation of

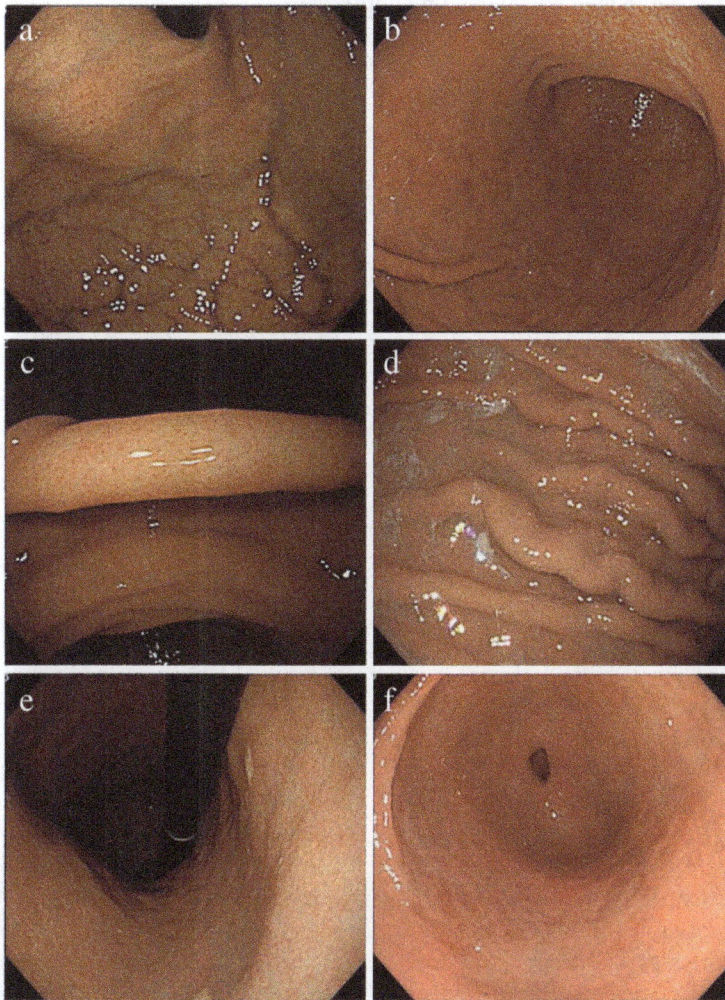

Figure 1 Different sites of the stomach showing *H. pylori* infection status. a. Cardia with hemorrhage. **b**. Lesser and greater curvature of lower body with atrophy, and spotty erythema. **c**. Angulus with regular arrangement of collecting venules. **d**. Greater curvature of the upper body with exudates, edema, and rugal hyperplasia. **e**. Lesser curvature of lower body with xanthoma. **f**. Antrum with motteled patchy erythema.

77 cases. To calculate the diagnostic yield of all six physicians, the results of the 77 cases were totaled, and 462 cases were used for analysis. Diagnostic yield was then compared among endoscopists with different levels of experience using the Chi-squared test. We calculated the value of intra- and inter-observer agreement using the kappa statistic [24] to clarify the reproducibility of the endoscopic diagnosis of *H. pylori* infection status. Kappa values (K) >0.80 denoted excellent, >0.60–0.80 good, >0.40–0.60 moderate, >0.20–0.40 fair, and ≤0.20 poor [24].

To determine intra-observer agreement, all six physicians reassessed the same endoscopic images one week after the first evaluation in a different order. Inter-observer agreement among all six endoscopists and between endoscopist pairs of different levels of experience (two each for beginner, intermediate, and advanced) was calculated. Inter-observer agreement of the 11 endoscopic

findings was calculated in the same manner. After training the beginners for two years, diagnostic yield and inter-observer agreement were reassessed and compared against the values of the initial diagnosis using the McNemar test.

Values of $p < 0.05$ were considered significant. All statistical analysis was performed using Stata version 10 software (StataCorp, Lakeway Drive College Station, TX).

Results
Patient characteristics
A total of 77 patients (32 men and 45 women; mean age (SD), 39.7 (13.4) years) and 462 images were assessed. Of them, 28 were *H. pylori*-uninfected, 28 were -infected, and 21 were -eradicated. Of the 21 eradicated cases, 18 had information on the date of eradication therapy. The mean (SD) period from eradication therapy to endoscopy of these 18 cases was 28 (32) months.

Table 1 Diagnostic yield of *H. pylori* infection status on endoscopy

	H. pylori-uninfected	*H. pylori*-infected	*H. pylori*-eradicated
All physicians* (n = 6)	88.9% (82.3–93.6%)	62.1% (55.3–68.7%)	55.8% (46.1–65.1%)
Individual physicians**			
Beginner 1	82.6% (61.2–95.0%)	55.3% (38.3–71.4%)	37.5% (15.2–64.6%)
Beginner 2	90.9% (70.8–98.9%)	54.8% (36.0–72.7%)	50.0% (29.1–70.9%)
Intermediate 1	91.3% (72.0–98.9%)	67.6% (49.5–82.6%)	65.0% (40.8–84.6%)
Intermediate 2	82.6% (61.2–95.0%)	66.7% (49.0–81.4%)	66.7% (49.0–81.4%)
Advanced 1	90.5% (69.6–98.8%)	63.9% (46.2–79.2%)	50.0% (27.2–72.8%)
Advanced 2	95.7% (78.1–99.9%)	64.1% (47.2–78.8%)	80.0% (51.9–95.7%)

*Analyzed cases: n = 462. **Analyzed cases: n = 77. 95% confidence interval values are given in parentheses.
Abbreviation: *H. pylori*, Helicobacter pylori.

Diagnostic yield of endoscopic diagnosis of H. pylori infection status

The yield of endoscopic diagnosis of *H. pylori* infection status is shown in Table 1. The yield was highest for *H. pylori*-uninfected (88.9%), followed by *H. pylori*-infected (62.1%), and *H. pylori*-eradicated (55.8%) for all six endoscopists. The same order of yield for *H. pylori* infection status was also found within each level of endoscopic experience: the yield of *H. pylori*-infected and -eradicated was lower in the beginner group than in the intermediate and advanced groups, but differences were not statistically significant (p > 0.05).

Intra- and inter-observer agreement of endoscopic diagnosis of H. pylori infection status

Intra-observer agreement of all six physicians was relatively good (K > 0.6) irrespective of endoscopic experience (Table 2). Inter-observer agreement was moderate (K = 0.46) in the beginner group but high in the intermediate and advanced groups (K > 0.6) (Table 2).

Inter-observer agreement of endoscopic findings associated with H. pylori infection status

The inter-observer agreement of the endoscopic findings is shown in Table 3. A high agreement among the six endoscopists was found for atrophic change (K = 0.63), hemorrhage (K = 0.62), and RAC (K = 0.63). Of the different levels of endoscopic experience, beginners showed the lowest inter-observer agreement for all findings, except for exudate and xanthoma.

Change in endoscopic diagnostic yield and endoscopic findings after two years of training

Figure 2 shows the diagnostic yield of all cases of *H. pylori* infection status on endoscopy before and after training. A significant increase was noted in diagnostic yield of *H. pylori*-uninfected (82.6% and 88.6%, p < 0.05) and *H. pylori*-eradicated (37.5% and 46.2%, p < 0.05) in beginner 1. Slight increases were also evident for the diagnostic yield of *H. pylori*-infected (55.3% and 58.6%, P = 0.41) in

beginner 1, *H. pylori*-infected (54.8% and 68.6%, P = 0.25) in beginner 2, and *H. pylori*-eradicated (50.0% and 65.0%, P = 0.25) in beginner 2. In contrast, the diagnostic yield of *H. pylori*-uninfected in beginner 2 remained high (90.0% and 90.9%) after training.

Discussion

In previous studies on endoscopic diagnosis for *H. pylori* infection, one or two tests were regarded as the gold standard. However accurate diagnosis of *H. pylori* infection is difficult; thus combining several diagnostic approaches is preferable [25,26]. In our study, we used histology, serology, and the urea breast test to diagnose *H. pylori* infection status accurately, making the results highly reliable.

The low diagnostic yield for *H. pylori*-eradicated cases (55.8%) may reflect insufficient knowledge of typical endoscopic images of *H. pylori*-eradicated mucosa because few studies have reported such endoscopic findings [19,27]. However, this value is still considered relatively good, because it is not easy to discriminate between *H. pylori*-eradicated and -uninfected cases, even when using serological or UBT testing [28,29]. *H. pylori* eradication is currently recommended worldwide, so the number of eradicated patients is expected to increase. However, gastric cancer is sometimes detected on endoscopy even after eradication [3,4],

Table 2 Intra- and inter-observer agreement of *H. pylori* infection status on endoscopy

	Intra-observer agreement	Inter-observer agreement
Beginner 1	0.65	0.46
Beginner 2	0.62	
Intermediate 1	0.72	0.78
Intermediate 2	0.74	
Advanced 1	0.67	0.65
Advanced 2	0.82	

Note: All values calculated using kappa statistics.

Table 3 Inter-observer agreement of endoscopic findings

	All physicians	Beginner	Intermediate	Advanced	Beginner (two years later)
Atrophic change	0.69	0.54	0.75	0.81	0.77
RAC	0.63	0.58	0.87	0.50	0.81
Hemorrhage	0.62	0.29	0.77	0.81	0.64
Fundic gland polyp	0.55	0.17	0.58	0.67	0.75
Rugal hyperplasia	0.51	0.42	0.65	0.54	0.84
Spotty erythema	0.51	0.53	0.54	0.72	0.57
Linear erythema	0.51	0.15	0.80	0.72	0.55
Exudate	0.48	0.51	0.58	0.38	0.59
MPE	0.48	0.27	0.67	0.47	0.63
Edema	0.46	0.27	0.58	0.53	0.38
Xanthoma	0.35	0.22	0.06	0.75	0.55

Note: All values calculated using kappa statistics.

therefore, it is important that *H. pylori*-eradicated cases can be endoscopically distinguished from *H. pylori*-uninfected ones.

Although a number of endoscopic studies on *H. pylori* infection (uninfected versus infected) have been reported, results have been contradictory. Khaloo et al. evaluated the updated Sydney system (USS) on endoscopy and obtained a low diagnostic yield of 41.8% [8], and Belair et al. concluded that endoscopic diagnosis of *H. pylori* infection is not useful because of a low ROC of 0.55 [9]. Redeen et al. also reported a low diagnostic yield (43–53%) [10], while a slightly higher diagnostic yield of 64% was obtained by Bah et al. [7].

In contrast, a study of *H. pylori* infection in highly endemic areas by Mihara et al. obtained a high diagnostic yield of 79.5% in accordance with the USS [11]. The inconsistency in diagnostic yields might have been caused by differences in regional disease prevalence. In the present study, diagnostic yield was relatively low compared with previous studies, as reflected by the difficulty in distinguishing between *H. pylori*-infected and *H. pylori*-eradicated cases.

The diagnostic yield in *H. pylori*-uninfected cases was high. We believe this is because many of the endoscopists correctly identified RAC [16], hemorrhage [20], and fundic gland polyps [21], all of which are characteristic of *H. pylori*-uninfected mucosa. These findings in fact attained good inter-observer agreement.

We hypothesized that diagnostic yield is influenced by endoscopist experience and found that scores for *H. pylori*-infected and -eradicated cases were low for beginners compared with intermediate and advanced endoscopists. In addition, inter-observer agreement on *H. pylori* infection status between beginners was noticeably inconsistent, presumably because endoscopic findings by beginners varied among cases compared with intermediate and advanced

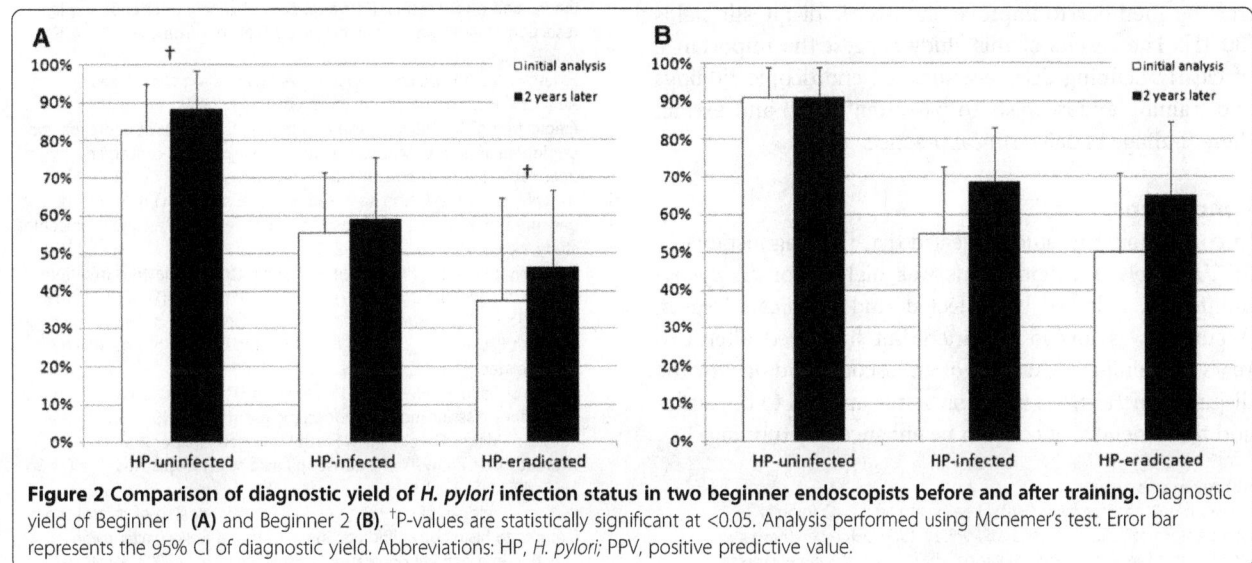

Figure 2 Comparison of diagnostic yield of *H. pylori* infection status in two beginner endoscopists before and after training. Diagnostic yield of Beginner 1 **(A)** and Beginner 2 **(B)**. †P-values are statistically significant at <0.05. Analysis performed using Mcnemer's test. Error bar represents the 95% CI of diagnostic yield. Abbreviations: HP, *H. pylori*; PPV, positive predictive value.

endoscopists. In intermediate and advanced endoscopists, the definition of endoscopic findings appears to have been well established, and thus the extraction was consistent.

Lastly, the diagnostic yield for *H. pylori*-infected and -eradicated gastric mucosa was increased in the two beginners after two years of training, and subsequently, their post-training inter-observer agreement has also improved. We believe that training improved their understanding of individual endoscopic findings that defined different states of *H. pylori* infection, resulting in consistent inter-observer agreement and higher diagnostic yield.

Because no video-based evaluation was performed, we could not observe detailed mucosal patterns and some local findings that may have been present, which is a limitation of our study. Endoscopists may not spend sufficient time performing detailed observation of the gastric mucosa in *H. pylori*-uninfected cases, whereas examination of *H. pylori*-infected gastric mucosa with inflammation is expected to be time-consuming and detailed. Therefore, we believe that blindness is maintained better with the use of photographic images.

Our diagnostic yield of approximately 90% for *H. pylori*-uninfected cases suggests that patients with a low risk of gastric cancer can be determined through screening endoscopy. Although, the diagnostic yield for *H. pylori*-infected and -eradicated cases was lower than that for uninfected cases, more than half of the patients who underwent screening endoscopy were determined to be at high risk of gastric cancer, so we performed careful observation of the gastric mucosa during endoscopy. In addition, we recommend additional tests such as a UBT or serology test for these patients. This diagnostic strategy may be efficient and cost-effective for the early detection of gastric cancer, which is an important clinical aspect of this study. Only a few studies have reported training methods to improve endoscopic diagnostic fields [30,31]. The results of this study suggest the importance of clearly defining disease-associated endoscopic findings and training endoscopists to pay attention to and extract these findings in daily clinical practice.

Conclusions

In conclusion, this study revealed that the diagnostic yield for *H. pylori* infection status was highest for *H. pylori*-uninfected, followed by -infected, and -eradicated cases. Accuracy was low in beginners but improved after two years of training. Extraction of endoscopic findings for the diagnosis of *H. pylori* infection status appears to be useful, and the beneficial effects can be enhanced by training.

Abbreviations

H. pylori: Helicobacter pylori; UBT: Urea breath test; RAC: Regular arrangement of collecting venules; MPE: Mottled patchy erythema; PPV: Positive predictive value; K: Kappa; USS: Updated Sydney system.

Competing interests

The authors declare that they have no competing interests.

Authors' contributions

KW participated in data acquisition and interpretation and wrote the manuscript. NN participated in the design of the study, data interpretation, performed endoscopy, and contributed to the writing of the manuscript. TS participated in the design of the study and contributed to statistical analysis. RN helped with data acquisition. EF, TS, NA, CY, and MK performed endoscopic assessment. JA and NU advised on the design of the study and contributed to the writing of the manuscript. MM advised on the content of the revised manuscript and contributed to the writing of the revised manuscript. All authors discussed the content and commented on the manuscript. All authors read and approved the final manuscript.

Acknowledgements

We wish to express our gratitude to Hisae Kawashiro, Clinical Research Coordinator, for help with data collection. This study was supported in part by a Grant-in-Aid from the Ministry of Health Labor and Welfare of Japan, a Grant-in-Aid from the Ministry of Education, Culture, Sports, Science and Technology of Japan (271000), and The Grant of National Center for Global Health and Medicine (22–302). The funders had no role in study design, data collection and analysis, decision to publish, or preparation of the manuscript.

Author details

[1]Department of Gastroenterology and Hepatology, National Center for Global Health and Medicine, 1-21-1 Toyama, Shinjuku-ku, Tokyo 162-8655, Japan. [2]Department of Clinical Research and Informatics, National Center for Global Health and Medicine, 1-21-1 ToyamaShinjuku-ku, Tokyo 162-8655, Japan. [3]Research Center for Hepatitis and Immunology, National Center for Global Health and Medicine, Kohnodai Hospital, 1-7-1 Kohnodai, Ichikawa City, Chiba 272-8516, Japan. [4]Department of Gastroenterology and Hepatology, National Center for Global Health and Medicine, Kohnodai Hospital, 1-7-1 Kohnodai, Ichikawa City, Chiba 272-8516, Japan.

References

1. Marshall BJ, Warren JR: **Unidentified curved bacilli in the stomach of patients with gastritis and peptic ulceration.** *Lancet* 1984, **1:**1311–1315.
2. Uemura N, Okamoto S, Yamamoto S, Matsumura N, Yamaguchi S, Yamakido M, Taniyama K, Sasaki N, Schlemper RJ: **Helicobacter pylori infection and the development of gastric cancer.** *N Engl J Med* 2001, **345:**784–789.
3. Uemura N, Mukai T, Okamoto S, Yamaguchi S, Mashiba H, Taniyama K, Sasaki N, Haruma K, Sumii K, Kajiyama G: **Effect of Helicobacter pylori eradication on subsequent development of cancer after endoscopic resection of early gastric cancer.** *Cancer Epidemiol Biomarkers Prev* 1997, **6:**639–642.
4. Fukase K, Kato M, Kikuchi S, Inoue K, Uemura N, Okamoto S, Terao S, Amagai K, Hayashi S, Asaka M, Japan Gast Study Group: **Effect of eradication of Helicobacter pylori on incidence of metachronous gastric carcinoma after endoscopic resection of early gastric cancer: an open-label, randomised controlled trial.** *Lancet* 2008, **372:**392–397.
5. Asaka M, Sugiyama T, Nobuta A, Kato M, Takeda H, Graham DY: **Atrophic gastritis and intestinal metaplasia in Japan: results of a large multicenter study.** *Helicobacter* 2001, **6:**294–299.
6. Weck MN, Brenner H: **Prevalence of chronic atrophic gastritis in different parts of the world.** *Cancer Epidemiol Biomarkers Prev* 2006, **15:**1083–1094.
7. Bah A, Saraga E, Armstrong D, Vouillamoz D, Dorta G, Duroux P, Weber B, Froehlich F, Blum AL, Schnegg JF: **Endoscopic features of Helicobacter pylori-related gastritis.** *Endoscopy* 1995, **27:**593–596.
8. Khakoo SI, Lobo AJ, Shepherd NA, Wilkinson SP: **Histological assessment of the Sydney classification of endoscopic gastritis.** *Gut* 1994, **35:**1172–1175.
9. Belair PA, Metz DC, Faigel DO, Furth EE: **Receiver operator characteristic analysis of endoscopy as a test for gastritis.** *Dig Dis Sci* 1997, **42:**2227–2233.
10. Redeen S, Petersson F, Jonsson KA, Borch K: **Relationship of gastroscopic features to histological findings in gastritis and Helicobacter pylori infection in a general population sample.** *Endoscopy* 2003, **35:**946–950.

11. Mihara M, Haruma K, Kamada T, Komoto K, Yoshihara M, Sumii K, Kajiyama G: The role of endoscopic findings for the diagnosis of *Helicobacter pylori* infection: evaluation in a country with high prevalence of atrophic gastritis. *Helicobacter* 1999, **4**:40–48.

12. Primignani M, Carpinelli L, Preatoni P, Battaglia G, Carta A, Prada A, Cestari R, Angeli P, Gatta A, Rossi A, Spinzi G, De Franchis R: **Natural history of portal hypertensive gastropathy in patients with liver cirrhosis. The New Italian Endoscopic Club for the study and treatment of esophageal varices (NIEC).** *Gastroenterology* 2000, **119**:181–187.

13. Laine L: Review article: the effect of *Helicobacter pylori* infection on nonsteroidal anti-inflammatory drug-induced upper gastrointestinal tract injury. *Aliment Pharmacol Ther* 2002, **16**(Suppl 1):34–39.

14. Sotoudehmanesh R, Ali Asgari A, Ansari R, Nouraie M: **Endoscopic findings in end-stage renal disease.** *Endoscopy* 2003, **35**:502–505.

15. Kawai T, Watanabe M, Yamashina A: Impact of upper gastrointestinal lesions in patients on low-dose aspirin therapy: preliminary study. *J Gastroenterol Hepatol* 2010, **25**(Suppl 1):S23–S30.

16. Yagi K, Nakamura A, Sekine A: **Characteristic endoscopic and magnified endoscopic findings in the normal stomach without *Helicobacter pylori* infection.** *J Gastroenterol Hepatol* 2002, **17**:39–45.

17. Kimura K, Takemoto T: **An Endoscopic Recognition of the Atrophic Border and its Significance in Chronic Gastritis.** *Endoscopy* 1969, **1**:87–97.

18. Kawaguchi H, Haruma K, Komoto K, Yoshihara M, Sumii K, Kajiyama G: *Helicobacter pylori* infection is the major risk factor for atrophic gastritis. *Am J Gastroenterol* 1996, **91**:959–962.

19. Yasunaga Y, Shinomura Y, Kanayama S, Yabu M, Nakanishi T, Miyazaki Y, Murayama Y, Bonilla-Palacios JJ, Matsuzawa Y: **Improved fold width and increased acid secretion after eradication of the organism in *Helicobacter pylori* associated enlarged fold gastritis.** *Gut* 1994, **35**:1571–1574.

20. Kaminishi M, Yamaguchi H, Nomura S, Oohara T, Sakai S, Fukutomi H, Nakahara A, Kashimura H, Oda M, Kitahora T, Ichikawa H, Yabana T, Yagawa Y, Sugiyama T, Itabashi M, Unakami M, Oguro Y, Sakita T: **Endoscopic classification of chronic gastritis based on a pilot study by the research society for gastritis.** *Digestive Endoscopy* 2002, **14**:138–151.

21. Watanabe N, Seno H, Nakajima T, Yazumi S, Miyamoto S, Matsumoto S, Itoh T, Kawanami C, Okazaki K, Chiba T: **Regression of fundic gland polyps following acquisition of *Helicobacter pylori*.** *Gut* 2002, **51**:742–745.

22. Isomoto H, Mizuta Y, Inoue K, Matsuo T, Hayakawa T, Miyazaki M, Onita K, Takeshima F, Murase K, Shimokawa I, Kohno S: **A close relationship between *Helicobacter pylori* infection and gastric xanthoma.** *Scand J Gastroenterol* 1999, **34**:346–352.

23. Nagata N, Shimbo T, Akiyama J, Nakashima R, Kim HH, Yoshida T, Hoshimoto K, Uemura N: **Predictability of Gastric Intestinal Metaplasia by Mottled Patchy Erythema Seen on Endoscopy.** *Gastroenterology Research* 2011, **5**:203–209.

24. Sim J, Wright CC: **The kappa statistic in reliability studies: use, interpretation, and sample size requirements.** *Phys Ther* 2005, **85**:257–268.

25. Thijs JC, van Zwet AA, Thijs WJ, Oey HB, Karrenbeld A, Stellaard F, Luijt DS, Meyer BC, Kleibeuker JH: **Diagnostic tests for *Helicobacter pylori*: a prospective evaluation of their accuracy, without selecting a single test as the gold standard.** *Am J Gastroenterol* 1996, **91**:2125–2129.

26. Ricci C, Holton J, Vaira D: **Diagnosis of *Helicobacter pylori*: invasive and non-invasive tests.** *Best Pract Res Clin Gastroenterol* 2007, **21**:299–313.

27. Avunduk C, Navab F, Hampf F, Coughlin B: **Prevalence of *Helicobacter pylori* infection in patients with large gastric folds: evaluation and follow-up with endoscopic ultrasound before and after antimicrobial therapy.** *Am J Gastroenterol* 1995, **90**:1969–1973.

28. Kosunen TU, Seppala K, Sarna S, Sipponen P: **Diagnostic value of decreasing IgG, IgA, and IgM antibody titres after eradication of *Helicobacter pylori*.** *Lancet* 1992, **339**:893–895.

29. Miwa H, Ohkura R, Nagahara A, Murai T, Ogihara T, Watanabe S, Hirai S, Sato N: 13C]-urea breath test for assessment of cure of *Helicobacter pylori* infection at 1 month after treatment. *J Clin Gastroenterol* 1998, **27**(Suppl 1):S150–S153.

30. Sidhu R, Sakellariou P, McAlindon ME, Leeds JS, Shafiq K, Hoeroldt BS, Hopper AD, Karmo M, Salmon C, Elphick D, Ali A, Sanders DS: **Is formal training necessary for capsule endoscopy? The largest gastroenterology trainee study with controls.** *Dig Liver Dis* 2008, **40**:298–302.

31. Yamazato T, Oyama T, Yoshida T, Baba Y, Yamanouchi K, Ishii Y, Inoue F, Toda S, Mannen K, Shimoda R, Iwakiri R, Fujimoto K: **Two years' intensive training in endoscopic diagnosis facilitates detection of early gastric cancer.** *Intern Med* 2012, **51**:1461–1465.

Study of *Helicobacter pylori* genotype status in cows, sheep, goats and human beings

Hassan Momtaz[1], Hossein Dabiri[2], Negar Souod[3*] and Mohsen Gholami[4]

Abstract

Background: *Helicobacter pylori* is one of the most controversial bacteria in the world causing diverse gastrointestinal diseases. The transmission way of this bacterium still remains unknown. The possibility of zoonotic transmission of *H. pylori* has been suggested, but is not proven in nonprimate reservoirs. In the current survey, we investigate the presence of *H. pylori* in cow, sheep and goat stomach, determine the bacterium virulence factors and finally compare the human *H. pylori* virulence factors and animals in order to examine whether *H. pylori* might be transmitted from these animals to human beings.

Methods: This cross- sectional study was performed on 800 gastric biopsy specimens of cows, sheep, goats and human beings. The PCR assays was performed to detection of *H. pylori*, *vacA* and *cagA* genes. The PCR products of Ruminant's samples with positive *H. pylori* were subjected to DNA sequencing analysis. Statistical tests were applied for data analysis.

Results: Overall 6 (3%) cows, 32 (16%) sheep and 164 (82%) human beings specimens were confirmed to be *H. pylori* positive; however we were not able to detect this bacterium in all 200 goat samples. The *vacA s1a/m1a* was the predominant *H. pylori* genotype in all three kinds of studied population. There was 3.4–8.4% variability and 92.9-98.5% homology between sheep and human samples.

Conclusions: Considering the high sequence homology among DNA of *H. pylori* isolated from sheep and human, our data suggest that sheep may act as a reservoir for *H. pylori* and in the some extent share the ancestral host for the bacteria with human.

Keywords: *Helicobacter pylori*, Virulence genes, Cow, Sheep, Goat, Human being

Background

Helicobacter pylori is a gram negative, spiral shaped bacterium which its main reservoir is humans, particularly the human stomach. It colonizes most of the population, making it one of the most controversial bacteria in the world that cause gastritis, peptic ulcer, duodenal ulcer, lymphoma and gastric cancer [1].

According to the reports the main routs of infection has not been clarified yet [2]. However it is likely that *H. pylori* infection occurs during childhood or adolescence both in developing and developed countries [3] and its transmission occurs by person to person, either by fecal-oral or oral-oral routes [4]. The possibility of zoonotic transmission of *H. pylori* has been suggested, but is not

proven in nonprimate reservoirs [4]. Some reports indicated that there is a high prevalence of antibody against this bacterium in veterinarians, butchers and slaughters rather than other people, so it suggests that *H. pylori* might be transmitted from animals to human [5,6]. Recently some researchers have been isolated *H. pylori* from cow, sheep, camel, pigs and dogs milk [7,8]. Therefore, it seems that these animals can be a reservoir of this bacterium. The severity of clinical manifestations varies depends on several factors such as host genetic, immune system, bacterial load and virulence factors [9]. This bacterium has several virulence factor genes which are generally classified into three categories: I) strain-specific genes, such as *cag* pathogenesity island (PAI) and genes located in plasticity island region (e.g. *jhp0947* and *dupA* genes), which are present in only some *H. pylori* strains. II) phase-variable genes which change during different

* Correspondence: negarsouod@yahoo.com
[3]Young Researchers and Elite club, Central Tehran Branch, Islamic Azad University, P.O.Box: 13185-768, Tehran, Iran

growth conditions. Based on comparison of three completed genomes of *H. pylori*, six genes encoding outer-membrane proteins (*babB*, *oipA*, *hopZ sabA*, *sabB* and *babC*) are supposed to have phase variation. III) The genes with polymorphisms, for instance, specific *vacA* genotypes have been associated with different clinical outcomes [10]. The *cag* pathogenicity island (PAI) which belongs to the first category, encodes a type IV secretion system [2,3]. The *cagA* gene is located in the end of the *cag* PAI and has been proposed as a marker for the *cag*PAI. Different type of the *cagA* gene in some region is associated with diverse clinical outcomes; for instance *cagA1a* in East Asian Strains, is associated with more severe clinical manifestations than the absence of the gene [11]. The other important virulence factor of *H. pylori* is a vacuolating cytotoxin (VacA), which belongs to the last category and is associated with injury to epithelial cells. The *vacA* gene is present in virtually all strains of *H. pylori* but it is polymorphic, comprising variable signal regions (type *s1* or *s2*) and mid-regions (type *m1* or *m2*). Type *s1/m1 vacA* contribute with more epithelial cell damage rather than type *s1/m2*, whereas type *s2/m2* and the rare *s2/m1* are supposed to be non-toxic due to the presence of a short 12-residue hydrophilic extension on the *s2* form [12,13]. The s-region is classified into *s1* and *s2* types and the m-region into *m1* and *m2* types. The *s1* type is further subtyped into *s1a*, *s1b* and *s1c* subtypes, and the *m1* into *m1a* and *m1b* subtypes. The mosaic combination of s and m-region allelic types determines the particular cytotoxin and, consequently, the pathogenicity of the bacterium [2,14].

In the current survey, we investigated the presence of *H. pylori* in cow, sheep and goat stomach, as well as bacterium virulence factors distribution among human and other studied population.

Methods

Population and sampling

Over all 800 samples; 200 from human and 600 from ruminant were included in the current study. In the ruminants group, over all 600 healthy domestic animals; 200 cows, 200 sheep and 200 goats referring for Zarrinshahr slaughterhouse in Isfahan, center of Iran, during February to August of 2012 were selected randomly. Considering sterile conditions, the sample from the rumen in size of 2 mm to 3 mm was obtained immediately after slaughtering. Samples were placed in 0.1 ml of sterile saline solution and were transported rapidly to the laboratory. The histological examinations were performed by the specialized veterinarians of Shahrekord Azad University. For analysis of *H. pylori* DNA from human origin, regardless to career of patients, two hundred patients with dyspepsia symptoms referring to gastroenterology department of Hajar Hospital Shahrekord, Iran, from December 2011

to April 2012 were selected and gastric biopsies from antrum were obtained during endoscopy by endoscopist. All patients provided written informed consent prior to endoscopy. All the specimens were placed in 0.1 ml of sterile saline solution and were transported to the laboratory immediately and were stored at -70°C until further investigation.

DNA analysis

From all of biopsy specimens, DNA was extracted by using Genomic DNA purification kit (DNP™, CinnaGen, Iran) considering sterile condition according to manufacture recommendations. The *H. pylori* presence in studied samples was detected by PCR method using housekeeping gene; *glmM* gene as a target gene. Due to low sensitivity and difficulty of *H. pylori* culture particularly from animal sources, the samples were not cultured. The primers sequences for *glmM* gene amplification were as follows: GlmM-F (5'- GCTTACTTTCTAACACT AACGCGC-3') and GlmM-R (5'- GGATAAGCTTTTA GGGGTGTTAGGGG-3') [2]. Primers were used for PCR assays of *vacA* allels and *cagA* genes has been described before [15,16]. DNA samples *H. pylori* (D0008, Genekam, Germany) were used as positive control of *cagA* and *vacA* genes, and sterile distilled water was used as negative control. PCR was done in 20 μL (for *glmM*) or 25 μL (for *vacA* and *cagA*) of total reaction volume containing 1.5 mM $MgCl_2$ (2.0 mM for *cagA*), 50 mM KCl, 10 mM Tris–HCl (pH 9.0), 0.1% Triton X-100, 200 μM dNTPs each (Fermentas), 0.4 μM primers, 0.3 U of Taq DNA polymerase (Fermentas), and 2 μL (40–260 ng/μL) of DNA. PCR was performed in a DNA Thermal Cycler (Eppendrof Mastercycler 5330, Eppendorf-Nethel-Hinz GmbH, Hamburg, Germany), with 40 cycles for GlmM primer and 35 cycles for *vacA* and *cagA* primers. Each cycle consisted of denaturation at 95°C/45 seconds; annealing at 59°C/30 seconds for *glmM*, 52°C/45 seconds for *vacA*, and 58°C/45 seconds for *cagA*; and extension at 72°C/45 seconds [16]. There was another longer extension of 6 minute at 72°C. PCR products were visualized by electrophoresis in 1% agarose gel, were stained with ethidium bromide, and were examined under ultraviolet illumination.

DNA sequencing analysis

DNA sequencing analysis was performed on 6 *H. pylori* positive sample; 3 samples from cows and 3 samples from sheep which were selected randomly. Due to limitations we were not able to do sequence on all positive samples for *glmM* gene. For this purpose the DNA extraction was done by the same method as mentioned before for PCR. The amplified 296-bp PCR products (*glmM* gene) from 6 positive samples were purified with High pure PCR product purification kit (Roche Applied

Science), according to manufacturer's recommendations. Single DNA strands were sequenced with ABI 3730 XL device and Sanger sequencing method (Macrogen, Korea).

After the sequence of 6 isolates were trimmed by using Edit View v.1.0.1 (Applied Bioscience, Australia), the sequences of 8 isolate with human source, which has been stored in GenBank with accession numbers: FN598874, CP003476, DQ462665, M60398, NC017361, GU445163, DQ141576, AB664954 were aligned separately against obtained animal isolate sequences using the Clustal W v1.81 in order to obtain a consensus sequence for the gene, glmM (*H. pylori ureC*). BioEdit Pakage V.7.0.4.1 was used to edit all sequence alignments. The nucleotide sequences of the Iranian ruminant *H. pylori glmM (ureC)* gene was compared with the correspond sequences reported from other regions via NCBI. By using Njplot software and 1000 bootstrap replicate, an unrooted dendrogramme was constructed.

Ethical considerations

The present study was accepted by the ethical committee of the Hajar Hospital of Shahrekord, Iran and Microbiology and Infectious Diseases Center of the Islamic Azad University of Shahrekord Branch, Iran. Written informed consent was obtained from all of the study patients or their parents.

Results

Totally 600 ruminants and 200 human gastric samples were collected in the current investigation. According to clinical and histopathological examinations, 10 cows and 2 sheep had moderate gastric inflammations while all goats were healthy, however none of the animals showed clinical manifestations. Based on gastroendoscopic and histopathologic finding, out of 200 human biopsy specimens, sixteen patients (11.8%) had gastric ulcers, 22 (16.2%) had duodenal ulcers, 194 (97.5%) had chronic gastritis and 3 (2.2%) had gastric cancer. Among 200 cow samples and 200 sheep samples, 6 (3%) and 32 (16%) were confirmed to be *H. pylori* positive; however, we were not able to find any *H. pylori* in goat samples. Out of 200 humans samples, 164 (82%) were infected with this bacterium.

When we came to analyze the *cagA* gene in the positive samples, out of 6 cow, 32 sheep and 164 human samples, positive for *H. pylori*, 4 (66.66%), 24 (75%) and 151 (92.08%) were *cagA*-positive respectively, however the *cagA* gene frequency among studied cow, sheep and human isolates was not statically significant (p = 0.7).In case of the *vacA* gene alleles, according to cow specimen results, the frequency of *vacA s1a, s1b, m1a* and *m2* were 5 (83.33%), 1 (16.66%), 2 (33.33%) and 4 (66.66%) respectively. We were not able to detect *vacA s1c, s2,* and *m1b* in the cows' population. The frequency of *vacA*

s1a, s1b, s2, m1a and *m2* were 16 (50%), 11 (34.37%), 5 (15.66%), 14 (43.75%) and 18 (56.25%) respectively in sheep's population. The *s1c* and *m1b* did not amplify any band in PCR assay for sheep samples (Table 1). As it was indicated in Table 1, in isolates from human samples, 79 (48.17%) *s1a*, 21 (12.80%) *s1b*, 35 (21.34%) *s1c*, 29 (17.68%) *s2* were observed while for *vacA* m region, 52 (31.70%), 15 (9.14%) and 97 (59.14%) isolates showed *m1a, m1b* and *m2* genotype respectively. There was a statistically significant differences in prevalence of the *s1b* allele among human beings and cows isolates ($P = 0.025$) as well as *s1a/m2* genotypes among human beings and sheep strains ($P = 0.04$). There was no statically significant relation between genotypes of *H. pylori* recovered from cows compare to sheep ($P = 0.81$) (Table 2). The nucleotide sequences of *H. pylori glmM* gene, obtained from 6 Iranian ruminants; 3 cows and 3 sheep were compared with those from the known human reference sequences obtained from the GenBank nucleotide sequence database (8 sequences corresponding to *H. pylori*). The nucleotide sequence analyses showed a variability of 0.7–1.4% for the *ureC* gene between sheep and cows samples (Table 3) and variations was consisted only in nucleotide sub-situation. Frame shift, deletion, insertion and nonsense mutations were not observed. When we compared the sequences of the *ureC* gene in sheep and human *H. pylori* isolates; there was 3.4–8.4% variability and 92.9-98.5% homology. The greatest sequence similarity (98.5%,) was found between *H. pylori* isolates of Iranian sheep and German human (FN598874), while the lowest relationship (91.6%) between Iranian cow *ureC* sequence and South Africa (NC017361) was observed (Figure 1).

Discussion

Human is known as the main host of *H. pylori*; however the histopathology of this bacterium is in contrasts with many other gastric *Helicobacter* spp. In which their natural host response against bacteria involve mild or even no inflammatory response [4], so it is possible that *H. pylori* has originated from another mammalian host in the distant past [17]. In the current survey we evaluated whether cow, sheep and goat can be the original host of this bacterium. In order to achieve this goal we collected 600 gastric specimens from healthy cows, sheep, goats and 200 gastric biopsy from human with dyspepsia in west of Iran where the prevalence of *H. pylori* is higher than 70% [18]. In our investigation, the prevalence of *H. pylori* in cows and sheep's population was 3% and 16% respectively, we were not able to detect it in goat's gastric tissue samples whereas the Italian survey on 400 milk samples by nested PCR assay, indicated that the prevalence of this bacterium in cow, sheep and goat populations were 50%, 33% and 25.6% respectively [8]. Scandinavian researchers found *H. pylori* in 60% of 38 sheep gastric tissue [4]. Also

Table 1 The frequency of *cagA* and *vacA* alleles in *Helicobacter pylori* of ruminants and human samples

Positive samples	cagA	s1a	s1b	s1c	s2	m1a	m1b	m2
Cow	4	5	1	0	0	2	0	4
6 (3%)	(66.66%)	(83.33%)	(16.66%)			(33.33%)		(66.66%)
Sheep	24	16	11	0	5	14	0	18
32 (16%)	(75%)	(50%)	(34.37%)		(15.62%)	(43.75%)		(56.25%)
Human	151	79	21	35	29	52	15	97
164 (82%)	(92.08%)	(48.17%)	(12.80%)	(21.34%)	(17.68%)	(31.70%)	(9.14%)	(59.14%)

Rahimi and Kheirabadi declared *H. pylori* existed in 12.2% of sheep, 8.7% of goat and 14.1% of cow milk by PCR method [19]. In the other study which was conducted in Japan, *H. pylori* was found in 72.2% of cow raw milk specimens [20]. The diversity of *H. pylori* frequency in various hosts and regions may relate to animal, microbe and environmental factors. The prevalence of this bacterium in Iranian patients was 82% which is similar to previous reports from Iran and also Japan, South America, Turkey and Pakistan where more than 80% of dyspepsia patients were *H. pylori* positive, however in Scandinavia and England the prevalence ranges between 20% to 40% [21,22]. According to our results, screening of goats' stomach for *H. pylori* was negative which is in accordance with Gueneau et al. study in 2003 in which they failed to detect *H.pylori* in studied goats [23]. This finding may support by two possible reasons: Ones that goats are an exception among ruminants in having particular natural mechanisms of resistance to this bacterium. Another hypothesis is that some other microorganisms like *Candidatus H. bovis* may colonize the goat's stomach and establish the extent of the resistance of goats to the super infection with *H. pylori* [23]. *H. pylori* strains with the *cagA* gene is supposed to be more virulent rather than *cagA*-negative strains [12] however this is not constant [2]. The prevalence of *cagA*-positive *H. pylori* varies from one geographic region to another, e.g., 97% in Korea, 94% in Malaysia, 90% in China, 78% in Turkey, 53% in Kuwait, 85% North America and 65% in Slovenia [14,24-27]. In the current study *cagA* gene was found in 92% of Iranian populations which is in accordance with previous local report [18]. Since the most of *H. pylori* isolated from human samples regardless to clinical outcomes harbor the *cagA* gene ($P > 0.05$), thereby as it was declared previously, our finding did not support the role of the *cagA* as predictive marker for increased virulence feature of *H. pylori* in Iranian dyspepsia patients [1]. The *cagA* gene was found in 66%, 75% of cow and sheep populations respectively, which was not studied on animals' samples yet. There was no statically meaningful difference in status of the *cagA* in human and animal samples, which may reflect that all *H. pylori* recovered from human and animals have same ancestors. According to our results for the *vacA*, all of our samples with positive PCR for *H. pylori*, irrespective to source of strains was positive for *vacA*. Although Dore et al. [4] in 2001 detected *vacA* gene in 60.3% and 7.9% of *H. pylori* strains isolated from sheep tissue and sheep milk samples respectively; now it is supposed that all *H. pylori* strains should possess the *vacA* gene, as it was supported by many studies around the world [12,26,27]. The *vacA s1a/m2* were predominant *vacA* alles among all three studied population including human, cow and sheep.

Based on statistical analyses, there was a significant correlation between *s1a/m2* genotype of *H. pylori* in sheep and human beings. Also *s1a* allele was significantly prevalent among cow and human. To our knowledge, this is the first comparison study of *H pylori* DNA sequence among specimens from cow, sheep and human in Middle East. As it was shown in Table 3 there was a high DNA sequence homology between *H. pylori* strains of sheep and human however this homology was low between cows

Table 2 The frequency of *vacA* genotypes in *Helicobacter pylori* of ruminants and human samples

Positive samples	s1a/m1a	s1a/m1b	s1a/m2	s1b/m1a	s1b/m1b	s1b/m2	s1c/m1a	s1c/m1b	s1c/m2	s2/m1a	s2/m1b	s2/m2
Cow	2	0	3	0	0	1	0	0	0	0	0	0
6 (3%)	(33.33%)		(50%)			(16.66%)						
Sheep	6	0	10	5	0	6	0	0	0	1	0	4
32 (16%)	(18.75%)		(31.25%)	(15.62%)		(18.75%)				(3.12%)		(12.5%)
Human	27	8	45	7	5	10	12	4	18	6	0	22
164 (82%)	(16.46%)	(4.87%)	(27.43%)	(4.26%)	(3.04%)	(6.09%)	(7.31%)	(2.43%)	(10.97%)	(3.65%)		(13.41%)

Table 3 Sequence identity matrix of partial *ureC* gene of Iranian ruminant *Helicobacter pylori* in comparison with 8 known human reference sequences

Seq	Cow-1	Cow-2	Cow-3	Sheep-1	Sheep-2	Sheep-3	FN598874-Germany	CP003476-USA	DQ462665-Iran	GU445163-Iran	M60398-France	NC017361-S Africa	DQ141576-China	AB664954-Japan
Cow-1	ID	0.999	1	0.989	0.987	0.991	0.953	0.962	0.932	0.941	0.928	0.920	0.926	0.926
Cow-2	0.999	ID	0.999	0.987	0.988	0.986	0.950	0.966	0.936	0.940	0.929	0.918	0.924	0.923
Cow-3	1	0.999	ID	0.992	0.986	0.993	0.927	0.964	0.932	0.944	0.930	0.916	0.922	0.923
Sheep-1	0.989	0.987	0.991	ID	1	0.998	0.983	0.979	0.976	0.973	0.967	0.937	0.952	0.954
Sheep-2	0.987	0.988	0.986	1	ID	0.999	0.985	0.981	0.978	0.981	0.966	0.934	0.958	0.959
Sheep-3	0.991	0.986	0.993	0.998	0.999	ID	0.980	0.983	0.969	0.980	0.964	0.929	0.961	0.962
FN598874-Germany	0.953	0.950	0.957	0.983	0.985	0.980	ID	0.986	0.992	0.991	0.985	0.983	0.976	0.984
CP003476-USA	0.962	0.966	0.964	0.979	0.981	0.983	0.986	ID	0.990	0.993	0.984	0.979	0.980	0.983
DQ462665-Iran	0.932	0.936	0.932	0.976	0.978	0.969	0.992	0.990	ID	1	0.982	0.969	0.983	0.986
GU445163-Iran	0.941	0.940	0.944	0.973	0.981	0.980	0.991	0.993	1	ID	0.985	0.970	0.986	0.989
M60398-France	0.928	0.929	0.930	0.967	0.966	0.964	0.985	0.984	0.982	0.985	ID	0.975	0.990	0.991
NC017361-S Africa	0.920	0.918	0.916	0.937	0.934	0.929	0.983	0.979	0.969	0.970	0.975	ID	0.993	0.989
DQ141576-China	0.926	0.924	0.922	0.952	0.958	0.961	0.976	0.980	0.983	0.986	0.990	0.993	ID	0.994
AB664954-Japan	0.926	0.923	0.923	0.954	0.959	0.962	0.984	0.983	0.986	0.989	0.991	0.989	0.994	ID

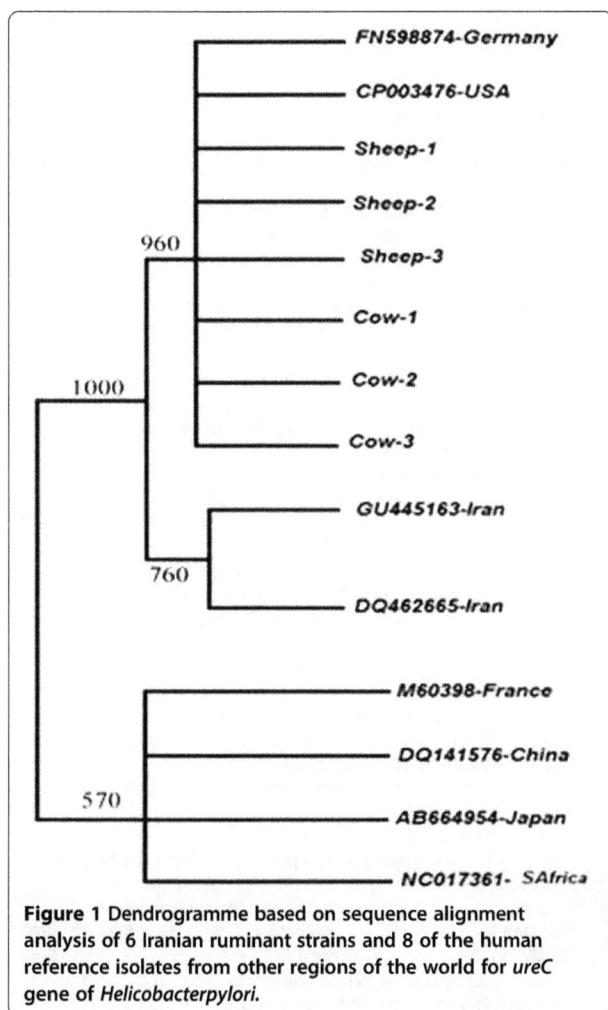

Figure 1 Dendrogramme based on sequence alignment analysis of 6 Iranian ruminant strains and 8 of the human reference isolates from other regions of the world for *ureC* gene of *Helicobacterpylori*.

and humans. The rate of homology was low between cow and sheep too. Since considerable number of studied sheep carried *H. pylori* without any pathological evidence, it seems that sheep may are natural host for *H. pylori*. Besides DNA sequence homology among sheep and human *H. pylori* strains suggest that sheep may serve as a reservoir for this bacteria. Our findings are consistent with Dore et al. study which has hypothesized sheep is the ancestor host of *H. pylori* [4]. Although high prevalence of *H. pylori* among human population in comparison with other mammalian, indicating *H. pylori* is more adapted to human body, the main role of sheep in *H. pylori* evolution story is supported by our study in company with some other studies. Dore et al. showed that nearly all of Sardinian shepherds carried *H. pylori*. Morris et al. has reported the higher prevalence of antibodies against *H. pylori* in abattoir workers, such as veterinarians, butchers, and slaughterers [28]. Mégraud and Broutet study showed a number of animals, mostly living in human environment, had *H. pylori* in their stomach and therefore to be

involved in the transmission of this bacterium [29]. Some other reports also support zoonotic transmission of *H. pylori via* close contact with domestic animals [4,30-33]. These studies, along with those have been shown that *H. pylori* can survive in sheep milk [4,19,34-36] are supportive for reservoir role of sheep for human infection. Due to lack of any recorded sequence for *H. pylori* with animal source in Gene bank, we compared our isolates sequences with recorded human isolates sequences. Despite the little diversity in studied sequences, we were able to justify the genetic diversity of the bacterium based on its diverse hosts. As the origin of many Iranian noble cows and sheep refer to the America and Germany, so the perceived genetic similarities among sequences of *H. pylori* FN598874-Germany and CP003476-USA with those of Iranian cow and sheep isolates in this research can justify this claim. On the other hand, transportation of livestock between Far-East Countries (Japan and China) and South Africa and Iran basically does not have historical background [37]. Thus, placing of Japanese, Chinese and South Africans strains in other branches of phylogenetic tree is indicating more differences in the sequence of *H. pylori* between Iran and mentioned countries.

Conclusion

In conclusion cows and sheep in Iran harbor *H. pylori* in their gastric tissue similar in genotype of the *cagA* and *vacA* alleles with isolates recovered from human. Also since there was a high homology sequence of *H. pylori* DNA among sheep and human, suggest that sheep may are the natural reservoir of the bacteria and can transmit *H. pylori* to human community.

Competing interests
The authors declare that they have no competing interests.

Authors' contributions
The DNA extraction, PCR techniques and supporting of project were performed by HM and HD. MG collected the Samples, Statistical analysis and writing of manuscript were performed by NS, All authors read and approved the final manuscript.

Acknowledgment
The authors would like to thank Mr. M. Momeni, Dr. Sh. Nejat, and Mr. Gh. Ramezani at the Biotechnology Research Center of the Islamic Azad University of Shahrekord and Endoscopy Unit of Hajar Hospital of Shahrekord, for their sincere technical and clinical support.

Author details
[1]Department of Microbiology, Faculty of Veterinary Medicine, ShahreKord Branch, Islamic Azad University, ShahreKord, Iran. [2]Department of Medical Microbiology, Faculty of Medicine, Shahid Beheshti University of Medical Science, Tehran, Iran. [3]Young Researchers and Elite club, Central Tehran Branch, Islamic Azad University, P.O.Box: 13185-768, Tehran, Iran. [4]Graduated of Veterinary Medicine, Faculty of Veterinary Medicine, ShahreKord Branch, Islamic Azad University, ShahreKord, Iran.

References

1. Kargar M, Souod N, Ghorbani-Dalini S, Doosti A, Rezaian AA: **Evaluation of cagA tyrosin phosphorylation DNA motifs in Helicobacter pylori isolates from gastric disorder patients in west of Iran.** Sci Res Essays 2011, 6:6454–6458.

2. Momtaz H, Souod N, Dabiri H: **Comparison of the virulence factors of Helicobacter pylori isolated in stomach and saliva in Iran.** Am J Med Sci 2010, 340:345–349.

3. Tabatabaei M: **Application of molecular and central cultural methods for identification of Helicobacter spp in different animal sources.** Global Vet 2012, 8:292–297.

4. Dore MP, Sepulveda AR, El-Zimaity H, Yamaoka Y, Osato MS, Mototsugu K, Nieddu AM, Realdi G, Graham DY: **Isolation of Helicobacter pylori from sheep-implications for transmission to humans.** Am J Gastroenterol 2001, 96:1396–1401.

5. Mohamed AA, El- Gohari AH: **Epidemiological aspects of Helicobacter pylori infections as an emergence zoonotic disease: Animal reservoirs and public health implications (A review article).** 7th Int Sci Conf, MANSOURA 2012:17–25.

6. Husson MO, Vincent P, Grabiaud MH, Furon D, Leclerc H: **Anti-Helicobacter pylori IgG levels in abattoir workers.** Gastroenterol Clin Biol 1991, 15:723–726.

7. Kolodzieyski L, Kim B, Park H, Yoon HS, Lim CW: **Prevalence of gastrospirillum-like organisms in pigs, cattle, and dogs: a comparison of diagnostic methods between species.** Vet Med 2008, 53:193–202.

8. Quaglia NC, Dambrosio A, Normanno G, Parisi A, Patrono R, Ranieri G, Rella A, Celano GV: **High occurrence of Helicobacter pylori in raw goat, sheep and cow milk inferred by glmM gene: a risk of food-borne infection?** Int J. Food Microbiol 2008, 124:43–47.

9. Kargar M, Ghorbani-Dalini S, Doosti A, Souod N: **Real-time PCR for Helicobacter pylori quantification and detection of clarithromycin resistance in gastric tissue from patients with gastrointestinal disorders.** Res Microbiol 2012, 163:109–113.

10. Yamaoka Y: **Roles of the plasticity regions of Helicobacter pylori in gastroduodenal pathogenesis.** J Med Microbiol 2008, 57:545–553.

11. Momtaz H, Souod N, Dabiri H, Sarshar M: **Study of Helicobacter pylori genotype status in saliva, dental plaques, stool and gastric biopsy samples.** World J Gastroenterol 2012, 18:2105–2111.

12. Jafari F, Shokrzadeh L, Dabiri H, Baghaei K, Yamaoka Y, Zojaji H, Haghazali M, Molaei M, Zali MR: **vacA genotypes of Helicobacter pylori in relation to cagA status and clinical outcomes in Iranian populations.** Jpn J Infect Dis 2008, 61:290–293.

13. Argent RH, Thomas RJ, Letley DP, Rittig MG, Hardie KR, Atherton JC: **Functional association between the Helicobacter pylori virulence factors VacA and CagA.** J Med Microbiol 2008, 57:145–150.

14. Torres LE, Melián K, Moreno A, Alonso J, Sabatier CA, Hernández M, Bermúdez L, Rodríguez BL: **Prevalence of vacA, cagA and babA2 genes in Cuban Helicobacter pylori isolates.** World J Gastroenterol 2009, 15:204–210.

15. Yamazaki S, Yamakawa A, Okuda T, Ohtani M, Suto H, Ito Y, Yamazaki Y, Keida Y, Higashi H, Hatakeyama M, Azuma T: **Distinct diversity of vacA, cagA, and cagE genes of Helicobacter pylori associated with peptic ulcer in Japan.** J Clin Microbiol 2005, 43:3906–3916.

16. Wang J, Chi DS, Laffan JJ, Li C, Ferguson DA Jr, Litchfield P, Thomas E: **Comparison of cytotoxin genotypes of Helicobacter pylori in stomach and saliva.** Dig Dis Sci 2002, 47:1850–1856.

17. Solnick JV, Schauer DB: **Emergence of diverse Helicobacter species in the pathogenesis of gastric and enterohepatic diseases.** Clin Microbiol Rev 2001, 14:59–97.

18. Farshad S, Japoni A, Alborzi A, Zarenezhad M, Ranjbar R: **Changing prevalence of Helicobacter pylori in south of Iran.** Iranian J Clin Infect Dis 2010, 5:65–69.

19. Rahimi E, Kheirabadi EK: **Detection of Helicobacter pylori in bovine, buffalo, camel, ovine, and caprine milk in Iran.** Foodborne Pathog Dis 2012, 9:453–456.

20. Fujimura S, Kawamura T, Kato S, Tateno H, Watanabe A: **Detection of Helicobacter pylori in cow's milk.** Lett Appl Microbiol 2002, 35:504–507.

21. Hunt RH, Xiao SD, Megraud F, Leon-Barua R, Bazzoli F, van der Merwe S, Vaz Coelho LG, Fock M, Fedail S, Cohen H, Malfertheiner P, Vakil N, Hamid S, Goh KL, Wong BC, Krabshuis J, Le Mair A: **Helicobacter pylori in developing countries: world gastroenterology organisation global guideline.** J Gastrointestin Liver Dis 2011, 20:299–304.

22. Javed M, Amin K, Muhammad D, Husain A, Mahmood N: **Prevalence of H. Pylori.** Professional Med Sep 2010, 17:431–439.

23. Gueneau P, Fuenmayor J, Aristimuño OC, Cedeño S, Báez E, Reyes N, Michelangeli F, Domínguez-Bello MG: **Are goats naturally resistant to gastric Helicobacter infection?** Vet Microbiol 2002, 84:115–121.

24. Albert MJ, Al-Akbal HM, Dhar R, De R, Mukhopadhyay AK: **Genetic affinities of Helicobacter pylori isolates from ethnic Arabs in Kuwait.** Gut Pathog 2010, 2:6.

25. Zhang Z, Zheng Q, Chen X, Xiao S, Liu W, Lu H: **The Helicobacter pylori duodenal ulcer promoting gene, dupA in China.** BMC Gastroenterol 2008, 8:49.

26. Homan M, Luzar B, Kocjan BJ, Orel R, Mocilnik T, Shrestha M, Kveder M, Poljak M: **Prevalence and clinical relevance of cagA, vacA, and iceA genotypes of Helicobacter pylori isolated from Slovenian children.** J Pediatr Gastroenterol Nutr 2009, 49:289–296.

27. Miernyk K, Morris J, Bruden D, McMahon B, Hurlburt D, Sacco F, Parkinson A, Hennessy T, Bruce M: **Characterization of Helicobacter pylori cagA and vacA genotypes among Alaskans and their correlation with clinical disease.** J Clin Microbiol 2011, 49:3114–3121.

28. Morris A, Nicholson G, Lloyd G, Haines D, Rogers A, Taylor D: **Seroepidemiology of Campylobacter pyloridis.** NZ Med J 1986, 99:657–659.

29. Mégraud F, Broutet N: **Have we found the source of Helicobacter pylori?** Aliment Pharmacol Ther 2000, 14(Suppl 3):7–12.

30. Vaira D, Ferron P, Negrini R, Cavazzini L, Holton J, Ainley C, Londei M, Vergura M, Dei R, Colecchia A: **Detection of Helicobacter pylori-like organisms in the stomach of some food-source animals using a monoclonal antibody.** Ital J Gastroenterol 1992, 24:181–184.

31. Fox JG: **Non-human reservoirs of Helicobacter pylori.** Aliment Pharmacol Ther 1995, 9(Suppl. 2):93–103.

32. Safaei GH, Rahimi E, Zandib A, Rashidipour A: **Helicobacter pylori as a zoonotic infection: the detection of H. pylori antigens in the milk and faeces of cows.** JRMS 2011, 16(2):184–187.

33. Dunn BE, Cohen H, Blaser MJ: **Helicobacter pylori.** Clin Microbiol Rev 1997, 10:720–741.

34. Dore MP, Bilotta M, Vaira D, Manca A, Massarelli G, Leandro G, Atzei A, Pisanu G, Graham DY, Realdi G: **High prevalence of helicobacter pylori infection in shepherds.** Dig Dis Sci 1999, 44(6):1161–1164.

35. Turutoglu H, Mudul S: **Investigation of helicobacter pylori in raw sheep milk samples.** J Vet Med B Infect Dis Vet Public Health 2002, 49(6):308–309.

36. Quaglia NC, Dambrosio A, Normanno G, Parisi A, Patrono R, Ranieri G, Rella A, Celano GV: **High occurrence of helicobacter pylori in raw goat, sheep and cow milk inferred by glmM gene: a risk of food-borne infection?** Int J Food Microbiol 2008, 124(1):43–47.

37. Rahman SA, Walker L, Ricketts W: **Global perspectives on animal welfare: Asia, the Far East, and Oceania.** Rev Sci Tech 2005, 24:597–612.

4

Occurrence of *Helicobacter pylori* and Epstein-Barr virus infection in endoscopic and gastric cancer patients from Northern Brazil

Carolina Rosal Teixeira de Souza[1*†], Kátia Soares de Oliveira[2†], Jefferson José Sodré Ferraz[3], Mariana Ferreira Leal[4,5], Danielle Queiroz Calcagno[6], Aline Damasceno Seabra[1], André Salim Khayat[6], Raquel Carvalho Montenegro[1], Ana Paula Negreiros Nunes Alves[7], Paulo Pimentel Assumpção[6], Marília Cardoso Smith[5] and Rommel Rodríguez Burbano[1]

Abstract

Background: *Helicobacter pylori* (HP) and *Epstein-Barr virus* (EBV) have been associated with cancer development. We evaluated the prevalence of HP, HP *CagA*+ and EBV infection in gastric cancer (GC) samples from adults and in gastric tissues from patients who underwent upper endoscopy (UE).

Methods: Samples from UE and GC were collected to investigate the presence of HP infection and the HP virulence factor *CagA* by a urease test and PCR. The presence of EBV was detected by *Eber-1 in situ* hybridization.

Results: In UE, 85.5% of juvenile patients showed some degree of gastritis (45.3% of patients with mild gastritis and 54.7% with moderate/severe gastritis) and patients with mild gastritis were younger than patients with moderate/severe gastritis. Among adults, 48.7% presented mild gastritis and 51.3% moderate/severe gastritis. HP infection was detected in 0% of normal mucosa, 58.5% of juvenile gastritis patients, 69.2% of adult gastritis patients and 88% of GC patients. In these same groups, HP *CagA*+ was detected in 0%, 37.7%, 61.5% and 67.2% of tissue samples, respectively. In juvenile patients, HP infection was more common in those with gastritis than in normal samples (p = 0.004). The patients with either HP or HP *CagA*+ were older than patients without these pathogens (p < 0.05). In juvenile patients, HP infection was more frequent in cases of moderate/severe gastritis than in cases of mild gastritis (p = 0.026). Moreover, in patients with GC, HP infection was more frequent in males than in females (p = 0.023). GC patients with HP *CagA*+ were older than patients with HP *CagA*- (p = 0.027). HP *CagA*+ was more common in intestinal-type than diffuse-type GC (p = 0.012). HP *CagA*+ was also associated with lymph-node (p = 0.024) and distal (p = 0.005) metastasis. No association between EBV infection and HP infection or any clinicopathological variable was detected.

Conclusions: Our results suggest that HP is involved in the pathophysiology of severe gastric lesions and in the development of GC, particularly when *CagA*+ is present. EBV was not the primary pathogenic factor in our samples.

Keywords: *Helicobacter pylori*, *Epstein-Barr virus*, Gastritis, Gastric cancer

* Correspondence: carolrosalts@gmail.com
†Equal contributors
[1]Laboratório de Citogenética Humana, Instituto de Ciências Biológicas, Universidade Federal do Pará, Rua Augusto Corrêa, 01 – Guamá. CEP 66075-110. Caixa postal 479, Belém, PA, Brasil
Full list of author information is available at the end of the article

Background

Gastric cancer (GC) and other gastrointestinal diseases occur at high rates worldwide [1], and infections involving viruses and bacteria have been associated with these diseases. Recently, several studies have been performed to understand the role of pathogens that infect the human stomach, particularly *Helicobacter pylori* (HP) and *Epstein-Barr virus* (EBV), in gastric carcinogenesis [2-5].

HP, a Gram-negative spiral bacterium, is considered a public health problem. In 1994, the International Agency for Research on Cancer (IARC) defined HP as a group 1 carcinogen [6,7]. This bacterium colonizes the gastric mucosa of more than 50% of the world's population [8]. However, only approximately 20% of infected individuals develop severe gastric diseases such as GC. Among the factors- that have been suggested to contribute to development of gastric disease in HP-infected patients are the virulence of HP strains, the permissiveness of the gastric environment and the host genetic background [9]. The HP cytotoxicity associated gene A (*CagA*) is one of the most significant virulence factors of this bacteria, and it has been associated with risk for GC [10].

EBV infects more than 90% of the global adult population, and most individuals are infected during childhood. Upon infection, the virus remains latent in B lymphocytes throughout life [5]. To be oncogenic, EBV must maintain its genome inside host cells to avoid cell death and to evade recognition by the immune system. The contribution of EBV to gastric carcinogenesis has not been fully elucidated [11,12]. EBV infects epithelial cells from the oropharynx and subsequently spreads to the lymphoid tissues where it infects B lymphocytes [13-15]. Atrophic gastritis may induce the infiltration of EBV-carrying lymphocytes and increase the chance of their contact with the gastric epithelial cells. On the other hand, the gastric inflammation may also produce a cytokine-rich microenvironment to support clonal growth of EBV-infected epithelial cells [16].

In developing countries such as Brazil, HP and EBV infections are particularly prevalent within lower socioeconomic populations. Furthermore, infection occurs at earlier ages in these populations compared to developed countries [17-19]. Studies are needed to determine these pathogens' association with and influence on the development of gastric diseases at earlier ages, where they could initiate or promote carcinogenic processes. Additionally, the role of HP and EBV in the development of gastric adenocarcinoma in the elderly, the population where this disease is most prevalent, remains unclear.

Therefore, this study aimed to assess the prevalence of HP and EBV infection, as well as the *CagA*-positive status of HP, in gastric tissues from juvenile and adult patients undergoing upper endoscopy (UE) and in tumor specimens from adult patients with GC.

Methods

Samples

The present study included: (i) gastric tissue samples from 62 juvenile patients ranging from 12 months to 18 years old, referred for UE to clarify clinical manifestations within the upper gastrointestinal tract, (ii) gastric tissue samples from 39 adult patients ranging from 19 to 61 years old, referred for UE to clarify clinical manifestations within the upper gastrointestinal tract, and (iii) tumor samples from 125 adults, 26 to 89 years old, with primary gastric adenocarcinoma. Samples were randomly collected during the period of 2005-2013 in Belém city of Pará State, Northern Brazil. Informed consent was obtained prior to sample collection from all adult patients or from the parents or guardians of all juvenile patients. Sample collection was carried out with the approval of the ethics committee of the Human Institute of Health Sciences of the Federal University of Pará (Protocol #35/2010) and João de Barros Barreto University Hospital (Protocol #142004). All patients had negative histories of exposure to chemotherapy and radiotherapy prior to sample collection, and no patient presented with co-occurrence of diagnosed cancers. Data on the clinical features of patients were collected from medical records.

Histopathology

Endoscopic findings were classified according to the updated Sydney System [20] which considers the degree of inflammation, activity, atrophy and intestinal metaplasia. For each patient, 5 biopsies of gastric tissues were evaluated: 2 from the antral region of the stomach, 1 from the *incisura angularis*, and 2 from the oxyntic mucosa. Chronic gastritis was designated as mild, moderate or severe.

Gastric tumors were classified according to the Lauren classification [21] and staged using standard criteria by pTNM staging [22]. Tables 1 and 2 show the clinicopathological features of gastritis and GC samples, respectively.

HP and *CagA* detection

The presence of HP was detected by a commercially available rapid urease test (Promedical, Brazil), and the negative results were confirmed by PCR using the oligonucleotides described by Covacci *et al.* [23]. All gastric samples were placed in a tube containing 2% Christensen's urea agar and examined for urea hydrolysis after 24 h of incubation at 37°C. In the presence of urease produced by HP, the urea is converted to ammonia, resulting in a change of pH and, consequently, the color of the solution.

The detection of the *CagA* gene was carried out by PCR in the gastric mucosa of all patients, using the oligonucleotides described by Covacci *et al.* [23]. All reactions were performed in duplicate. A sample was considered positive

Table 1 Clinicopathological features, *H. pylori* and EBV infection in gastritis samples of juvenile patients

Variable	H. pylori			CagA			EBV		
	Negative	Positive	p-value	Negative[c]	Positive	p-value	Negative	Positive	p-value
Age (years, Mean ± SD)	7.45 ± 3.88	12.19 ± 4.09	<0.001*	8.88 ± 4.49	12.45 ± 4.01	0.005*	9.96 ± 4.5	17 ± 1.41	0.033*
Gender [N(%)]									
Female	14 (42.4)	19 (57.6)	0.685[a]	23 (69.7)	10 (30.3)	0.096[a]	32 (97.0)	1 (3.0)	0.626[a]
Male	8 (40.0)	12 (60.0)		10 (50.0)	10 (50.0)		19 (95.0)	1 (5.0)	
Histological subtype [N(%)]									
Mild	16 (66.7)	8 (33.3)	0.026*[b]	20 (83.3)	4 (16.7)	0.108[b]	23 (95.8)	1 (4.2)	0.136[b]
Moderate/Severe	6 (20.7)	23 (79.3)		13 (44.8)	16 (55.2)		28 (96.6)	1 (3.4)	
EBV infection [N(%)]									
Absent	21 (41.2)	30 (58.8)	0.242[b]	31 (60.8)	20 (39.2)	0.998[b]			
Present	1 (50)	1 (50)		2 (100)	0 (0)				

*Significant difference between groups, p < 0.05. [a]p value after adjustment for age; [b]p value after adjustment for age and gender; [c]Negative samples for *H. pylori* and samples with *H. pylori* infection but without CagA virulence factor; EBV: *Epstein-Barr virus*; SD: standard deviation.

if a visible and clear band was observed on a 2% agarose electrophoresis gel.

EBV detection

EBV was detected by RNA in situ hybridization (ISH) with a 30-bp biotinylated probe (5'-AGACACCGTC CTCACCACCCGGGACTTGTA-3') complementary to EBV-encoded small RNA-1 (*Eber1*), the most abundant viral product in latently infected cells [24]. Signal amplification was achieved with a mouse anti-biotin antibody (clone BK, 1:20 dilution; DakoCytomation®, CA, USA) and biotinylated rabbit anti-immunoglobulin antibody (polyclonal, 1:100 dilution; DakoCytomation®, CA, USA). The reaction was detected with streptavidin-biotin peroxidase complex (DakoCytomation®, CA, USA) and diaminobenzidine chromogen (DakoCytomation®, CA, USA). The slides were counterstained with Harris's hematoxylin. Cell analysis was performed by 2 independent investigators

using light microscopy, at 40x or 20x magnification. A total of 10 representative microscopic fields were evaluated, and fields containing less than 5 cells were not considered. A gastric cancer sample positive for EBV was included as a positive control, and two slides treated without probe were used as negative controls. Samples where 5% or more of the epithelial cells contained brown/red staining were considered positive. Although lymphocytes were also found to be infected by EBV, we did not include infected lymphoid cells in our analysis.

Statistical analyses

The Shapiro-Wilk test was used to evaluate the distribution of age data and to determine the appropriate subsequent test for statistical comparison. The Mann-Whitney test (non-parametric) or T-test for independent samples (parametric) was used to compare ages between the groups. Associations between HP or EBV

Table 2 Clinicopathological features, *H. pylori* and EBV infection in gastritis samples of adults patients

Variable	H. pylori			CagA			EBV		
	Negative	Positive	p-value	Negative[c]	Positive	p-value	Negative	Positive	p-value
Age (Mean ± SD)	35.58 ± 7.82	45.00 ± 10.89	0.011*	37.6 ± 7.67	44.92 ± 11.75	0.039*	42.24 ± 11.14	39.50 ± 3.54	0.733
Gender [N(%)]									
Female	3 (21.4)	11 (78.6)	0.410[a]	5 (35.7)	9 (64.3)	0.915[a]	14 (100)	0 (0)	0.999[a]
Male	9 (36.0)	16 (64.0)		10 (40.0)	15 (60.0)		23 (92.0)	2 (8.0)	
Histological subtype [N(%)]									
Mild	7 (36.8)	12 (63.2)	0.715[b]	9 (47.4)	10 (52.6)	0.820[b]	17 (89.5)	2 (10.5)	0.999[b]
Moderate/Severe	5 (25.0)	15 (75.0)		6 (30.0)	14 (70.0)		20 (100)	0 (0)	
EBV infection [N(%)]									
Absent	12 (32.4)	25 (67.6)	0.999[b]	14 (37.8)	23 (62.2)	0.810[b]			
Present	0 (0)	2 (100)		1 (50.0)	1 (50.0)				

*Significant difference between groups, p < 0.05. [a]p value after adjustment for age; [b]p value after adjustment for age and gender; [c]Negative samples for *H. pylori* and samples with *H. pylori* infection but without CagA virulence factor; EBV: *Epstein-Barr virus*; SD: standard deviation.

and other clinicopathological features were analyzed using chi-square (χ^2) and logistic regression. A p-value less than 0.05 was considered significant, and the confidence interval was 95%.

Results

We investigated 226 individuals, including 92 women and 134 men, divided into three groups. The percentage of men was 38.7%, 64.1% and 68% for juvenile UE patients, adult UE patients and GC patients, respectively. The proportion of males was higher in the cohort of GC patients (p < 0.001, OR = 3.365, 95% CI = 1.784 – 6.345) and adult UE patients (p = 0.014, OR = 2.827, 95% CI = 1.233 – 6.485) than among juvenile UE patients.

Among juvenile UE patients, 40 patients presented gastritis by UE. However, 59% of patients without UE-diagnosed gastritis presented mild gastritis by histopathological analysis. Therefore, 53 (85.5%) patients showed some degree of gastritis in the group of juvenile UE patients. The age of patients without gastritis did not differ from that of patients with gastritis [median ± interquartile range (IQR): 7.33 ± 8 vs 10.23 ± 8 years old; p = 0.080, Mann-Whitney test]. However, patients with mild gastritis were younger than patients with moderate or severe gastritis (mean ± standard deviation (SD): 8.25 ± 4.30.90 vs 11.86 ± 4.27 years old; p = 0.004, T-test). The gender breakdown did not differ between juvenile patients with and without gastritis (p = 0.725), as well as between juvenile patients with mild gastritis and moderate or severe gastritis (p = 0.097).

Among adult UE patients, all of the evaluated individuals presented gastritis, including 19 (48.7%) with mild gastritis and 20 (51.3%) with moderate or severe gastritis. Patients with mild gastritis were younger than patients with moderate or severe gastritis (mean ± SD: 37.47 ± 7.20 vs 46.50 ± 12.07 years old; p = 0.003, T-test). The gender breakdown did not differ between juveniles patients with

mild gastritis and moderate or severe gastritis (p = 1) in this group of analysis.

HP infection was detected in 0% of normal gastric mucosa samples, 58.5% of samples from juvenile gastritis patients, 69.2% of adult gastritis samples and 88% of GC patients (Figure 1a). In juvenile individuals, HP infection was more frequently observed in gastritis samples than in normal samples (p = 0.004, Yates correction). The frequency of HP in adult gastritis did not differ from the observed frequency of gastritis in juvenile patients (p = 1.000, after adjustment for age and gender) or in the GC samples (p = 0.335, after adjustment for age and gender).

HP $CagA^+$ was detected in 0% of normal gastric mucosa samples, 37.7% of samples from juvenile gastritis patients, 61.5% of adult gastritis samples and 67.2% of GC patients (Figure 1b). The frequency of infection by HP $CagA^+$ did not differ between samples from juvenile patients with gastritis and normal gastric mucosa (p = 0.064, Yates correcton). Moreover, the frequency of HP $CagA^+$ in adult gastritis tissue samples did not differ from that observed in juvenile gastritis patients (p = 1, after adjustment for age and gender) or in GC samples (p = 0.500, after adjustment for age and gender).

The frequency of HP infection did not differ between males and females in the samples from juvenile or adult patients evaluated by UE (p > 0.05, after adjustment for age; Tables 1 and 2). However, in GC samples, HP infection was detected more frequently in males than in females (p = 0.023 OR = 3.651, 95% CI = 1.190 – 11.199, after adjustment for age; Table 3).

In juvenile patients who underwent UE, gastritis patients with HP infection and with HP $CagA^+$ were older than those without this pathogen (p < 0.001 and p = 0.005, respectively, T-test; Table 1). In this group of patients, HP infection was more prevalent in cases of moderate or severe gastritis than in those of mild gastritis (p = 0.026; OR = 5.136, 95% CI = 1.220 – 21.611, after adjustment for

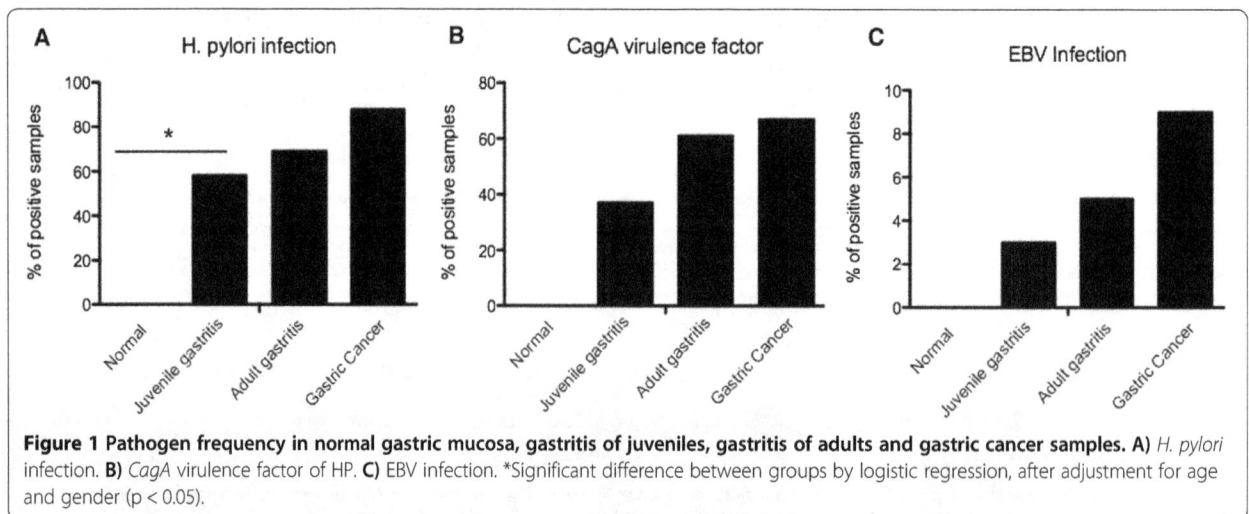

Figure 1 **Pathogen frequency in normal gastric mucosa, gastritis of juveniles, gastritis of adults and gastric cancer samples. A)** *H. pylori* infection. **B)** *CagA* virulence factor of HP. **C)** EBV infection. *Significant difference between groups by logistic regression, after adjustment for age and gender (p < 0.05).

Table 3 Clinicopathological features, *H. pylori* and EBV infection in gastric tumors

Variable	H. pylori			CagA			EBV		
	Negative	Positive	p-value	Negative[c]	Positive	p-value	Negative	Positive	p-value
Age (Median ± IQR)	57 ± 25	64 ± 16.75	0.027*	57 ± 22	64.5 ± 16.5	0.027*	63 ± 20	67 ± 21.5	0.192
Gender [N(%)]									
Female	9 (22.5)	31 (77.5)	0.023*[a]	15 (37.5)	25 (62.5)	0.307[a]	39 (97.5)	1 (2.5)	0.115[a]
Male	6 (7.1)	79 (92.9)		26 (30.6)	59 (69.4)		74 (87.1)	11 (12.9)	
Tumor location [N(%)]									
Non-cardia	12 (16.4)	61 (83.6)	0.080[b]	26 (35.6)	47 (64.4)	0.519[b]	67 (91.8)	6 (8.2)	0.592[b]
Cardia	3 (5.8)	49 (94.2)		15 (28.8)	37 (71.2)		46 (88.5)	6 (11.5)	
Histological subtype [N(%)]									
Intestinal-type	6 (8.5)	65 (91.5)	0.247[b]	25 (46.3)	29 (53.7)	0.012*[b]	63(88.7)	8 (11.3)	0.650[b]
Diffuse-type	9 (16.7)	45 (83.3)		16 (22.5)	55 (77.5)		50 (92.6)	4 (7.4)	
Stage [N(%)]									
Early	7 (15.9)	37 (84.1)	0.680[b]	25 (56.8)	19 (43.2)	0.000*[b]	41 (93.2)	3 (6.8)	0.999[b]
Advanced	6 (8.3)	66 (91.7)		14 (19.4)	58 (80.6)		64 (88.9)	8 (11.1)	
Tumor invasion [N(%)]									
T1/T2	4 (13.3)	26 (86.7)	0.453[b]	13 (43.3)	17 (56.7)	0.616[b]	29 (96.7)	1 (3.3)	0.560[b]
T3/T4	11 (11.6)	84 (88.4)		28 (29.5)	67 (70.5)		84 (88.4)	11 (11.6)	
Lymph node metastasis [N(%)]									
Absent	3 (25)	9 (75.0)	0.193[b]	8 (66.7)	4 (33.3)	0.024*[b]	12 (100)	0(0)	0.999[b]
Present	12 (10.6)	101 (89.4)		33 (29.2)	80 (70.8)		101 (89.4)	12 (10.6)	
Distant metastasis [N(%)]									
Absent	11 (16.7)	55 (83.3)	0.136[b]	30 (45.5)	36 (54.5)	0.005*[b]	62 (93.9)	4 (6.1)	0.258[b]
Present	4 (6.8)	55 (93.2)		11 (18.6)	48 (81.4)		51 (86.4)	8 (13.6)	
EBV infection [N(%)]									
Absent	15 (13.3)	98 (86.7)	0.998[b]	39 (34.5)	74 (65.5)	0.358[b]			
Present	0 (0)	12 (100)		2 (16.7)	10 (83.3)				

*Significant difference between groups, $p < 0.05$. [a]p value after adjustment for age; [b]p value after adjustment for age and gender; [c]Negative samples for *H. pylori* and samples with *H. pylori* infection but without CagA virulence factor; EBV: *Epstein-Barr virus*; IQR: interquartile range.

age and gender; Table 1). As observed in juvenile patients, adults with gastritis who were also positive for HP infection and HP *CagA*[+] were older than those without this pathogen (p = 0.011 and p = 0.039, respectively, T-test; Table 2).

In tumor samples, patients with HP *CagA*[+] were older than patients without HP *CagA*[-] (p = 0.027, Mann-Whitney test; Table 3). HP *CagA*[+] was more prevalent in intestinal-type than diffuse-type GC (p = 0.012; OR = 2.741, 95% CI 1.252 – 6.001, after adjustment for age and gender; Table 3). The presence of HP *CagA* + was also associated with lymph node metastasis (p = 0.024; OR = 5.611, 95% CI = 1.255 – 25.097, after adjustment for age and gender) and distal metastasis (p = 0.005; OR 3.299, 95% CI = 1.441 – 7.556, after adjustment for age and gender; Table 3).

EBV infection was detected in 0% of normal gastric mucosa samples, 3.8% of samples from juvenile gastritis patients, 5.1% of samples from adult gastritis patients and 9.6% of GC patients (Figure 1c and Figure 2). In the gastric mucosa, we found that 5-15% of cells were infected. Rates of EBV infection did not differ among normal gastric mucosa and mucosa from juvenile patients with gastritis (p > 0.05, Yates correction). Moreover, the frequency of EBV infection in the gastritis of adults did not differ from that observed in the gastritis of juvenile patients and GC samples (p > 0.05, after adjustment for age and gender). No association between EBV infection and HP infection or any clinicopathological variable was found (p > 0.05, Table 1, 2 and 3).

Although we did not observe a statistically significant association between the two pathogens, only one EBV-positive case was found without concomitant HP infection. This case was an 18-year-old female with no sign of gastric disease by UE evaluation and mild gastritis by histopathological analysis.

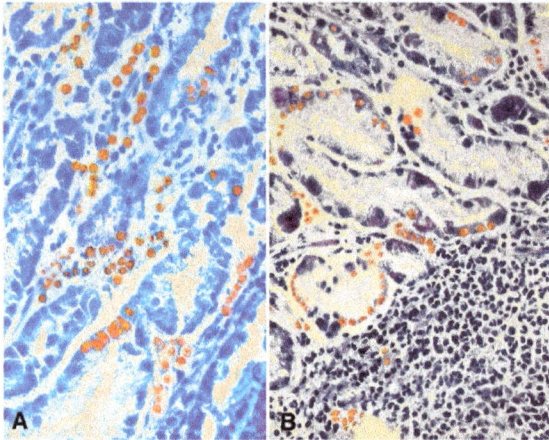

Figure 2 Detection of EBV by *in situ* hybridization. Strong nuclear staining was observed in infected nuclei in a **A)** mild gastritis (40x) and **B)** adult moderate gastritis.

Discussion

Infection by HP and EBV occurs most often during childhood, and both viruses can synergistically enhance the alteration of gastric mucosa to chronic gastritis and GC [6,17,19,25].

Gastritis is more likely to occur in older adults but can affect people of all ages, including children. Many studies [26,27] have attempted to understand the development of gastritis in children. Souza *et al.* [28], identified endoscopic abnormalities in 74% of the children and adolescents studied. Among these, 26% (7/21) had gastritis as determined by UE. In our study, gastritis was identified by UE in a larger number of juvenile patients (40/62). However, finding an apparently normal mucosa by endoscopy does not exclude the possibility of pathological change, as biopsy is required for a definitive determination. Our results confirm this assertion because in 22 normal endoscopic exams, only 9 showed a normal histological pattern. In addition, patients with mild gastritis were younger than patients with moderate or severe gastritis, perhaps because they had not yet been exposed to many aggressive agents that can lead to gastritis [6].

In the present study, HP infection was detected in most of the UE patients and GC samples, although the techniques used may underestimate the presence of the bacteria. Other studies in Brazil, such as those by Gatti *et al.* [29] and Souza *et al.* [28], reported the prevalence of HP infection in juveniles to be 51% and 60%, respectively. These results are consistent with our findings. An investigation in other developing countries also showed a similar frequency (61.8%) [30]. In adults, a slightly higher frequency was found in other studies in Brazilian (88.4%) [31] and African (70–97%) populations [32]. These numbers most likely reflect the social and health conditions of the studied populations because infections by HP are more common in developing countries than in developed countries [19].

In our study, HP infection was more common in cases of moderate or severe gastritis than in juveniles with mild gastritis. Similarly, Álvarez *et al.* [31] found a higher frequency of moderate and severe gastritis in patients infected by HP. Additionally, we observed that the prevalence of HP, particularly HP $CagA^+$, increased with age, corroborating previous investigations in populations from northeastern Brazil, China, and Japan [31-33]. It has been suggested that the earlier HP infection occurs, the greater the risk for GC due to chronic inflammatory reactions to the infection [34]. In the population studied here, the frequency of infection by HP or HP $CagA^+$ in GC patients did not differ from that observed in adults patients with gastritis. However, some studies have found that the spontaneous disappearance of HP during malignant transformation of gastric epithelia is possible [35,36]. Nevertheless, cancer still occurs after successful eradication of HP; therefore, eradication of HP does not lead to a significant decrease in the incidence of gastric cancer [37]. Furthermore, it has been observed that the eradication of HP must occur before carcinomatous change develops [38]. This finding highlights the necessity of epidemiological studies to understand the incidence and prevalence of HP in a population and to help in the development of population-specific strategies to prevent and control HP.

The prevalence of HP in gastric tumors varies with the country being analyzed [39]. In Brazil, a previous study detected this bacteria in 85.7% of gastric tumor samples [40], which is similar to the frequency observed in our study (88%). In addition, we observed that the frequency of HP was 1.5-times greater in GC samples than in juvenile gastritis samples, and almost ninety times higher than in normal gastric mucosa, highlighting a strong association between HP and the process of gastric carcinogenesis. After initial infection by HP, patients develop acute gastritis. This may resolve spontaneously, but the majority of cases progress to chronic gastritis [41]. The clinical outcome of HP infection is determined by the complex interaction between host factors and bacteria [42]. *CagA* is likely the most significant virulence factor [43] and is strongly associated with the risk for GC [42]. It is known that the basic *CagA* genotype acquired in childhood remains throughout life [44].

HP $CagA^+$ strains have been associated with more intense inflammation and greater bacterial density, as well as progression to gastric atrophy, peptic ulcer and gastric cancer [43]. However, the involvement of HP $CagA^+$ in gastric carcinogenesis in Brazilian individuals is still controversial. Oliveira *et al.* [45] found an association between the presence of *CagA* with more marked antral inflammation in duodenal ulcers (90%) and gastric carcinoma (94.23%) in Brazilian adults. In another study of the Brazilian population, Gatti et al. [29] found a slightly greater frequency (69%) of CagA$^+$ in patients with chronic gastritis. However, the authors did not find any association between CagA$^+$ strains and chronic gastritis, suggesting that other bacterial factors are involved in disease genesis. Consistent with this, in our study we did not find an association between HP CagA$^+$ and the presence of gastritis. However, HP CagA$^+$ was associated with poor prognostic variables in GC cancer.

Here, the CagA$^+$ genotype was associated with the age, histological subtype and metastatic process of GC patients. Unlike Kuo et al. [46], we found a higher frequency of CagA$^+$ patients in the older cohort of our Brazilian population. Moreover, the presence of HP CagA$^+$ was higher in intestinal-type than in diffuse-type GC. The transformation in gastric mucosa induced by HP CagA$^+$ is similar to the alterations that occur in the intestinal-type of GC [2,47]; thus, finding the highest frequency (84.6%) of CagA$^+$ in intestinal-type GC is reasonable. Additionally, the presence of HP CagA$^+$ may induce tumor alterations that lead to metastasis. Kong et al. [48] observed that HP stimulates the synthesis of CACUL1 in a gastric tumor cell line, which in turn promotes the expression of matrix metalloproteinase 9 and increases invasion and metastasis.

Approximately 7% of our patients presented EBV infection in gastric tissue samples. None of these patients presented symptoms of mononucleosis. Therefore, EBV infection in gastric mucosa is not necessarily associated with infection in lymph nodes or tonsils.

The frequency of infection by EBV in GC (9.6%) was similar to the frequency previously described in other populations (approximately 7.3 – 13%) [49-51]. However, the prevalence of EBV infection in patients with gastritis (3.8% among juvenile and 5.1% among adults) was reduced in comparison to the prevalence reported in the literature. Ryan et al. [25] found EBV sequences in 83% (5/6) of adult and 30% (15/50) of pediatric gastritis lesions. The low frequency identified in gastric mucosa of the younger patients may be because the stomach is not the primary location for B lymphocytes immortalized by EBV infection. The gastric mucosa does not seem to possess the necessary homing mechanism for settlement by these infected lymphocytes [5].

Although our results suggest that EBV is not critical for the initial steps of gastric mucosal injury in the Brazilian population, the presence of EBV genomes and their expression in gastric carcinoma cells raises the possibility that this virus may contribute to neoplastic transformation. Notably, EBV was found within the malignant cells in approximately 10% of gastric adenocarcinomas, and this infection seems to precede malignant transformation [52]. Additionally, a previous in vitro study reported that reactive products from HP infection trigger EBV reactivation in latently infected gastric epithelial cells [53]. Inflammatory stress that occurs during the malignization of gastric cells may lead to infiltration of lymphocytes carrying EBV. This process may increase the possibility of contact with epithelial cells, or it may produce a rich medium that supports the cytokine-stimulated clonal replication of EBV-infected epithelial cells [16].

Recently, Cárdenas-Mondragón [54] reported that co-infection with EBV and HP CagA$^+$ was associated with the presence of severe gastritis, reveling a critical role for EBV in gastric mucosal alterations. Here, we did not find an association between EBV and HP or the presence of CagA in our gastritis or cancer samples, most likely due to the low frequency of EBV.

The main limitation of this study is its relatively small sample size. Therefore, some of the statistical analyses presented reduced the power to detect significant differences between groups. Therefore, further investigations are still necessary to fully understand the roles of EBV and HP in gastric carcinogenesis in the Brazilian population.

Conclusion

Our results strongly suggest that HP is involved in the pathophysiology of severe gastric lesions and development of GC in infected juveniles and adults. Furthermore, the frequency of these pathologies increases with age. HP CagA$^+$ was associated with greater inflammation and more advanced stage of cancer. EBV was not the primary pathogenic factor in our sample. Additionally, a better understanding of the most prevalent strains of pathogens, and their associated antigens, will be valuable for the development of vaccines clinical protocols for screening and treating infection.

Abbreviations
HP: *Helicobacter pylori*; EBV: *Epstein-Barr virus*; UE: Upper endoscopy; GC: Gastric cancer; IARC: International agency for research on cancer; CagA: Cytotoxin associated gene A.

Competing interest
The authors declare that they have no competing interests.

Authors' contributions
CRTS: acquired data, analyzed and interpreted data, performed statistical analysis, wrote and revised the manuscript; KSO: acquired data, analyzed and interpreted data, wrote and revised the manuscript; JJSF: acquired data and revising it critically for important intellectual content; MFL: designed the study and performed the statistical analysis; DQC: designed the study, assisted with revision of the manuscript through contribution of important intellectual content; ADS: performed the statistical analysis and revised the manuscript; ASK: performed the statistical and revised the manuscript ; RCM: analyzed and interpreted data, revised the manuscript; APNNA: pathological analysis; PPA: acquisition of funding and acquired data; MCS: re-analyzed and re-interpreted data, and revised the manuscript; RRB: conceived of the study, participated in its design and coordination and helped to draft the manuscript. All authors read and approved the final manuscript.

Authors' information

CRTS: Biomedical research with PhD in Genetic and Molecular Biology, experience in Human Genetics with an emphasis on carcinogenesis and molecular markers, as well as experience in diagnostic imaging; KSO: professor at School of Medicine - UFPA; JJSF: pharmaceutical assistant professor at University Center of Pará (CESUPA) with a PhD in Cell Biology; MFL: researcher at the Department of Orthopedics and Traumatology and at the Department of Morphology and Genetics -UNIFESP, with experience in genetics and gastric cancer; DQC: visiting professor at the Center for Research in Oncology-UFPA, with experience in genetics and gastric cancer; ADS: PhD student in Genetics and Molecular Biology at UFPA; ASK: associate professor at the Institute of Biological Sciences and Center for Research in Oncology-UFPA, with experience in genetics with an emphasis on Human and Medical Genetics; RCM: assistant professor at UFPA, experience in pharmacology with an emphasis on oncology; APNNA: pathologist and professor at UFC; PPA: surgeon at University Hospital João de Barros Barreto-UFPA, experience in oncology and gastroenterology; MCS: Full professor of genetics, Head of Genetics Division, experience in Human Genetics and cancer; RRB: associate professor at the Institute of Biological Sciences-UFPA, experience in Human Genetics with an emphasis on carcinogenesis and mutagenesis.

Acknowledgements

The authors are thankful to Conselho Nacional de Desenvolvimento Científico e Tecnológico (CNPq; CRTS, ASK, RCM and RRB); Fundação de Amparo à Pesquisa do Estado de São Paulo (FAPESP; MFL and DQC); Coordenação de Aperfeiçoamento de Pessoal de Nível Superior (CAPES; ADS), which supported this study through grants and fellowships.

Author details

[1]Laboratório de Citogenética Humana, Instituto de Ciências Biológicas, Universidade Federal do Pará, Rua Augusto Corrêa, 01 – Guamá. CEP 66075-110. Caixa postal 479, Belém, PA, Brasil. [2]Instituto de Ciências da Saúde, Universidade Federal do Pará, Belém, PA, Brasil. [3]Centro Universitário do Pará, Belém, PA, Brasil. [4]Departamento de Ortopedia e Traumatologia, Universidade Federal de São Paulo, São Paulo, SP, Brazil. [5]Disciplina de Genética, Departamento de Morfologia e Genética, Universidade Federal de São Paulo, São Paulo, SP, Brasil. [6]Núcleo de Pesquisa em Oncologia, Universidade Federal do Pará, Belém, PA, Brasil. [7]Departamento de Patologia Oral, Faculdade de Odontologia, Universidade Federal do Ceará, Fortaleza, CE, Brasil.

References

1. Boyle P, Levin B: **World CanCer report 2008.** *Cancer Control* 2008, **199**(Book, Edited):512.
2. Ding S, Goldberg J, Hatakeyama M: **Helicobacter pylori infection, oncogenic pathways and epigenetic mechanisms in gastric carcinogenesis.** *Future Oncol* 2010, **6**:851–862.
3. Eslick G-D: **Helicobacter pylori infection causes gastric cancer? A review of the epidemiological, meta-analytic, and experimental evidence.** *World J Gastroenterol* 2006, **12**:2991–2999.
4. Fukayama M, Ushiku T: **Epstein-Barr virus-associated gastric carcinoma.** *Pathol Res Pract* 2011, **207**:529–537.
5. Thompson MP: **Epstein-Barr Virus and Cancer.** *Clin Cancer Res* 2004, **10**:803–821.
6. Nagini S: **Carcinoma of the stomach: A review of epidemiology, pathogenesis, molecular genetics and chemoprevention.** *World J Gastrointest Oncol* 2012, **4**:156–169.
7. IARC: **Schistosomes, liver flukes and Helicobacter pylori. IARC Working Group on the Evaluation of Carcinogenic Risks to Humans.** *IARC Monogr Eval Carcinog Risks Hum* 1994, **61**:1–241.
8. Bücker R, Azevedo-Vethacke M, Groll C, Garten D, Josenhans C, Suerbaum S, Schreiber S: **Helicobacter pylori colonization critically depends on postprandial gastric conditions.** *Sci Rep* 2012, **2**:994.
9. Das JCPN: **Epidemiology and pathophisiology of helicobacter pylori infection children.** *Indian J Pediatr* 2007, **74**:287–290.
10. Delahay RM, Rugge M: **Pathogenesis of Helicobacter pylori infection.** *Helicobacter* 2012, **17**(Sup 1):9–15.
11. Imai S, Koizumi S, Sugiura M, Tokunaga M, Uemura Y, Yamamoto N, Tanaka S, Sato E, Osato T: **Gastric carcinoma: monoclonal epithelial malignant cells expressing Epstein-Barr virus latent infection protein.** *Sci USA* 1994, **91**:9131–9135.
12. Oda K, Tamaru J, Takenouchi T, Mikata A, Nunomura M, Saitoh N: **Association of Epstein-Barr virus with gastric carcinoma with lymphoid stroma.** *Am J Pathol* 1993, **143**:1063–1071.
13. Iezzoni J, Gaffey M, Weiss L: **The role of Epstein-Barr virus in lymphoepithelioma-like carcinomas.** *Am J Clin Pathol* 1995, **103**:308–315.
14. Wu MS, Shun CT, Wu CC, Hsu TY, Lin MT, Chang MC, Wang HP, Lin JT: **Epstein-Barr virus-associated gastric carcinomas: relation to H. pylori infection and genetic alterations.** *Gastroenterology* 2000, **118**:1031–1038.
15. Tsuchiya S: **Diagnosis of Epstein–Barr virus-associated diseases.** *Crit Rev Oncol Hematol* 2002, **44**:227–238.
16. Saiki Y, Otani H, Naito Y, Miyazawa M, Nagura H: **Immunophenotypic characterization of Epstein-Barr virus-associated gastric carcinoma: mas- sive infiltration by proliferating CD8+ T-lymphocytes.** *Lab Invest* 1996, **75**:67–76.
17. Rodrigues O, Moraes E, Fernandes M, Sassi R, Rodrigues F, Pinheiro H: **Prevalência do *Helicobacter pylori* em adolescentes submetidos à esofagogastroduodenoscopia.** *Vitalle* 2009, **21**:51–58.
18. De Oliveira AM, Rocha GA, Queiroz DM, Mendes EN, de Carvalho AS, Ferrari TC, Nogueira AM: **Evaluation of enzyme-linked immunosorbent assay for the diagnosis of Helicobacter pylori infection in children from different age groups with and without duodenal ulcer.** *J Pediatr Gastroenterol Nutr* 1999, **28**:157–161.
19. Hunt RH, Xiao SD, Megraud F, Leon-Barua R, Bazzoli F, van der Merwe S, Coelho LGV, Fock M, Fedail S, Cohen H, Malfertheiner P, Vakil N, Hamid S, Goh KL, Wong BCY, Krabshuis J, Le MA: *Helicobacter Pylori in Developing Countries.* 2010:1–15.
20. Dixon MF, Genta RM, Yardley JH, Correa P: **Classification and grading of gastritis: the Updated Sydney System.** *Am J Surg Pathol* 1996, **20**:1161–1181.
21. Lauren P: **The two histological main types of gastric carcinoma: diffuse and so-called intestinal-type carcinoma. An attempt at a histo-clinical classification.** *Acta Pathol Microbiol Scand* 1965, **64**:31–49.
22. Washington K: **7th edition of the AJCC cancer staging manual: stomach.** *Ann Surg Oncol* 2010, **17**:3077–3079.
23. Covacci A, Rappuolu R: **PCR amplification of gene sequences form Helicobacter pylori strains.** In *Helicobacter pylori techniques for clinical diagnosis and basic research.* Edited by Lee and F Mégraud. London: WB Saunders Company Ltda; 1996:94–109.
24. Bacchi CE, Bacchi MM, Rabenhorst SH, Soares FA, Fonseca LE Jr, Barbosa HS, Weiss LMGA: **AIDS-related lymphoma in Brazil: histopathology, immunophenotype, and association with Epstein-Barr virus.** *Am J Clin Pathol* 1996, **105**:230–237.
25. Ryan JL, Shen Y, Morgan DR, Leigh B, Kenney SC, Dominguez RL, Margaret L: **Epstein-Barr Virus Infection is Common in Inflamed Gastrointestinal Mucosa.** *Dig Dis Sci* 2012, **57**:1887–1898.
26. Uhlig HH, Tannapfel A, Mössner J, Jedwilayties S, Deutscher J, Müller DM, Kiess WRT: **Histopathological parameters of Helicobacter pylori-associated gastritis in children and adolescents: comparison with findings in adults.** *Scand J Gastroenterol* 2003, **38**:701–706.
27. Whitney A, Guarner J, Hutwagner L, Gold B: **Helicobacter pylori Gastritis in Children and Adults: Comparative Histopathologic Study.** *Ann Diagn Pathol* 2000, **4**:279–285.
28. Souza D, Cipolotti R, Filho M: **Achados das endoscopias digestivas altas em crianças e adolescentes de Sergipe.** *Rev Paul Pediatr* 2008, **26**:361–364.
29. Gatti LL, Lábio R, Silva LC, Smith Mde APS: **CagAPositive Helicobacter pylori in Brazilian Children Related to Chronic Gastritis.** *Braz J Infect Dis* 2006, **10**:254–258.
30. Ricuarte O, Gutierrez O, Cardona H, Kim JG, Graham DY, El-Zimaity HMT: **Atrophic gastritis in young children and adolescents.** *J Clin Pathol* 2005, **58**:1189–1193.
31. Álvares MMD, Marino M, de Oliveira CA, Mendes CC, de Costa ACF, Guerra J, Queiroz, Dulciene Maria de Magalhães Nogueira AMMF: **Características da gastrite crônica associada a Helicobacter pylori : aspectos topográficos, doenças associadas e correlação com o status cag A.** *J Bras Patol e Med Lab* 2006, **42**:51–59.
32. Holcombe C: **Helicobacter pylori: the African Enigma.** *Gut* 1992, **33**:429–431.

33. Xu X, Liu F, Zhang S, Zhao J, Shi J: **Analysis on Helicobacter pylori infection and its related diseases in 1,442 children in Tianjin city.** *Zhonghua Liu Xing Bing Xue Za Zhi* 2000, **21**:100–102.

34. Recavarren-Arce S, Gilman RH, Leon-Barua R, Salazar G, McDonald J, Lozano R, Diaz F, Ramirez-Ramos A, Berendson R: **Chronic atrophic gastritis: early diagnosis in a population where Helicobacter pylori infection is frequent.** *Clin Infect Dis* 1997, **25**:1006–1012.

35. Kokkola A, Kosunen TU, Puolakkainen P, Sipponen P, Harkonen M, Laxen F, Virtamo J, Haapiainen R, Rautelin H: **Spontaneous disappearance of Helicobacter pylori antibodies in patients with advanced atrophic corpus gastritis.** *APMIS* 2003, **111**:619–624.

36. Perri F, Pastore M, Clemente R, Festa V, Quitadamo M, Niro G, Conoscitore P, Rutgeerts P, Andriulli A: **Helicobacter pylori infection may undergo spontaneous eradication in children: a 2-year follow-up study.** *J Pediatr Gastroenterol Nutr* 1998, **27**:181–183.

37. Wong BC-Y, Lam SK, Wong WM, Chen JS, Zheng TT, Feng RE, Lai KC, Hu WHC, Yuen ST, Leung SY, Fong DYT, Ho J, Ching CK, Chen JS: **Helicobacter Pylori Eradication to Prevent Gastric Cancer in a High-Risk Region of China: a Randomized Controlled Trial.** *APMIS* 2003, **111**(6):619–624.

38. Kato M, Asaka M: **Recent knowledge of the relationship between Helicobacter pylori and gastric cancer and recent progress of gastroendoscopic diagnosis and treatment for gastric cancer.** *Jpn J Clin Oncol* 2010, **40**:828–837.

39. Helicobacter A: **Gastric cancer and Helicobacter pylori: a combined analysis of 12 case control studies nested within prospective cohorts.** *Gut* 2001, **49**:347–353.

40. Thomazini CM, Aparecida M, Rodrigues M: **Infecção por Helicobacter pylori e câncer gástrico : freqüência de cepas patogênicas cagA e vacA em pacientes com câncer gástrico.** *J Bras Patol Med Lab* 2006, **42**:25–30.

41. Tan VP, Wong BC: **Helicobacter pylori and gastritis: untangling a complex relationship 27 years on.** *J Gastroenterol Hepatol* 2011, **26**(SUp 1):42–45.

42. Ladeira M, Salvadori D, Rodrigues M: **Biopatologia do Helicobacter pylori.** *J Bras Patol Med Lab* 2003, **39**:335–342.

43. Stein M, Ruggiero P, Rappuoli R, Bagnoli F: **Helicobacter pylori CagA: From Pathogenic Mechanisms to Its Use as an Anti-Cancer Vaccine.** *Front Immunol* 2013, **4**(October):328.

44. Yamaoka Y, Reddy R, Graham DY: **Helicobacter pylori virulence factor genotypes in children in the United States: clues about genotype and outcome relationships.** *J Clin Microbiol* 2010, **48**:2550–2551.

45. Oliveira AG, Santos A, Guerra JB, Rocha GA, Rocha AMC, Oliveira CA, Cabral MMDA, Nogueira AMMF, Queiroz DMM: **babA2- and cagA-positive Helicobacter pylori strains are associated with duodenal ulcer and gastric carcinoma in Brazil.** *J Clin Microbiol* 2003, **41**:3964–3966.

46. Kuo SH, Chen LT, Lin CW, Wu MS, Hsu PN, Tsai HJ, Chu CY, Tzeng YS, Wang HP, Yeh KH, Cheng A: **Detection of the Helicobacter pylori CagA protein in gastric mucosa-associated lymphoid tissue lymphoma cells: clinical and biological significance.** *Blood Cancer J* 2013, **3**:e125.

47. Wroblewski LE, Peek RM, Wilson KT: **Helicobacter pylori and gastric cancer: factors that modulate disease risk.** *Clin Microbiol Rev* 2010, **23**:713–739.

48. Kong Y, Ma LQ, Bai PS, Da R, Sun H, Qi XG, Ma JQ, Zhao RM, Chen NZNK: **Helicobacter pylori promotes invasion and metastasis of gastric cancer cells through activation of AP-1 and up-regulation of CACUL1.** *Int J Biochem Cell Biol* 2013, **45**:2666–2678.

49. Campos FI, Koriyama C, Akiba S, Carrasquilla G, Serra M, Carrascal E, Itoh T, Minakami Y, Eizuru Y: **Environmental factors related to gastric cancer associated with Epstein-Barr virus in Colombia.** *Asian Pac J Cancer Prev* 2006, **7**:633–637.

50. Herrera-Goepfert R, Akiba S, Koriyama C, Ding S, Reyes E, Itoh T, Minakami Y, Eizuru Y: **Epstein-Barr virus-associated gastric carcinoma: Evidence of age-dependence among a Mexican population.** *World J Gastroenterol* 2005, **11**:6096–6103.

51. Hao Z, Koriyama C, Akiba S, Li J, Luo X, Itoh T, Eizuru Y, Zou J: **The Epstein-Barr virus-associated gastric carcinoma in Southern and Northern China.** *Oncol Rep* 2002, **9**:1293–1298.

52. Gulley ML, Pulitzer DR, Eagan PA, Schneider BG: **Epstein-Barr virus infection is an early event in gastric carcinogenesis and is independent of bcl-2 expression and p53 accumulation.** *Hum Pathol* 1996, **27**:20–27.

53. Minoura-Etoh J, Gotoh K, Sato R, Ogata M, Kaku N, Fujioka T, Nishizono A: **Helicobacter pylori-associated oxidant monochloramine induces reactivation of Epstein-Barr virus (EBV) in gastric epithelial cells latently infected with EBV.** *J Med Microbiol* 2006, **55**:905–911.

54. Cárdenas-Mondragón MG, Carreón-Talavera R, Camorlinga-Ponce M, Gomez-Delgado A, Torres J, Fuentes-Pananá EM: **Epstein Barr virus and Helicobacter pylori co-infection are positively associated with severe gastritis in pediatric patients.** *PLoS One* 2013, **8**:e62850.

5

Beyond Maastricht IV: are standard empiric triple therapies for *Helicobacter pylori* still useful in a South-European country?

Nuno Almeida[1*], Maria Manuel Donato[2], José Manuel Romãozinho[1,2], Cristina Luxo[3], Olga Cardoso[3], Maria Augusta Cipriano[4], Carol Marinho[4], Alexandra Fernandes[1], Carlos Calhau[2] and Carlos Sofia[1,2]

Abstract

Background: Empiric triple treatments for *Helicobacter pylori* (*H. pylori*) are increasingly unsuccessful. We evaluated factors associated with failure of these treatments in the central region of Portugal.

Methods: This single-center, prospective study included 154 patients with positive ^{13}C-urea breath test (UBT). Patients with no previous *H. pylori* treatments (Group A, n = 103) received pantoprazole 40 mg 2×/day, amoxicillin 1000 mg 12/12 h and clarithromycin (CLARI) 500 mg 12/12 h, for 14 days. Patients with previous failed treatments (Group B, n = 51) and no history of levofloxacin (LVX) consumption were prescribed pantoprazole 40 mg 2×/day, amoxicillin 1000 mg 12/12 h and LVX 250 mg 12/12 h, for 10 days. *H. pylori* eradication was assessed by UBT 6–10 weeks after treatment. Compliance and adverse events were assessed by verbal and written questionnaires. Risk factors for eradication failure were determined by multivariate analysis.

Results: Intention-to-treat and per-protocol eradication rates were Group A: 68.9% (95% CI: 59.4–77.1%) and 68.8% (95% CI: 58.9–77.2%); Group B: 52.9% (95% CI: 39.5–66%) and 55.1% (95% CI: 41.3–68.2%), with 43.7% of Group A and 31.4% of Group B reporting adverse events. Main risk factors for failure were *H. pylori* resistance to CLARI and LVX in Groups A and B, respectively. Another independent risk factor in Group A was history of frequent infections (OR = 4.24; 95% CI 1.04–17.24). For patients with no *H. pylori* resistance to CLARI, a history of frequent infections (OR = 4.76; 95% CI 1.24–18.27) and active tobacco consumption (OR = 5.25; 95% CI 1.22–22.69) were also associated with eradication failure.

Conclusions: Empiric first and second-line triple treatments have unacceptable eradication rates in the central region of Portugal and cannot be used, according to Maastricht recommendations. Even for cases with no *H. pylori* resistance to the used antibiotics, results were unacceptable and, at least for CLARI, are influenced by history of frequent infections and tobacco consumption.

Keywords: Clarithromycin, Compliance, *Helicobacter pylori*, Levofloxacin, Treatment failure

Background

Approximately 50% of the world population is infected by *Helicobacter pylori* (*H. pylori*). This bacterium is responsible for multiple gastric diseases, including gastroduodenal ulcer, gastric adenocarcinoma and mucosa-associated lymphoid tissue lymphoma [1-3]. After almost thirty years of treating *H. pylori*, the ideal regimen has not been found. Some consensus conferences have recommended treatments with cure rates of ≥80% on an intention-to-treat (ITT) basis [4]. More recently, regimens of at least 90–95% efficacy, and preferably 95–100%, have been suggested as the standard of care [5].

Although meta-analyses have reported a decreased effectiveness for triple regimens containing clarithromycin (CLARI), the so-called "legacy triple therapy" is still widely used in several countries; the last Maastricht consensus maintained it as a first-line treatment under certain conditions [2,5,6]. The main reason for failure of this regimen is

* Correspondence: nunoperesalmeida@gmail.com
[1]Gastroenterology Department, Centro Hospitalar e Universitário de Coimbra, Praceta Mota Pinto e Avenida Bissaya Barreto, 3000-075 Coimbra, Portugal

increased resistance to CLARI [2,7]. In Europe, primary *H. pylori* resistance to this drug increased from 9.9% to 17.5% in one decade [8,9]. In fact, *H. pylori* infections refractory to first treatment attempts are becoming more frequent with expanding use of antibiotics for multiple infections and the rising number of patients who undergo *H. pylori* treatment.

After failure of a therapy containing proton pump inhibitor (PPI) and CLARI, either bismuth-based quadruple therapy or PPI–levofloxacin (LVX) triple therapy is recommended by the most recent Maastricht consensus (2012) [2]. Multiple studies and meta-analysis have shown LVX to be a valid alternative to standard antimicrobial agents in first- and second-line regimens [10-12]. It is active even in *H. pylori* strains resistant to CLARI and metronidazole. Eradication rates of patients who harbor these doubly resistant strains are reportedly 92% if the isolates are sensitive to LVX [13]. Levofloxacin-based therapy can be used as second-line treatment in countries with low prevalence of LVX-resistant strains, but should probably be used only as third-line therapy if resistance to this fluoroquinolone is higher than 15% [14].

The *H. pylori* prevalence rate in Portuguese adults is 84.2% [15]. Although the aforementioned empirical triple-therapies are regularly used in the central region of Portugal, to our knowledge, there is no information about the efficacy of these treatments.

This study evaluated eradication rates of a 14-day triple therapy with PPI, amoxicillin and CLARI as empiric first-line therapy and a 10-day triple treatment with PPI, amoxicillin and LVX as a rescue therapy. As secondary aim, we intended to identify clinical and bacterial factors associated with treatment failure.

Methods

Patients

In this single-center study, patients with dyspepsia, iron-deficient anemia, need for chronic therapy with PPI and/or first-degree relatives with gastric carcinoma were prospectively considered for inclusion. Each had a recent positive ^{13}C-urea breath test (UBT) and indication for upper endoscopy. Exclusion criteria were: age <18 years; pregnancy; lactating and/or fertile women who were not using safe contraceptive methods; history of allergy/hypersensitivity to any antibiotic or PPI; previous gastric malignancy and/or gastric surgery; current use of anticoagulants; marked thrombocytopenia; systemic severe disease (hepatic, cardio-respiratory or renal disease; uncontrolled diabetes; active malignant diseases, coagulopathies); use of antibiotics in the last 4 weeks; use of PPI in the last 2 weeks; intolerance/refusal to undergo upper endoscopy; previous *H. pylori* eradication treatments including fluoroquinolones or known use of this antibiotic for other infections.

They were divided in two groups: Group A—patients who had never received eradication treatments ($n = 103$; 73 female; mean age: 41.6 ± 12.9 years); Group B—patients who failed ≥ 1 eradication attempts that did not include LVX ($n = 51$; 39 female; mean age: 45.2 ± 13.9 years) and had no documented history of treatment with fluoroquinolones.

Empiric triple treatments and efficacy assessment

After undergoing upper endoscopies, patients in Group A were immediately prescribed pantoprazole 40 mg 2×/day, amoxicillin 1000 mg 12/12 h and CLARI 500 mg 12/12 h, for 14 days. Patients in Group B were prescribed pantoprazole 40 mg 2×/day, amoxicillin 1000 mg 12/12 h, and LVX 250 mg 12/12 h, for 10 days. We provided detailed explanation of the therapies and potential secondary effects to patients and their families, who were given diaries to record all administrations, side effects and symptoms during therapy. Patients were phoned immediately after treatment to register compliance and any potential symptoms or side effects. They underwent UBT 6–10 weeks after treatment to assess *H. pylori* status. At this time, compliance was confirmed by counting tablets returned by each patient. Treatment was considered complete if all medication was taken. Poor compliance was assumed if <80% of the prescribed drugs were taken.

Patients also returned the diaries they maintained during treatment and were asked to assess tolerability and efficacy of treatment in resolving symptoms by visual scales from 0 to 10 (0: not tolerable at all, 10: excellent tolerability; and 0: not efficacious, 10: fully efficacious, respectively). Adverse events were scored as mild, moderate or severe by their effect on daily activities (daily activities not limited, limited to some extent, or not possible at all, respectively) and need to discontinue treatment. The scoring system was based on that proposed by de Boer et al., with minor modifications [16]. During the study, patients could directly telephone an investigator to resolve any doubts or problems that occurred. Patients were allowed no antibiotics or antisecretory drugs 4 and 2 weeks, respectively, before their UBTs, which were considered positive if δ above baseline was $\geq 4‰$.

Microbiological studies

As this was a research protocol and patients each had indication for upper endoscopy, we took biopsies for *H. pylori* culture, susceptibility testing and genotyping. Minimum inhibitory concentrations (MIC) for amoxicillin, CLARI and LVX, and point mutations in gene *23S rRNA* and in the quinolones resistance-determining region of the *gyrA* gene were determined by a previously published protocol [17]. The *cagA* and *vacA* genotypes were obtained with real-time PCR by using specific primers selected from previously published works [18,19].

Stopping rules

Efficacy assessment was performed in each group for every 50 included patients. Inclusion was halted if this preliminary analysis revealed eradication rates <80%.

Statistics

Categorical variables are shown with their relative and absolute values; quantitative variables are expressed as mean ± standard deviation or median + range. The *H. pylori* eradication success was analyzed on both an ITT basis (including all eligible enrolled patients, regardless of compliance with study protocol; patients with unavailable data were assumed to be unsuccessfully treated) and "per protocol" (PP) (including only patients with good compliance and whose data was all evaluable at end of treatment).

Univariate analyses with Student's *t* test, Mann–Whitney and Fisher's exact test were used to evaluate associations between treatment effectiveness and age, sex, ethnicity, symptoms/indication for *H. pylori* treatment, body mass index (BMI), location of residence, education level, olive oil, alcohol and tobacco consumption, frequent infections, use of antibiotics in the last 12 months, family history of gastric pathology, *H. pylori* genotype, adverse events during treatment and compliance. Significant variables were subsequently included in a binomial logistic regression that assumed *H. pylori* eradication as the dependent variable. We used the statistical software package SPSS 20.0 (IBM Corp., Armonk, NY, USA).

Ethics

The study was approved by the ethical committee of our hospital and the Faculty of Medicine, and performed in accordance with the Declaration of Helsinki, the International Conference on Harmonisation of Good Clinical Practice Guidelines, and applicable local laws and regulations. Signed informed consent was obtained from each patient.

Results

Demographic variables

During the 4-year period, we included 154 patients (Group A: *n* = 103; Group B: *n* = 51; Table 1). Group B patients received a median of one eradication (range: 1 to 5) before inclusion with the following drugs: amoxicillin: 100%; CLARI: 92.2%; nitroimidazoles: 29.4%. The most common regimen was triple therapy with PPI, amoxicillin and CLARI, followed by PPI, CLARI and nitroimidazoles, and by PPI, amoxicillin and nitroimidazoles.

Table 1 Patients' demographic and clinical characteristics

	Group A n = 103	Group B n = 51
Mean age (years)	41.6 ± 12.9	45.2 ± 13.9
	(range 19–77)	(range 18–85)
Sex		
- Male	30 (29.1%)	12 (23.5%)
- Female	73 (70.9%)	39 (76.5%)
Ethnic background		
- European	99 (96.1%)	50 (98%)
- African	4 (3.9%)	1 (2%)
Education level		
- Level 1	30 (29.1%)	19 (37.3%)
- Level 2	73 (70.9%)	32 (62.8%)
Residence		
- Rural	55 (53.4%)	30 (58.8%)
- Urban	48 (46.6%)	21 (31.2%)
Indication(s) for *H. pylori* eradication		
- Non-ulcer dyspepsia	63 (61.2%)	34 (66.7%)
- Iron-deficient anemia	25 (24.3%)	7 (13.7%)
- GERD/Chronic therapy with PPI	24 (23.3%)	17 (33.3%)
- First-degree relatives with gastric cancer	14 (13.6%)	7 (13.7%)
- Peptic ulcer	9 (8.7%)	4 (7.8%)
BMI (Kg/m^2)	24.6 ± 4.2	25 ± 4
	(range 17.1–37.8)	(range 17.1–33.8)
Alcohol consumption	21 (20.4%)	10 (19.6%)
Smoking	13 (12.6%)	11 (21.6%)
Olive oil consumption ≥1 dl/week	53 (51.5%)	27 (52.9%)
History of frequent infections	20 (19.4%)	13 (25.5%)
Antibiotic consumption in the last 12 months	28 (27.2%)	40 (78.4%)
Family history of gastric diseases	49 (47.6%)	29 (56.9%)

BMI: body mass index; GERD: gastroesophageal reflux disease; PPI: proton pump inhibitors; Level 1: no education or primary school; Level 2: high-school or university grade.

Compliance, tolerability/adverse events and follow-up losses

Of the 103 patients in Group A, 25 (24.3%) failed to take at least one pill during treatment but only 7 (6.8%) were noncompliant; and 45 Group A patients (43.7%) experienced adverse events (mild: 36; moderate: 8; severe: 1). The patient with severe side effects had an allergic reaction with diffuse rash. Patients' median assessments of the regimens according to a visual scale, were tolerability: 8 (range: 2–10); efficacy: 8 (range: 0–10). Of the 51 patients in Group B, 3 (5.9%) failed to take at least one pill during treatment but only 2 (3.9%) were noncompliant;

and 16 (31.4%) experienced adverse events (mild: 13; moderate: 2; severe: 1). The patient with severe side effects had intractable nausea, vomiting and diarrhea. Patients' median assessments of treatment according to a visual scale, were tolerability: 8 (range: 2–10) and efficacy: 7 (range :2–9). No patient was lost to follow-up in either group.

Microbiological studies

Endoscopies with biopsies and culture were successfully and safely performed in all patients. *H. pylori* resistance to CLARI was detected in 22 isolates (21.4%) in Group A, and resistance to LVX in 13 (25.5%) isolates of Group B. Only one case showed resistance to amoxicillin, with a MIC level of 2 mg/L.

Twenty isolates of Group A had point mutations in the *23S rRNA* gene (A2143G/A2142G), and 9 isolates of Group B in the *gyrA* gene. All isolates with mutations had *in vitro* resistance to antibiotics related with those genetic patterns. *H. pylori cagA* and *vacA* genotypes are presented in Table 2.

Efficacy of eradication therapy

For Group A, the eradication rate was 68.9% (95% CI 59.4–77.1%) on ITT and 68.8% (95% CI: 58.9–77.2%) on PP analysis. For Group B eradication rate was 52.9% (95% CI: 39.5–66%) on ITT and 55.1% (95% CI: 41.3–68.2%) on PP analysis.

Factors associated with eradication failure

We successfully treated 85.2% of patients with CLARI-susceptible *H. pylori*, but only 9.1% of patients with CLARI-resistant *H. pylori* (P <0.0001). None (0%) of the Group B patients with LVX-resistant infections had successful therapy, compared with 71.1% of patients with LVX-susceptible infections (P <0.0001). Antibiotic resistance was independently associated with treatment failure in both groups (Table 3); however multivariate analysis showed only history of frequent infections to independently predict treatment failure in Group A (odds ratio [OR]: 4.24; 95% CI: 1.04–17.24).

We then repeated the analysis excluding patients with CLARI-resistant strains in Group A and LVX-resistant

strains in Group B. In susceptible-only Group A, history of frequent infections (OR: 4.76; 95% CI: 1.24–18.27) and active tobacco consumption (OR: 5.25; 95% CI: 1.22–22.69) were associated with treatment failure. In susceptible-only Group B, noncompliance was higher in patients with treatment failure but not significantly so (18.2% *vs* 0%; P = 0.078).

Discussion

Over the last two decades, widespread use of certain antibiotics has progressively decreased *H. pylori* antimicrobial susceptibility [20-22]. Resistance to CLARI and fluoroquinolones develops rapidly and cannot be overcome by increasing dose or duration of therapy [23]. The only way to identify effective drug combinations is to regularly monitor the success of *H. pylori* eradication and antibiotic resistance in every region.

Although PPI-CLARI-amoxicillin is probably the most common anti-*H. pylori* treatment, its eradication rates have decreased as resistance to antibiotics, particularly macrolides, rises. Almost all consensus statements and reviews still recommend it [2,4,20,24], although some authors suggest longer therapy duration (10–14 days instead of 7 days) or avoiding this regimen in regions where *H. pylori* resistance to CLARI is higher than 15–20% [2,20].

Levofloxacin-based second-line therapies are an encouraging strategy for addressing eradication failures. Multiple studies and meta-analyses show that combined PPI, amoxicillin and LVX regimens have better results, even in patients with more than one failed eradication attempt and CLARI- and metronidazole-resistant strains [10,12,25-27]. Unfortunately, fluoroquinolone resistance is rapidly increasing in many countries [9,28].

The *H. pylori* prevalence rate in Portugal is > 80% [15]. Multiple drugs commonly used for this infection, such as bismuth salts, tetracycline, furazolidone and rifabutin, are not easily available in Portugal, and doxycycline has disappointing results [17]. Although quadruple non-bismuth, sequential and hybrid therapies have been proposed as alternative first-line options, these treatments are complex. Empiric triple-therapy with CLARI is still the preferred first-line treatment and was recommended by the Portuguese Society of Gastroenterology in 2008 [29], with LVX-based treatment recently assuming a major second-line or rescue position. Although by 2000, Cabrita et al. reported *H. pylori* resistance to be 14.6% to CLARI and 11.1% to ciprofloxacin among adults from the Lisbon area [30], and a European multicenter study found resistance rates in the same population of 20.7% for CLARI and 33.3% for metronidazole, the empiric triple treatment remained the most common first-line regimen. In 2013, Megraud et al. reported primary resistance as 31.5% to CLARI and 26.3% to LVX in Portugal [9], and reportedly,

Table 2 *H. pylori* **genotypes**

Genotype	Group A (n = 103)	Group B (n = 51)
cagA positive	44 (42.7%)	10 (19.6%)
vacA s1m1	24 (23.3%)	4 (7.8%)
vacA s1m2	28 (27.2%)	12 (23.5%)
vacA s2m1	1 (1%)	2 (3.9%)
vacA s2m2	50 (48.5%)	33 (64.7%)

Table 3 Risk factors for eradication failure in univariate analysis

	Triple therapy with clarithromycin			Triple therapy with levofloxacin		
	Failure (n = 32)	Success (n = 71)	P/OR (95% CI)	Failure (n = 24)	Success (n = 27)	OR (95% CI); P
Female	**27 (84.4%)**	**46 (64.8%)**	**0.043/2.94 (1.01–8.57)**	19 (79.2%)	20 (74.1%)	0.749
Age	41.5 ± 13.7	41.7 ± 12.6	0.967	45.2 ± 10.4	45.3 ± 16.6	0.678
>50 years	9 (28.1%)	22 (31%)	0.820	9 (37.5%)	10 (37%)	1
Caucasian	30 (93.8%)	69 (97.2%)	0.586	23 (95.8%)	27 (100%)	0.471
No education or primary school	20 (62.5%)	53 (74.6%)	0.245	8 (33.3%)	11 (40.7%)	0.772
Urban residence	11 (34.4%)	37 (52.1%)	0.135	12 (50%)	9 (33.3%)	0.265
Non-ulcer dyspepsia	22 (68.8%)	41 (57.7%)	0.383	13 (54.2%)	21 (77.8%)	0.136
GERD/Chronic therapy with PPI	6 (18.8%)	18 (25.4%)	0.616	9 (37.5%)	8 (29.6%)	0.569
First-degree relatives with gastric cancer	5 (15.6%)	9 (12.7%)	0.759	3 (12.5%)	4 (14.8%)	1
Iron-deficient anemia	6 (18.8%)	19 (26.8%)	0.462	4 (16.7%)	3 (11.1%)	0.693
Peptic ulcer	1 (3.1%)	8 (11.3%)	0.268	3 (12.5%)	1 (3.7%)	0.331
BMI	**23.3 ± 3.3**	**25.2 ± 4.4**	**0.035**	26.2 ± 4.4	23.9 ± 3.3	0.064
BMI < 26 kg/m^2	**29 (90.6%)**	**44 (62%)**	**0.004/5.92 (1.65–21.28)**	13 (54.2%)	21 (77.8%)	0.136
Smoking	7 (21.9%)	6 (8.5%)	0.104	6 (25%)	5 (18.5%)	0.736
Alcohol consumption	4 (12.5%)	17 (23.9%)	0.290	3 (12.5%)	7 (25.9%)	0.300
Olive oil consumption ≥1 dl/week	18 (56.2%)	35 (49.3%)	0.531	11 (45.8%)	16 (59.3%)	0.406
History of frequent infections	**11 (34.4%)**	**9 (12.7%)**	**0.015/3.61 (1.31–9.91)**	7 (29.2%)	6 (22.2%)	0.749
Antibiotic consumption in the last 12 months	12 (37.5%)	16 (22.5%)	0.151	19 (79.2%)	21 (77.8%)	1
Family history of gastric diseases	18 (56.2%)	31 (43.7%)	0.289	11 (45.8%)	18 (66.7%)	0.164
Adverse events	13 (40.6%)	32 (45.1%)	0.830	8 (33.3%)	8 (29.6%)	1
Incomplete treatment	6 (18.8%)	19 (26.8%)	0.462	3 (12.5%)	0 (0%)	0.097
No compliance	2 (6.2%)	5 (7%)	1	2 (8.3%)	0 (0%)	0.216
CagA negative	**24 (75%)**	**35 (49.3%)**	**0.018/3.09 (1.22–7.81)**	20 (83.3%)	21 (77.8%)	0.731
vacA s1m1	**3 (9.4%)**	**21 (29.6%)**	**0.026/0.25 (0.07–0.90)**	3 (12.5%)	1 (3.7%)	0.331
vacA s1m2	7 (21.9%)	21 (29.6%)	0,480	5 (20.8%)	7 (25.9%)	0.749
vacA s2m1	0 (0%)	1 (1.4%)	1	0 (0%)	2 (7.4%)	0.492
vacA s2m2	**22 (68.8%)**	**28 (39.4%)**	**0.01/3.38 (1.39–8.20)**	16 (66.7%)	17 (63%)	1

BMI: body mass index (kg/m^2); GERD: gastroesophageal reflux disease.
Significant relationships (i.e., P <0.05) are shown in boldface type. Age is shown in years. Odds ratios are shown for significant variables only.

obese patients proposed for bariatric surgery in northern Portugal have low eradication rates with CLARI- and LVX-based ITT triple therapies [31]. However, the efficacy of empiric *H. pylori* treatments in Portugal is little studied. To our knowledge, this is the first study of the efficacy of empiric triple regimens among patients in the central region of Portugal.

Our eradication rates were 68.9% for first-line ITT treatment with 14-day PPI-CLARI-amoxicillin and 52.9% for second-line/rescue treatment with 10-day PPI-LVX-amoxicillin. These first-line results are slightly better than the ones published by Cerqueira et al. for patients treated in 2009–2010, and our second-line/rescue results are similar [31].

The main risk factor for treatment failure is undoubtedly antibiotic resistance [7]. We found 21.4% of *H. pylori* isolates were for CLARI-resistant in Group A, and 25.5% were LVX-resistant in Group B. Only two patients with CLARI-resistant *H. pylori*, and none with LVX-resistant *H. pylori*, achieved eradication. Strains of *H. pylori* in Central Portugal are thus often resistant to CLARI and LVX. Notably, although Group B excluded patients with known histories of exposure to fluoroquinolones, its resistance rate to LVX was very high, probably due to common use and misuse of macrolides and fluoroquinolones for respiratory and urinary infections in Portugal and the cross-resistance of *H. pylori* to all macrolides and fluoroquinolones [9,32].

Macrolide-resistant *H. pylori* will certainly become more prevalent in the near future. A recent study of children found a primary resistance rate to CLARI of 34.7% [33]. Clearly macrolides and fluoroquinolones cannot be used to treat *H. pylori* in patients previously exposed to them, as resistance is practically universal in such circumstances [28].

Although we prescribed empiric treatments in patients for whom *H. pylori* susceptibility patterns were determined, this study was a research protocol, the main objective of which was to establish the efficacy of commonly used empiric treatments. Prescriptions were implemented immediately after the endoscopies, but we received antibiotic susceptibility results much later, 2–3 weeks after these procedures. Even among only those patients infected by *H. pylori* strains with no resistance to CLARI in Group A or LVX in Group B, eradication rates were 85.2% and 71.1%, respectively—well below the 90% accepted as the minimum efficacy rate for *H. pylori* treatment regimens [5]. As compliance and adverse event rates did not significantly differ, these factors cannot be considered as responsible for such failures. However, in Group B, treatment failure tended to be higher in noncompliant patients, although not significantly so, due to the limited number of patients.

History of frequent infections was a risk factor for eradication failure in all circumstances, even in patients with no *H. pylori* resistance to CLARI. One possible explanation is that our methodology underestimated *H. pylori* resistance to macrolides. Infection by multiple strains, with different resistance patterns, is common, but subculture testing might mask identification of resistant strains [34,35]. This is a potential cause of treatment failure and negative cultures; thus direct molecular studies of biopsy specimens might be more illuminating [36]. For CLARI, De Francesco et al. recently reported that the prevalence of usually identified point mutations A2143G, A2142G and A2142C might be decreasing [37]. However, we identified mutations in positions A2143G/A2142G of *23S rRNA* gene in 20 of the 22 resistant strains. Notably, the methodology we used does not distinguish A2143G from A2142G, but the clinical significance of this limitation is controversial, although some authors state that the A2143G mutation is the one that significantly lowers *H. pylori* eradication rate [7]. Point mutation A2142C was not detected and we did not search for other mutations; this can be a limitation of our work [37].

Active tobacco consumption was also a risk factor for failure in patients with CLARI-susceptible *H. pylori*. This negative effect is already known and may result from a reduction of antibiotic delivery due to a decreased gastric blood flow, lower intragastric pH or increased activity of the vacuolating toxin activity in gastric cells [2,38].

We had only one case of *H. pylori* resistance to amoxicillin, but that did not determine eradication failure. Resistance to this antibiotic has also been held responsible for treatment failure, but there is no accurate estimate of its effect [39,40].

H. pylori genotype can be important as it is reported to be strongly associated with eradication success, antibiotic susceptibility and *H. pylori* virulence factors [14,41,42]. Genotypes *cagA* negative and *vacA* s2m2 induce less inflammation and may contribute to reduced antibiotic delivery and decreased *H. pylori* eradication. Our univariate analysis also suggested this association but logistic regression did not confirm it, although the limited number of patients might have affected these results.

Another possible explanation for our results is that PPI and amoxicillin might have been prescribed in inadequate doses and/or intervals between administrations. Generally, Caucasians metabolize PPI quickly and might need higher doses and frequency of PPI administration [43]. The same might be needed for amoxicillin, as its bactericidal effect depends on % time above MIC and its plasma half-life is very short; thus frequent dosing for amoxicillin is necessary [44]. However, we prescribed the combinations traditionally supported in the literature. Different combinations, with four daily administrations of PPI and amoxicillin, could eventually be tested in future studies.

Various diseases can influence *H. pylori* eradication rates. Patients with peptic ulcers tend to respond better to treatment than patients with non-ulcer dyspepsia [2,45,46]. Although our study found no association between disease manifestations and therapeutic failure, relatively few patients with peptic ulcers were included. The predominance of non-ulcer dyspepsia in our series explains the high number of female patients, as non-ulcer dyspepsia is more common in women [47].

Another limitation of our study was the relatively small study cohort. First, we included only patients with previous positive UBT and indications for upper endoscopy, with very restrictive exclusion criteria, which limited the number of includible patients. Second, when our protocol was designed, no clear rules were in place on interrupting treatment of patients in prospective studies for *H. pylori* treatments. However, Maastricht III consensus established that proposed therapies must achieve eradication rates ≥80%. In following these recommendations, we decided to perform preliminary analyses of each 50 patients and to stop the study if eradication rate was less than 80%. That threshold occurred in the first analysis for Group B and in the second one for Group A. Even stricter stopping rules were more recently proposed by Graham (50 patients; eradication rate <90%) [48].

Finally, some recent studies suggest that 14-day LVX-based triple therapy can provide a >90% *H. pylori* eradication rate, but a 10-day duration may be suboptimal [49]. Although our LVX-treated patients in Group B received a 10-day regimen, 7- and 10-day regimens with LVX were acceptable when our protocol was designed; we chose the longer one specifically to optimize results. Another problem with LVX is lack of consensus about dosage: 250 mg 2×/day, 500 mg 1×/day, or 500 mg 2×/day. The 10-day 500 mg 2×/day dose reportedly has higher eradication rates, but still <80% [50]. Other authors still use a 10-day rescue regimen with PPI, amoxicillin 1 g and LVX 250 mg, all 2×/day [51].

Conclusions

Empiric triple-therapies with PPI-CLARI-amoxicillin and PPI-LVX-amoxicillin are ineffective as first- and second-line *H. pylori* regimens, respectively, in the central region of Portugal and they are now unacceptable as treatments. The main reason for treatment failure is high *H. pylori* resistance to CLARI and LVX.

History of frequent infections and active tobacco consumption contribute to unsuccessful treatments with CLARI for *H. pylori* strains with no resistance to this drug. In patients with these characteristics, another tailored first-line treatment is preferable.

For first-line empiric treatment, we suggest empiric concomitant or hybrid therapies for 14 days. However, study of the efficacy of these treatments in our region is urgently needed. In light of the scarcity of effective *H. pylori* antimicrobials in our country, if these regimens fail, it is our opinion that second-line treatments must be prescribed according to susceptibility testing.

Abbreviations

H. pylori: Helicobacter pylori; ITT: Intention-to-treat; PPI: Proton pump inhibitor(s); UBT: ^{13}C-urea breath test; MIC: Minimum inhibitory concentrations; PP: Per protocol; OR: Odds ratio.

Competing interests

The authors declare that they have no competing interests.

Authors' contributions

The involvement of each author was as follows: NA (1-8); MMD (1,2,5,7); JMR (1-8); CL (1,2,5); OC (1,2,5); MAC (1,2,5); CM (1,2,5); AF (2-6); CC (2,7); CS (5,8), [Key: (1) Study concept and design; (2) Acquisition of data; (3) Analysis and interpretation of data; (4) Drafting of the manuscript; (5) Critical revision of the manuscript for important intellectual content; (6) Statistical analysis; (7) Administrative, technical, or material support; (8) Study supervision.], All authors read the final version of this manuscript, approve its' content and submission for publication.

Acknowledgments

The authors are indebted to Dr. João Casalta for his help in the statistical analysis. This work was supported by a grant from the Portuguese Institute Fundação para a Ciência e Tecnologia (PIC/IC/83122/2007).

Author details
[1]Gastroenterology Department, Centro Hospitalar e Universitário de Coimbra, Praceta Mota Pinto e Avenida Bissaya Barreto, 3000-075 Coimbra, Portugal. [2]Gastroenterology Centre, Faculty of Medicine, Coimbra University, Praceta Mota Pinto e Avenida Bissaya Barreto, 3000-075 Coimbra, Portugal. [3]Laboratory of Microbiology, Faculty of Pharmacy, Coimbra University, Azinhaga de Santa Comba, 3000-548 Coimbra, Portugal. [4]Pathology Department, Coimbra University Hospital Centre, Praceta Mota Pinto e Avenida Bissaya Barreto, 3000-075 Coimbra, Portugal.

References

1. Correa P, Piazuelo MB. Natural history of Helicobacter pylori infection. Dig Liver Dis. 2008;40(7):490–6.
2. Malfertheiner P, Megraud F, O'Morain CA, Atherton J, Axon AT, Bazzoli F, et al. Management of Helicobacter pylori infection–the Maastricht IV/Florence Consensus Report. Gut. 2012;61(5):646–64.
3. Chuah SK, Tsay FW, Hsu PI, Wu DC. A new look at anti-Helicobacter pylori therapy. World J Gastroenterol. 2011;17(35):3971–5.
4. Malfertheiner P, Megraud F, O'Morain C, Bazzoli F, El-Omar E, Graham D, et al. Current concepts in the management of Helicobacter pylori infection: the Maastricht III Consensus Report. Gut. 2007;56(6):772–81.
5. Graham DY, Fischbach L. Helicobacter pylori treatment in the era of increasing antibiotic resistance. Gut. 2010;59(8):1143–53.
6. Fischbach LA, Goodman KJ, Feldman M, Aragaki C. Sources of variation of Helicobacter pylori treatment success in adults worldwide: a meta-analysis. Int J Epidemiol. 2002;31(1):128–39.
7. Giorgio F, Principi M, De Francesco V, Zullo A, Losurdo G, Di Leo A, et al. Primary clarithromycin resistance to Helicobacter pylori: is this the main reason for triple therapy failure? World J Gastrointest Pathophysiol. 2013;4(3):43–6.
8. Glupczynski Y, Megraud F, Lopez-Brea M, Andersen LP. European multicentre survey of in vitro antimicrobial resistance in Helicobacter pylori. Eur J Clin Microbiol Infect Dis. 2001;20(11):820–3.
9. Megraud F, Coenen S, Versporten A, Kist M, Lopez-Brea M, Hirschl AM, et al. Helicobacter pylori resistance to antibiotics in Europe and its relationship to antibiotic consumption. Gut. 2013;62(1):34–42.
10. Gisbert JP, Morena F. Systematic review and meta-analysis: levofloxacin-based rescue regimens after Helicobacter pylori treatment failure. Aliment Pharmacol Ther. 2006;23(1):35–44.
11. Gisbert JP, Pajares JM. Helicobacter pylori "rescue" therapy after failure of two eradication treatments. Helicobacter. 2005;10(5):363–72.
12. Saad RJ, Schoenfeld P, Kim HM, Chey WD. Levofloxacin-based triple therapy versus bismuth-based quadruple therapy for persistent Helicobacter pylori infection: a meta-analysis. Am J Gastroenterol. 2006;101(3):488–96.
13. Gatta L, Zullo A, Perna F, Ricci C, De Francesco V, Tampieri A, et al. A 10-day levofloxacin-based triple therapy in patients who have failed two eradication courses. Aliment Pharmacol Ther. 2005;22(1):45–9.
14. Sugimoto M, Yamaoka Y. Virulence factor genotypes of Helicobacter pylori affect cure rates of eradication therapy. Arch Immunol Ther Exp (Warsz). 2009;57(1):45–56.
15. Bastos J, Peleteiro B, Barros R, Alves L, Severo M, de Fatima PM, et al. Sociodemographic determinants of prevalence and incidence of Helicobacter pylori infection in Portuguese adults. Helicobacter. 2013;18(6):413–22.
16. de Boer WA, Thys JC, Borody TJ, Graham DY, O'Morain C, Tytgat GN. Proposal for use of a standard side effect scoring system in studies exploring Helicobacter pylori treatment regimens. Eur J Gastroenterol Hepatol. 1996;8(7):641–3.
17. Almeida N, Romaozinho JM, Donato MM, Luxo C, Cardoso O, Cipriano MA, et al. Triple therapy with high-dose proton-pump inhibitor, amoxicillin, and doxycycline is useless for Helicobacter pylori eradication: a proof-of-concept study. Helicobacter. 2014;19(2):90–7.
18. Atherton JC, Cao P, Peek Jr RM, Tummuru MK, Blaser MJ, Cover TL. Mosaicism in vacuolating cytotoxin alleles of Helicobacter pylori, association of specific vacA types with cytotoxin production and peptic ulceration. J Biol Chem. 1995;270(30):17771–7.

19. Santos A, Queiroz DM, Menard A, Marais A, Rocha GA, Oliveira CA, et al. New pathogenicity marker found in the plasticity region of the Helicobacter pylori genome. J Clin Microbiol. 2003;41(4):1651–5.

20. Vakil N, Megraud F. Eradication therapy for Helicobacter pylori. Gastroenterology. 2007;133(3):985–1001.

21. Boyanova L, Mitov I. Geographic map and evolution of primary Helicobacter pylori resistance to antibacterial agents. Expert Rev Anti Infect Ther. 2010;8(1):59–70.

22. De Francesco V, Giorgio F, Hassan C, Manes G, Vannella L, Panella C, et al. Worldwide H. pylori antibiotic resistance: a systematic review. J Gastrointestin Liver Dis. 2010;19(4):409–14.

23. Graham DY, Fischbach LA. Empiric therapies for Helicobacter pylori infections. CMAJ. 2011;183(9):E506–8.

24. Fock KM, Katelaris P, Sugano K, Ang TL, Hunt R, Talley NJ, et al. Second Asia-Pacific Consensus Guidelines for Helicobacter pylori infection. J Gastroenterol Hepatol. 2009;24(10):1587–600.

25. Gisbert JP. Rescue therapy for Helicobacter pylori infection 2012. Gastroenterol Res Pract. 2012;2012:974594.

26. Gisbert JP. "Rescue" regimens after Helicobacter pylori treatment failure. World J Gastroenterol. 2008;14(35):5385–402.

27. Gisbert JP, Gisbert JL, Marcos S, Jimenez-Alonso I, Moreno-Otero R, Pajares JM. Empirical rescue therapy after Helicobacter pylori treatment failure: a 10-year single-centre study of 500 patients. Aliment Pharmacol Ther. 2008;27(4):346–54.

28. Graham DY, Shiotani A. New concepts of resistance in the treatment of Helicobacter pylori infections. Nat Clin Pract Gastroenterol Hepatol. 2008;5(6):321–31.

29. Gastrenterologia SPd. Normas de orientação clínica - helicobacter pylori. GE - Jornal Português de Gastrenterologia. 2008;15:192–4.

30. Cabrita J, Oleastro M, Matos R, Manhente A, Cabral J, Barros R, et al. Features and trends in Helicobacter pylori antibiotic resistance in Lisbon area, Portugal (1990–1999). J Antimicrob Chemother. 2000;46(6):1029–31.

31. Cerqueira RM, Correia MR, Fernandes CD, Vilar H, Manso MC. Cumulative Helicobacter pylori eradication therapy in obese patients undergoing gastric bypass surgery. Obes Surg. 2013;23(2):145–9.

32. Adriaenssens N, Coenen S, Versporten A, Muller A, Minalu G, Faes C, et al. European surveillance of antimicrobial consumption (ESAC): outpatient antibiotic use in Europe (1997–2009). J Antimicrob Chemother. 2011;66 Suppl 6:vi3–vi12.

33. Oleastro M, Pelerito A, Nogueira P, Benoliel J, Santos A, Cabral J, et al. Prevalence and incidence of Helicobacter pylori Infection in a healthy pediatric population in the Lisbon area. Helicobacter. 2011;16(5):363–72.

34. Kim JJ, Kim JG, Kwon DH. Mixed-infection of antibiotic susceptible and resistant Helicobacter pylori isolates in a single patient and underestimation of antimicrobial susceptibility testing. Helicobacter. 2003;8(3):202–6.

35. Van Doorn LJ, Figueiredo C, Megraud F, Pena S, Midolo P, Queiroz DM, et al. Geographic distribution of vacA allelic types of Helicobacter pylori. Gastroenterology. 1999;116(4):823–30.

36. Kanizaj TF, Kunac N. Helicobacter pylori: future perspectives in therapy reflecting three decades of experience. World J Gastroenterol. 2014;20(3):699–705.

37. De Francesco V, Zullo A, Giorgio F, Saracino I, Zaccaro C, Hassan C, et al. Change of point mutations in Helicobacter pylori rRNA associated with clarithromycin resistance in Italy. J Med Microbiol. 2014;63(Pt 3):453–7.

38. Suzuki T, Matsuo K, Ito H, Sawaki A, Hirose K, Wakai K, et al. Smoking increases the treatment failure for Helicobacter pylori eradication. Am J Med. 2006;119(3):217–24.

39. Gerrits MM, van Vliet AH, Kuipers EJ, Kusters JG. Helicobacter pylori and antimicrobial resistance: molecular mechanisms and clinical implications. Lancet Infect Dis. 2006;6(11):699–709.

40. Han SR, Bhakdi S, Maeurer MJ, Schneider T, Gehring S. Stable and unstable amoxicillin resistance in Helicobacter pylori: should antibiotic resistance testing be performed prior to eradication therapy? J Clin Microbiol. 1999;37(8):2740–1.

41. Agudo S, Perez-Perez G, Alarcon T, Lopez-Brea M. High prevalence of clarithromycin-resistant Helicobacter pylori strains and risk factors associated with resistance in Madrid. Spain J Clin Microbiol. 2010;48(10):3703–7.

42. van Doorn LJ, Schneeberger PM, Nouhan N, Plaisier AP, Quint WG, de Boer WA. Importance of Helicobacter pylori cagA and vacA status for the efficacy of antibiotic treatment. Gut. 2000;46(3):321–6.

43. Miehlke S, Hansky K, Schneider-Brachert W, Kirsch C, Morgner A, Madisch A, et al. Randomized trial of rifabutin-based triple therapy and high-dose dual therapy for rescue treatment of Helicobacter pylori resistant to both metronidazole and clarithromycin. Aliment Pharmacol Ther. 2006;24(2):395–403.

44. Shirai N, Sugimoto M, Kodaira C, Nishino M, Ikuma M, Kajimura M, et al. Dual therapy with high doses of rabeprazole and amoxicillin versus triple therapy with rabeprazole, amoxicillin, and metronidazole as a rescue regimen for Helicobacter pylori infection after the standard triple therapy. Eur J Clin Pharmacol. 2007;63(8):743–9.

45. Broutet N, Tchamgoue S, Pereira E, Lamouliatte H, Salamon R, Megraud F. Risk factors for failure of Helicobacter pylori therapy–results of an individual data analysis of 2751 patients. Aliment Pharmacol Ther. 2003;17(1):99–109.

46. Wolle K, Malfertheiner P. Treatment of Helicobacter pylori. Best Pract Res Clin Gastroenterol. 2007;21(2):315–24.

47. Schmulson M, Adeyemo M, Gutierrez-Reyes G, Charua-Guindic L, Farfan-Labonne B, Ostrosky-Solis F, et al. Differences in gastrointestinal symptoms according to gender in Rome II positive IBS and dyspepsia in a Latin American population. Am J Gastroenterol. 2010;105(4):925–32.

48. Graham DY. Efficient identification and evaluation of effective Helicobacter pylori therapies. Clin Gastroenterol Hepatol. 2009;7(2):145–8.

49. Tai WC, Chiu CH, Liang CM, Chang KC, Kuo CM, Chiu YC, et al. Ten-Day versus 14-Day levofloxacin-containing triple therapy for second-line anti-Helicobacter pylori Eradication in Taiwan. Gastroenterol Res Pract. 2013;2013:932478.

50. Gisbert JP, Perez-Aisa A, Bermejo F, Castro-Fernandez M, Almela P, Barrio J, et al. Second-line therapy with levofloxacin after failure of treatment to eradicate helicobacter pylori infection: time trends in a Spanish Multicenter Study of 1000 patients. J Clin Gastroenterol. 2013;47(2):130–5.

51. De Francesco V, Hassan C, Ridola L, Giorgio F, Ierardi E, Zullo A. Sequential, concomitant and hybrid first-line therapies for Helicobacter pylori eradication: a prospective randomized study. J Med Microbiol. 2014;63(Pt 5):748–52.

6

Diagnostic accuracy of reused Pronto Dry® test and CLOtest® in the detection of *Helicobacter pylori* infection

Shahidi Jamaludin[1], Nazri Mustaffa[1*], Nor Aizal Che Hamzah[2], Syed Hassan Syed Abdul Aziz[1] and Yeong Yeh Lee[1]

Abstract

Background: Unchanged substrate in a negative rapid urease test may be reused to detect *Helicobacter pylori* (*H. pylori*). This could potentially reduce costs and wastage in low prevalence and resource-poor settings. We thus aimed to investigate the diagnostic accuracy of reused Pronto Dry® and CLOtest® kits, comparing this to the use of new Pronto Dry® test kits and histopathological evaluation of gastric mucosal biopsies.

Methods: Using a cross-sectional study design, subjects who presented for upper endoscopy due to various non-emergent causes had gastric biopsies obtained at three adjacent sites. Biopsy samples were tested for *H. pylori* using a reused Pronto Dry® test, a reused CLOtest®, a new Pronto Dry® test and histopathological examination. Concordance rates, sensitivity, specificity, positive predictive value (PPV), negative predictive value (NPV) and diagnostic accuracy were then determined.

Results: A total of 410 subjects were recruited. The sensitivity and diagnostic accuracy of reused Pronto Dry® tests were 72.60 % (95 % CI, 61.44 – 81.51) and 94.15 % (95 % CI, 91.44 – 96.04) respectively. For reused CLOtests®, the sensitivity and diagnostic accuracy were 93.15 % (95 % CI 85.95 – 97.04) and 98.29 % (95 % CI 96.52 – 99.17) respectively. There were more true positives for new and reused Pronto Dry® pallets as compared to new and reused CLOtests® when comparing colour change within 30 min vs. 31–60 min ($P < 0.001$ and $P = 0.7$ respectively).

Conclusion: Negative Pronto Dry® and CLOtest® kits may be reused in a low prevalence setting where cost issues remain paramount. Reused CLOtest® kits have better accuracy than reused Pronto Dry® tests. Reused Pronto Dry® tests however have a more rapid colour change whilst maintaining diagnostic accuracy.

Background

Since its identification in 1982 by Barry Marshall and Robyn Warren, the flagellated Gram-negative bacilli *Helicobacter pylori* (*H. pylori*) has been recognised as the predisposing factor for gastroduodenal diseases, particularly peptic ulcer disease, gastric malignancies and B-cell mucosa-associated lymphoid tissue (MALT) lymphomas [1–3]. Due to the availability of commercial test kits as well as solutions prepared in-house, the rapid urease test (RUT) has been widely used for the detection of *H. pylori*, with reported studies indicating high sensitivity (95–98 %) and specificity (92–100 %) [4–7]. RUT

assays exploit the fact that *H. pylori* produces large amounts of urease, which hydrolyses urea to ammonia thus enabling the organism to survive in a low pH environment [8, 9].

Theoretically, unchanged substrate in a negative RUT may be used again to test for the presence of *H. pylori* in a new gastric biopsy sample. This has been shown to be true for CLOtest® pallets, where some studies have concluded that diagnostic accuracy is maintained despite being reused up to 6 months from the initial test application [10–14]. The CLOtest® has a urea gel capsule that changes colour over time in the presence of specimens that contain *H. pylori*, whilst the Pronto Dry® kit consists of a dry filter paper that contains urea and an indicator that detects a rise in pH of specimens that are *H. pylori* positive. The main advantages of using Pronto Dry® over CLOtest® kits in the detection of *H. pylori* is the fact that Pronto Dry® kits may be stored at room temperature, with

* Correspondence: mustaffa.nazri@gmail.com
[1]School of Medical Sciences, Universiti Sains Malaysia, Kubang Kerian, Kelantan, Malaysia
Full list of author information is available at the end of the article

no need to incubate the applied specimen in a warm environment thus offering quicker results. There is also a linear correlation between the histological grading of *H. pylori* stomach mucosal colonisation density with the Pronto Dry® graded colour change index. In comparison to the various studies done on the reuse of CLOtest® kits, there is a paucity of information in the literature on the ability of reused Pronto Dry® tests to detect the presence of *H. pylori*. Bearing in mind the issue of potential cost-savings and reduction in wastage especially in a resource-poor setting, we thus sought to assess the diagnostic accuracy of re-using negative Pronto Dry® test and CLOtest® kits in comparison to *H. pylori* detection using new Pronto Dry® test kits as well as histological methods.

Methods

Study participants

This cross-sectional study was performed from March 2008 to June 2010 in Hospital Universiti Sains Malaysia, Kubang Kerian. Kelantan. This is a tertiary referral centre and a teaching hospital located at the northeastern region of Peninsular Malaysia. Inclusion criteria were subjects aged 18 and above who presented for upper GI endoscopy due to investigation of upper abdominal symptoms or suspected gastric pathology. Exclusion criteria were subjects who had recently taken antibiotics, bismuth salts and/or proton pump inhibitors within 2 weeks of their endoscopy date, were pregnant, had overt upper GI bleeding as well as those who could not tolerate upper gastrointestinal endoscopic examination.

Eligible participants were provided with an information sheet that contained relevant details of the study. A verbal explanation was also provided and informed consent obtained. Following this, clinical and demographic details of participants were recorded. Participants would then undergo upper GI endoscopy as per standard protocol, where after adequate endoscopic examination gastric biopsies would then be obtained for assessment of *H. pylori* infection. Four separate biopsies, each measuring approximately 2 – 3 mm were obtained using the same biopsy forceps from the same adjacent gastric area for *H. pylori* testing using a new Pronto Dry® kit, a reused Pronto Dry® kit, a reused CLOtest® as well as for histopathology assessment. Histological examination was performed by pathologists who were blinded to study outcomes where *H. pylori* was reported to be either present or absent. Relevant histological details were reported using the Sydney classification.

Ethical approval

Approval was obtained from the Human Research Ethics Committee (HREC), Universiti Sains Malaysia (Ref.: USMKK/PPP/JEPeM [200.4(2.5)]).

New and reused Pronto Dry® kits

The new as well as reused Pronto Dry® kits for this study were produced by Medical Instruments Corporation, France; and reused pallets that were used in this study varied from an interval period of 1–28 weeks after the first negative interpretation. Both new and reused Pronto Dry® kits were stored at room temperature (20–25 °C). There was no special precaution taken prior to using a new Pronto Dry® kit, however for a reused Pronto Dry® kit (i.e. no colour change at 1 h after the first use), the date of first use was noted prior to applying the second specimen adjacent to the previous tissue biopsy sample. The test kits were read at 1, 10, 15, and 30 min, then 1, 12 and 24 h, with the time taken for a positive result for each test kit recorded.

Reused CLOtest® kits

The reused CLOtest® in this study was manufactured by Ballard Medical Products, Utah, USA. A reused CLOtest® was one that had been used once previously but with a negative result after 24 h. The time interval between initial use and reuse of the pallets ranged from 1 to 24 weeks. These kits were stored in the refrigerator at 5 °C whilst awaiting reuse. The label for a reused kit was lifted far enough to expose the yellow gel to room temperature before second usage. For quicker test results, we allowed the gel to reach room temperature between 7 and 10 min prior to inserting the new biopsy specimen.

Data and statistical analysis

Sample size was calculated based on sensitivity and specificity of reused CLOtest® kits in a study by Lee et al. [10]. For a study power of 80 % and α of 0.05, 369 subjects were needed. Another 10 % was added to account for possible attrition, giving a final number of 410 subjects. The Statistical Package for Social Sciences Ver. 18 (SPSS Inc., Chicago, Illinois, USA), as well as OpenEpi Ver. 2.3 [15] was used for data entry and statistical analysis. Categorical variables were expressed as frequency with percentage and continuous data as mean with standard deviation (SD). For comparison purposes, *H. pylori* was considered present if either the new Pronto Dry® test or histology was positive and thus regarded as the 'standard test' in the current study. Performance of reused rapid urease tests vs. standard tests was assessed for sensitivity, specificity, positive predictive value (PPV), negative predictive value (NPV), accuracy and likelihood ratio (LR) at 95 % confidence intervals (CIs). Concordance between reused vs. new tests was assessed using the Kappa agreement test. A *P* value ≤ 0.05 was considered clinically significant.

Results

A total of 410 participants who presented between March 2008 and June 2010 for upper GI endoscopic assessment were recruited into this study. There were 236 male and 174 female participants (57.6 and 42.4 % respectively), with a mean age of 54.1 ± 15.4 years. The majority of participants who underwent upper endoscopy was for investigation of recurrent dyspepsia (n = 205, 41.2 %), whilst 133 (32.4 %) underwent an endoscopic reassessment due to a previous episode of upper GI tract bleed. Upon histological examination, 244 (59.5 %) participants were reported to have chronic gastritis, 124 (30.2 %) with gastric ulcers, 121 (29.5 %) with duodenal ulcers and 119 (29 %) had erosive oesophagitis. Other findings included gastroduodenitis, uraemic gastropathy and oesophageal varices with one case of gastric carcinoma. The overall prevalence of $H.$ $pylori$ infection was low i.e. 17.8 % (73/410) based on either a positive new Pronto Dry® test kit (68/73) or histology (73/73).

Diagnostic accuracy of reused Pronto Dry® test

For reused Pronto Dry® test vs. standard test, 53 tested positive and 333 were negative. Thus the concordance rate of reused Pronto Dry® tests was 94 % (n = 386) with the remaining 24 (5.8 %) having discrepant results. The discrepant results were observed in 20 reused Pronto Dry® negative pallets (i.e. false negatives) and four in reused Pronto Dry® positive pallets (i.e. false positives). Therefore, the sensitivity and specificity of the reused Pronto Dry® test kits were 72.60 % (95 % CI 61.44 – 81.51) and 98.81 % (95 % CI 96.99 – 99.54). The PPV was 92.98 % (95 % CI 83.30 – 97.24) and NPV was 94.33 % (95 % CI 91.41 – 96.30) with a diagnostic accuracy of 94.15 % (95 % CI 91.44 – 96.04) (Table 1). While the LR of a positive reused test is good i.e. 61.17 (95 % CI 36.95 – 101.20), the LR of a negative test is low i.e. 0.27 (95 % CI 0.25 – 0.31). The kappa agreement between reused Pronto Dry® and standard test at 1 h was 0.78 (95 % CI, 0.69 – 0.88). The majority of the reused Pronto Dry® pallets that were positive for $H.$ $pylori$ (88.7 % or n = 47/53) took less than 30 min to change colour, with 11.3 % (n = 6/53)

taking more than 30 min. In less than 30 min, 45 of new and reused Pronto Dry® pallets turned positive compared to 2 of new and reused pallets in 31 – 60 min; this was significantly different (P < 0.001) (Fig. 1).

Diagnostic accuracy of reused CLOtest®

For reused CLOtest® kits, 68 were reported as positive and 335 negative. The concordance rate was 98 % (n = 404) with 6 discrepant results, where 4 were observed in reused CLOtest® negative pallets (i.e. false negatives) and two in reused positive pallets (i.e. false positives). The sensitivity and specificity of reused CLOtest® kits were 93.15 % (95 % CI 84.95 – 97.04) and 99.41 % (95 % CI, 97.86 – 99.84) (Table 1). The PPV was 97.14 % (95 % CI 90.17 – 99.21) and NPV was 98.53 % (95 % CI 96.60 – 99.37) with a diagnostic accuracy of 98.29 % (95 % CI 96.52 – 99.17). The kappa agreement between reused CLOtest® vs. standard test at 24 h was 0.94 (95 % CI, 0.84 – 1.03). Most of the reused CLOtest® pallets took 31–60 min to change colour, indicating presence of $H.$ $pylori$ (44.1 % or 33/68 of the positive samples). For reused CLOtest® and new Pronto Dry® pallets, 17 became positive within 30 min whilst 12 took between 30 and 60 min. This however was not significantly different (P = 0.7) (Fig. 1).

Discussion

Various methods of $H.$ $pylori$ detection, either invasive or non-invasive in nature are available with each of them having different diagnostic accuracies. There have been many studies comparing these detection methods to ensure superiority in terms of diagnostic accuracy and qualitative characteristics between them. Cost however is always an issue to be reflected upon, especially in resource-poor circumstances. As it costs approximately $6 for a new Pronto Dry® or CLOtest® kit, reusing negative kits may bring about substantial cost savings. In fact, VH Chong calculated that at a CLOtest® price of $5.72 per kit a potential cost saving of $2.45 per patient was achievable

Table 1 Sensitivity, specificity, predictive values, diagnostic accuracy and likelihood ratios of reused Pronto Dry® test and reused CLOtest® for $H.$ $pylori$ infection

Parameter	Reused Pronto Dry® % (95 % CI[a])		Reused CLOtest® % (95 % CI[a])	
Sensitivity	72.60 %	(61.44, 81.51)	93.15 %	(84.95, 97.04)
Specificity	98.81 %	(96.99, 99.54)	99.41 %	(97.86, 99.84)
Positive predictive value	92.98 %	(83.30, 97.24)	97.14 %	(90.17, 99.21)
Negative predictive value	94.33 %	(91.41, 96.30)	98.53 %	(96.60, 99.37)
Diagnostic accuracy	94.15 %	(91.44, 96.04)	98.29 %	(96.52, 99.17)
Likelihood ratio of a positive test	61.17	(36.95 – 101.20)	157	(58.78 – 419.1)
Likelihood ratio of a negative test	0.27	(0.25 – 0.31)	0.07	(0.05 – 0.10)
Diagnostic odds	220.60	(72.56 – 670.70)	2278	(432.9 – 11990)
Cohen's kappa (Unweighted)	0.78	(0.69 – 0.88)	0.94	(0.84 – 1.03)

[a]Wilson score interval is used for estimation of 95 % confidence interval (95 % CI)

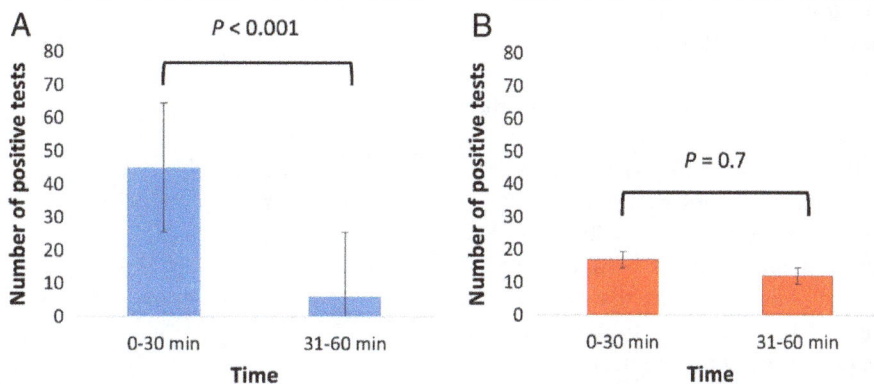

Fig. 1 Colour change time for 0–30 min vs. 31–60 min for reused Pronto Dry® (**a**) and reused CLOtest® (**b**) when paired with the new Pronto Dry® pallets (i.e. true positives), # P value significant if < 0.05

with maximal kit reuse. This translated to an annual cost savings of $2,941/year based on their patient population [13]. Also, based on the fact that unaltered substrate that has not been consumed in a negative rapid urease test may be reused, studies were done to assess the feasibility of re-using CLOtest® pallets. Results were encouraging, proving that these reused pallets had a high diagnostic accuracy with the ability to be used repeatedly over a period of months following an initial negative CLOtest® result. To our knowledge however, there is no published data on the diagnostic accuracy and qualitative characteristics of reused Pronto Dry® kits.

In our cross-sectional study of 410 adults who underwent upper GI endoscopy in a non-emergent setting, we found that the overall prevalence of *H. pylori* infection was low at 17.8 % (73/410). This prevalence was based on the results of using either a new Pronto Dry® kit or a positive histology examination for *H. pylori*, and is slightly higher compared to results quoted by Gurjeet and Naing (prevalence of 13.5 %) [16] but nevertheless reflecting the general prevalence of *H. pylori* infection in the northeastern coast of Peninsular Malaysia [17]. In comparison, based on rapid urease tests a much higher prevalence of *H. pylori* infection (49.0 %) was recorded among dyspeptic Malaysians in highly developed Kuala Lumpur, the capital city of Malaysia [18]. This disparity in *H. pylori* prevalence has been noted before in multiple studies, but despite theories ascribing this to differences in ethnicity and genetics as well as related socioeconomic plus dietary factors, no definite answer has been found [19–22]. An exceptionally low prevalence of *H .pylori* as seen in this population may mean possible wastage (and associated high costs) if an RUT is used for each and every patient during endoscopy. Reusing these tests could therefore be a preferable choice in a low prevalence and low resource setting.

With regards to re-using rapid urease tests, earlier studies have shown that reused CLOtest® kits have similar sensitivity and specificity as compared to new ones

[10, 12]. Our results support the validity of reusing CLO tests. On the other hand, reused Pronto Dry® had demonstrated a relatively lower sensitivity (72.60 %) in the detection of *H. pylori*, but specificity remained high at 98.81 %, with a diagnostic accuracy of 94.15 %. Several factors or limitations were identified that could have explained this difference in sensitivity for reused Pronto Dry® test. For instance, the time interval from initial use to re-use of the Pronto Dry® kit may have been too far apart, ranging from 7 days up to 7 months. Reagents may have deteriorated over this period, resulting in the high number of false negative results seen. At the same time due to the presence of the previous specimen there may be less media left for implantation on to the urea soaked paper of a reused Pronto Dry® test kit, leading to a poor chemical reaction. Alternatively there may be issues in sampling as *H. pylori* does not uniformly colonise the stomach lining causing varying population densities. Recent PPI use may also give a negative result; we however have excluded such patients from our study. Likelihood ratios (LR) may be used to compare between two diagnostic methods, and in our study (as stated in Table 1) there were good LR for positive reused Pronto Dry® and reused CLOtest® kits (61.17 and 157 respectively). As for the reused kits with negative results, LR for reused Pronto Dry® was 0.27 whilst for a reused CLOtest® this was 0.07 indicating that a reused CLOtest® was much better at indicating the absence of *H. pylori*.

Many factors affect the time taken for colour change in RUTs which include the urease testing process itself (warmed vs room temperature), bacterial load, biopsy location (antrum vs body), biopsy size as well as number of specimens [8, 23]. In our study 88 % of the positive reused Pronto Dry® pallets changed colour within 30 min, which was similar in duration to new Pronto Dry® tests. However, this was not the case with reused CLOtest®. Previous studies on the qualitative characteristic of new Pronto Dry® tests have been done [24], which showed that a new Pronto Dry® test offers a quicker diagnosis as compared to a new CLOtest® kit at 30 min with its chromatin grading correlating well with stomach mucosal *H. pylori* colonisation density. Hence we can conclude that the chemical in reused Pronto Dry® kits are still able to maintain their qualitative characteristics similar to a new test kit with regards to colour changing time of up to a seven month period. The same cannot be said for reused CLOtest® kits. Another main difference between reusing CLOtest® vs Pronto Dry® kits is the fact that the former needs to be in refrigerated storage prior to use, and then brought to room temperature prior to inserting the biopsy specimen. Pronto Dry® kits on the other hand have a practical advantage as it can be stored at room temperature and used immediately when needed. It must be cautioned though that a tropical climate might contribute to a more rapid deterioration of used Pronto Dry® and CLOtest® kits, as well as having a higher possibility of fungal growth and contamination.

Conclusion

Our study showed that reused Pronto Dry® test kits have a relatively lower diagnostic accuracy as compared to new Pronto Dry® test kits. Reused CLOtest® kits however were able to maintain its diagnostic accuracy. Plausible explanations or limitations for this study include a prolonged interval between initial use and reuse and a decreased media for specimen implantation. On the other hand, reused Pronto Dry® rather than CLOtest® offer a quicker diagnostic result despite being stored for a prolonged period. Therefore if accuracy is of concern a reused CLOtest® is preferable, alternatively a reused Pronto Dry® test may be a better choice for quick and reliable results.

Competing interests

Elements of this study have been presented as a poster at the Asian Pacific Monothematic Meeting on Helicobacter pylori 2012, 13–15 January 2012, Kuala Lumpur, Malaysia; and published as a conference-related abstract: S Jamaludin, N Mustaffa, NA Che Hamzah, YY Lee. Reused CLOtest® Are Better Than Reused ProntoDry® in Diagnosing Helicobacter pylori Infection. Journal of Gastroenterology and Hepatology. Volume:27, Supp 1, page 14. January 2012.

Authors' contributions

SJ carried out the study and drafted the initial manuscript. NM and NACH assisted in carrying out the study and drafting of the finalised manuscript. SHSAA participated in the design and coordination of the study. YYL conceived of the study, participated in its design and coordination, performed statistical analysis and helped to draft the finalised manuscript. All authors read and approved the final manuscript.

Acknowledgements

The authors wish to thank the subjects who were involved, as well as the staff of the Endoscopy Unit, Hospital Universiti Sains Malaysia for their assistance and contributions.

Author details

[1]School of Medical Sciences, Universiti Sains Malaysia, Kubang Kerian, Kelantan, Malaysia. [2]Pasir Gudang Specialist Hospital, Pasir Gudang, Johor, Malaysia.

References

1. Graham DY, Lew GM, Klein PD, Evans DG, Evans Jr DJ, Saeed ZA, et al. Effect of treatment of Helicobacter pylori infection on the long-term recurrence of gastric or duodenal ulcer. A randomized, controlled study. Ann Intern Med. 1992;116(9):705–8.
2. Marshall BJ, McGechie DB, Rogers PA, Glancy RJ. Pyloric Campylobacter infection and gastroduodenal disease. Med J Aust. 1985;142(8):439–44.
3. Parsonnet J, Hansen S, Rodriguez L, Gelb AB, Warnke RA, Jellum E, et al. Helicobacter pylori infection and gastric lymphoma. N Engl J Med. 1994;330(18):1267–71.
4. Yakoob J, Abid S, Jafri W, Abbas Z, Islam M, Ahmad Z. Comparison of biopsy-based methods for the detection of Helicobacter pylori infection. Br J Biomed Sci. 2006;63(4):159–62.
5. van Keeken N, van Hattum E, de Boer WA. Validation of a new, commercially available dry rapid urease test for the diagnosis of Helicobacter pylori infection in gastric biopsies. Neth J Med. 2006;64(9):329–33.
6. Chomvarin C, Kulsuntiwong P, Mairiang P, Sangchan A, Kulabkhow C, Chau-in S, et al. Detection of H. pylori in dyspeptic patients and correlation with clinical outcomes. Southeast Asian J Trop Med Public Health. 2005;36(4):917–22.
7. Said RM, Cheah PL, Chin SC, Goh KL. Evaluation of a new biopsy urease test: Pronto Dry, for the diagnosis of Helicobacter pylori infection. Eur J Gastroenterol Hepatol. 2004;16(2):195–9.
8. Laine L, Lewin D, Naritoku W, Estrada R, Cohen H. Prospective comparison of commercially available rapid urease tests for the diagnosis of Helicobacter pylori. Gastrointest Endosc. 1996;44(5):523–6.
9. Yousfi MM, el-Zimaity HM, Genta RM, Graham DY. Evaluation of a new reagent strip rapid urease test for detection of Helicobacter pylori infection. Gastrointest Endosc. 1996;44(5):519–22.
10. Lee CL, Tu TC, Dai YC, Wu CH, Chen TK, Ma VL, et al. Negative CLOtest pellet can be reused. Gastrointest Endosc. 1999;50(2):225–8.
11. Liu CC, Lee CL, Wu CH, Chen TK, Lai YC, Tu TC, et al. The optimal interval for the usage of reuse CLO test. Gastroenterol J Taiwan. 2000;17:73.
12. Tomtitchong P. Effectively Reusable CloTest. J Gastroenterol Hepatol. 1999;14:S67–80.
13. Chong VH, Jamaludin AZ, Jacob AP, Jalihal A. Feasibility of reusing negative rapid urease test (CLOtest) kit. Indian J Gastroenterol. 2007;26(2):99–100.
14. Elitsur Y, Neace C, Heitlinger L. Reuse of negative CLOtest kits in children. Gastrointest Endosc. 2001;53(2):169–71.
15. OpenEpi. Open Source Epidemiologic Statistics for Public Health, Version 2.3.1. [http://www.openepi.com/Menu/OE_Menu.htm]
16. Gurjeet K, Naing NN. Prevalence and ethnic distributionof Helicobacter pylori infection in North Eastern Peninsular Malaysia. Malays J Med Sci. 2003;10(2):68–72.
17. Lee YY, Mahendra Raj S, Graham DY. Helicobacter pylori infection—a boon or a bane: lessons from studies in a low-prevalence population. Helicobacter. 2013;18(5):338–46.
18. Goh KL. Prevalence of and risk factors for Helicobacter pylori infection in a multi-racial dyspeptic Malaysian population undergoing endoscopy. J Gastroenterol Hepatol. 1997;12(6):S29–35.
19. Rahim AA, Lee YY, Majid NA, Choo KE, Raj SM, Derakhshan MH, et al. Helicobacter pylori infection among Aborigines (the Orang Asli) in the northeastern region of Peninsular Malaysia. Am J Trop Med Hyg. 2010;83(5):1119–22.
20. Lee YY, Ismail AW, Mustaffa N, Musa KI, Majid NA, Choo KE, et al. Sociocultural and dietary practices among Malay subjects in the north-eastern region of Peninsular Malaysia: a region of low prevalence of Helicobacter pylori infection. Helicobacter. 2012;17(1):54–61.
21. Maran S, Lee YY, Xu SH, Raj MS, Abdul Majid N, Choo KE, et al. Towards understanding the low prevalence of Helicobacter pylori in Malays: genetic

variants among Helicobacter pylori-negative ethnic Malays in the north-eastern region of Peninsular Malaysia and Han Chinese and South Indians. J Dig Dis. 2013;14(4):196–202.

22. Maran S, Lee YY, Xu S, Rajab NS, Hasan N, Mustaffa N, et al. Deleted in Colorectal Cancer (DCC) gene polymorphism is associated with H. pylori infection among susceptible Malays from the north-eastern region of Peninsular Malaysia. Hepatogastroenterology. 2013;60(121):124–8.

23. El-Zimaity HM, Ota H, Scott S, Killen DE, Graham DY. A new triple stain for Helicobacter pylori suitable for the autostainer: carbol fuchsin/Alcian blue/hematoxylin-eosin. Arch Pathol Lab Med. 1998;122(8):732–6.

24. Tseng CA, Wang WM, Wu DC. Comparison of the clinical feasibility of three rapid urease tests in the diagnosis of Helicobacter pylori infection. Dig Dis Sci. 2005;50(3):449–52.

7

The distribution of *jhp0940, jhp0945, jhp0947, jhp0949* and *jhp0951* genes of *Helicobacter pylori* in China

Yanan Gong[1,2], Xianhui Peng[1,2], Lihua He[1,2], Hao Liang[1,2], Yuanhai You[1,2] and Jianzhong Zhang[1,2*]

Abstract

Background: The plasticity region of *Helicobacter pylori* (*H. pylori*) is a large chromosomal segment containing strain-specific genes. The prevalence of the plasticity region genes of the *H. pylori* strains in China remains unknown. The aim of this study was to examine the status of these genes and to assess the relationship between the genes and the diseases caused by *H. pylori* infection.

Methods: A total of 141 strains were isolated from patients with chronic active gastritis (CAG), peptic ulcer disease (PUD) and gastric carcinoma (GC). The prevalence of *jhp0940, jhp0945, jhp0947, jhp0949* and *jhp0951* was determined using PCR, and the results were analyzed using the chi-squared test.

Results: The prevalence rates of *jhp0940, jhp0945, jhp0947, jhp0949* and *jhp0951* in the *H. pylori* strains were 42.55, 51.06, 20.57, 56.03 and 63.12 %, respectively. The prevalence rates of *jhp0940* were similar in the isolates from the CAG, PUD and GC patients, and there was no association between the *jhp0940* status and any of the diseases. In contrast, the prevalence rates of *jhp0945, jhp0947, jhp0949* and *jhp0951* were significantly higher in the PUD and GC isolates than in the CAG isolates ($p < 0.01$). A univariate analysis showed that *jhp0945, jhp0947, jhp0949* and *jhp0951* increased the risk of PUD, while only *jhp0951* was significantly associated with PUD in the multivariate analysis ($p = 0.0149$). The *jhp0945*-positive isolates were significantly associated with an increased risk for GC ($p = 0.0097$).

Conclusion: The plasticity region genes are widely distributed in Chinese patients, and a high prevalence of these genes occurs in more serious diseases. Therefore, *jhp0951* status is an independent factor associated with the development of PUD, and *jhp0945* may predict the future development of GC in patients with CAG and is considered to be the best candidate disease marker for *H. pylori*-related diseases.

Background

H. pylori is the major cause of chronic gastritis, peptic ulcer disease, gastric carcinoma and mucosa-associated lymphoid tissue lymphoma [1, 2]. The majority of infected individuals remain asymptomatic throughout their lifetime, and only approximately 15 % develop gastroduodenal diseases. Variations in the clinical outcomes of these diseases have been attributed to differences in environmental factors, bacterial strains and host genetics [3, 4]. A number of bacterial virulence factors that are

* Correspondence: zhangjianzhong@icdc.cn
[1]State Key Laboratory of Infectious Disease Prevention and Control, National Institute for Communicable Disease Control and Prevention, Chinese Center for Disease Control and Prevention, 155 Changbai Road, Changping District, Beijing 102206, China
[2]Collaborative Innovation Center for Diagnosis and Treatment of Infectious Diseases, Hangzhou, China

associated with these diseases have been described for *H. pylori*, such as the *cag* pathogenicity island (*cag* PAI) [5, 6].

A comparison of the genomes of two *H. pylori* strains revealed that in addition to the *cag* PAI, a large region of approximately 45 kb in strain J99 and 68 kb in strain 26695 is present in both strains and has been termed the "plasticity region" [7, 8]. Up to 50 % of the strain-specific genes transferred from other species are located in the plasticity region [9]. Whether these strain-specific genes influence the severity of different diseases or the biological functions of the ORFs in the plasticity region still remains unknown. Recent studies have revealed that the *jhp0940, jhp0945, jhp0947, jhp0949* and *jhp0951* genes from *H. pylori* are associated with an increased risk for gastroduodenal diseases [3, 9–11]. In a Brazilian study, the *jhp0947* gene was found to be involved in the development of duodenal ulcers (DUs) and GC [11]. In addition, Romo-González et al. found that *jhp0951* is also associated with DUs [9]. In China, the number of *H. pylori* infections has exceeded 60 %, and the high-risk incidence of GC poses a serious health and economic burden. Moreover, there are no reports discussing the prevalence of these genes or the relationship between the genes and the severity of the clinical outcomes of the abovementioned diseases in China. The aim of this study was to assess the prevalence of *jhp0940*, *jhp0945*, *jhp0947*, *jhp0949* and *jhp0951* and to determine their association with *H. pylori*-related diseases.

Methods
Strains
A total of 141 *H. pylori* strains were selected from the *H. pylori* strain bank of China at the National Institute for Communicable Disease Control and Prevention, Chinese Center for Disease Control and Prevention. A total of 40 strains were isolated from patients in Heilongjiang (HLJ) Province (located in northern China), and another 101 strains were isolated from patients from Jiangxi (JX) Province (located in southeast China). These strains were related with CAG only ($n = 58$), PUD ($n = 45$) or GC ($n = 38$). Two strains with fully sequenced genomes, including strain 26695, which was isolated from a gastritis patient, and strain J99, which was isolated from a patient with a duodenal ulcer, were used as controls. This study was approved by the Ethics Committee of National Institute for Communicable Disease Control and Prevention, Chinese Center for Disease Control and Prevention. The written informed consent was obtained from all patients.

Culture and extraction of genomic DNA
The strains stored in brain heart infusion in −80 °C were recovered on Columbia agar plates (Oxoid) supplemented with 5 % fresh defibrinated sheep blood and kept under microaerophilic conditions (5 % O2, 10 % CO2 and 85 % N2) at 37 °C for 3 days. Colonies displaying typical *H. pylori* morphology were selected and identified by Gram staining and urease, oxidase, and catalase activity testing. The bacterial cells on chocolate agar plate were washed twice with phosphate buffer saline (PBS, pH7.5) and centrifuged at 5000 rpm for 10 min. The chromosomal DNA was extracted using the QIAamp DNA Mini Kit (Qiagen, Germany) according to the manufacturer's instructions.

Determination of the *jhp0940*, *jhp0945*, *jhp0947*, *jhp0949* and *jhp0951* status via PCR
The status of the genes was determined via PCR using the primer pairs shown in Table 1. The amplification of

Table 1 The primer sequences for the five genes

Primer name	Primer sequence (5'-3')	Product size	Reference
jhp0940-1	F5'-GAAATGTCCTATACCAATGG R5'-CCTAAGTAGTGCATCAAGG	591 bp	[3]
jhp0940-2	F5'-ATGCCAACCATTGATTTTACTTTT R5'-TTATCGTCTACGCTTAGGTGTG	978 bp	[12]
jhp0945	F5'-CAATGCGACTAACAGCATAG R5'-CGCATTTGCTGTCATCTTTG	1028 bp	[3]
jhp0947	F5'-GATAATCCTACGCAGAACG R5'-GCTAAAGTCATTTGGCTGTC	611 bp	[3]
jhp0949	F5'-TTCAAAAAGTCCCCGAAATG R5'-GGATGTCCTGGCATGTCTCT	235 bp	[10]
jhp0951	F5'-ATGCGTGGCTAAGCGATACT R5'-GACCCAACGCTCTTGAAGTT	243 bp	[19]

The primer sequences used for the five genes were the same as the references. There were two pairs of primers used for *jhp0940*
F, forward primer sequence; R, reverse primer sequence

the genes was performed in a volume of 25 µl containing 25 pmol of both forward and reverse primers. The PCR conditions were 95 °C for 5 min, followed by 35 cycles of 95 °C for 45 s, 52 °C for 45 s, and 72 °C for 45 s, and finally 72 °C for 5 min. Two primer sets were used for the *jhp0940* gene, and when the PCR using one pair was positive, the *jhp0940* status was determined to be positive. The status of the genes was positive in strain J99 and negative in strain 26695.

Statistical analysis
The prevalence rates of all five genes were evaluated. The association between each genotype and the clinical outcomes were quantified using the chi-squared test. A probability (p) value equal to or less than 0.05 was considered to be statistically significant, and a value of 0.001 or less was considered to be highly significant. Univariate analysis and a multivariate logistic regression model were used to calculate the odds ratios (ORs) of the clinical outcomes using SAS 9.3.

Results
Distribution of the *jhp0940*, *jhp0945*, *jhp0947*, *jhp0949* and *jhp0951* genes
The prevalence rates of *jhp0940*, *jhp0945*, *jhp0947*, *jhp0949* and *jhp0951* in the tested *H. pylori* were 42.55 % (60/141), 51.06 % (72/141), 20.57 % (29/141), 56.03 % (79/141) and 63.12 % (89/141), respectively (Table 2).

Geographic variation of plasticity region genes
The results were divided into two groups based on their geographic variation. By comparing the results of the strains from HLJ Province and JX Province, we

Table 2 The prevalence of the five genes in the CAG, PUD and GC isolates

Gene	No[a] (%) found			
	CAG[b]	PUD[c]	GC[d]	Total[e]
	HLJ (n = 20)	HLJ (n = 9)	HLJ (n = 11)	
	JX (n = 38)	JX (n = 36)	JX (n = 27)	
HLJ[f] *jhp0940* 6 (30 %)		3 (33.33 %)	7 (63.64 %)	16 (40 %)
n = 40				
jhp0945 5 (25 %)		4 (44.44 %)	8 (72.73 %)	17 (42.5 %)
jhp0947 2 (10 %)		0	2 (18.18 %)	4 (10 %)
jhp0949 8 (40 %)		7 (77.78 %)	6 (54.55 %)	21 (52.5 %)
jhp0951 11 (55 %)		6 (66.67 %)	6 (54.55 %)	23 (57.5 %)
JX[g] *jhp0940* 14 (36.84 %)		19 (52.78 %)	11 (40.74 %)	44 (43.56 %)
n = 101				
jhp0945 11 (28.95 %)		24 (66.67 %)	20 (74.07 %)	55 (54.46 %)
jhp0947 2 (5.26 %)		15 (41.67 %)	8 (29.63 %)	25 (24.75 %)
jhp0949 15 (39.47 %)		24 (66.67 %)	19 (70.37 %)	58 (57.43 %)
jhp0951 20 (52.63 %)		29 (80.56 %)	17 (62.96 %)	66 (65.35 %)

The positive rates of each gene in the CAG, PUD and GC patients from HLJ and JX Provinces
[a] *No* the number of positive isolates
[b] *CAG* chronic active gastritis
[c] *PUD* peptic ulcer disease
[d] *GC* gastric carcinoma
[e] *Total* the total positive rate of each gene
[f] *HL* Heilongjiang Province, China
[g] *JX* Jiangxi Province, China

found no significant differences in the prevalence of *jhp0940* (40 %, 16/40 and 43.56 %, 44/101, respectively, $p = 0.699$), *jhp0945* (42.5 %, 17/40 and 54.46 %, 55/101, $p = 0.201$), *jhp0947* (10 %, 4/40 and 24.75 %, 25/101, $p = 0.051$), *jhp0949* (52.5 %, 21/40 and 57.43 %, 58/101, $p = 0.595$), or *jhp0951* (57.5 %, 23/40 and 65.35 %, 66/101, $p = 0.384$).

Plasticity region genes and diseases
The prevalence rates of *jhp0940* in the strains from the CAG, PUD and GC patients were 34.48 % (20/58), 48.89 % (22/45) and 47.37 % (18/38), respectively, and there were no differences between the three diseases. The prevalence rates of *jhp0945* in the isolates from the patients with PUD (62.22 %, 28/45) and GC (73.68 %, 28/38) were significantly higher than from the CAG patients (27.59 %, 16/58; $p = 0.0004$ and $p < 0.0001$, respectively). The *jhp0947* gene occurred in only 4 (6.89 %) of the strains isolated from the CAG patients, and the occurrence was much lower than in the PUD and GC patients (33.33 %, 15/45 and 26.32 %, 10/38; $p = 0.0006$ and $p = 0.0084$, respectively). The prevalence of *jhp0949* was similar (68.89 %, 31/45 and 65.79 %, 25/38) in the PUD and GC isolates and was much higher than that in the CAG patients (39.66 %, 23/58; $p = 0.0032$ and $p = 0.0123$, respectively). For *jhp0951*, the prevalence rate in the PUD patients was

higher than that in the CAG patients (77.78 %, 35/45 and 53.45 %, 31/58, respectively; $p = 0.0107$); however, there was no difference between GC and CAG.

The relationship between *jhp0940*, *jhp0945*, *jhp0947*, *jhp0949* and *jhp0951*
The status of all of the genes showed that they are significantly associated with each other (Table 3). The status of *jhp0945* was associated with *jhp0949* ($p = 0.009$) and *jhp0951* ($p = 0.022$). All of the *jhp0947*-positive isolates possessed *jhp0949*, and both were significantly associated with *jhp0951* ($p = 0.0008$ and $p < 0.0001$, respectively).

When combining the five genes together, the majority of the genotypes were all negative or all positive (the −/−/−/−/− genotype or the +/+/+/+/+ genotype, 12.06 %, 17/141). The rates of the all-positive genotypes were 15.79 % (6/38), 20 % (9/45) and 3.45 % (2/58) in the isolates from the patients with GC, PUD and CAG only, respectively. In contrast, the rates of the all-negative genotypes were 5.26 % (2/38), 2.22 % (1/45) and 24.14 % (14/58) for GC, PUD, and CAG, respectively.

The relationship between the gene status and the clinical outcomes
A univariate analysis showed that there was no significant association between the *jhp0940* status and the selected diseases (Table 4), but the status of *jhp0945*, *jhp0947*, *jhp0949* and *jhp0951* was significantly associated with a lower risk for CAG (odds ratio (OR), [95 % confidence interval (CI)], 0.176 [0.081 to 0.381]; 0.116 [0.035 to 0.389]; 0.300 [0.145 to 0.623] and 0.445 [0.214 to 0.928], respectively). On the converse, they were also related to an increased risk for PUD (OR [95 % CI], 2.306 [1.08 to 4.927]; 2.835 [1.191 to 6.751]; 2.452 [1.126 to 5.336] and 2.825 [1.226 to 6.51], respectively). Moreover, only the *jhp0945*-positive isolates were associated with an increased risk for GC (OR, 5.9259; 95 % CI, 1.267 to 27.714).

A multivariate analysis, including age and *jhp0940*, *jhp0945*, *jhp0947*, *jhp0949* and *jhp0951* status, was performed to determine the factors that were related to the

Table 3 The relationship between the different plasticity region genes

gene	Relationship (coefficient value[a]/p value)			
	jhp0945	*jhp0947*	*jhp0949*	*jhp0951*
jhp0940	0.183/0.03	0.236/0.005	0.184/0.029	0.182/0.031
jhp0945	—	0.358/<0.0001	0.219/0.009	0.193/0.022
jhp0947	—	—	0.415/<0.0001	0.280/0.0008
jhp0949	—	—	—	0.478/<0.0001

The coefficient value for assessing the association between each pair of genes. A *p* value of 0.001 or less was considered to be highly significant
The coefficient value[a] was analyzed using Fisher's test

Table 4 The relationship between each gene and the clinical outcomes

gene	ORd	CAGa 95 % CIe	p	OR	PUDb 95 % CI	p	GCc OR	95 % CI	p
jhp0940	0.488	0.235–1.013	0.054	1.449	0.694–3.026	0.323	1.822	0.734–4.523	0.196
jhp0945	0.176	0.081–0.381	<0.0001	2.306	1.08–4.927	0.031	3.542	1.362–9.209	0.009
jhp0947	0.116	0.035–0.389	0.0005	2.835	1.191–6.751	0.019	2.307	0.765–6.952	0.134
jhp0949	0.300	0.145–0.623	0.0012	2.452	1.126–5.336	0.024	2.067	0.812–5.26	0.128
jhp0951	0.445	0.214–0.928	0.031	2.825	1.226–6.51	0.015	1.008	0.403–2.517	0.987

The univariate analysis showing the association between each gene status and the indicated disease
[a]CAG chronic active gastritis
[b]PUD peptic ulcer disease
[c]GC gastric carcinoma
[d]OR odds ratio
[e]CI confidence interval

clinical outcomes of the selected diseases (Table 5). The *jhp0945* status for GC and the *jhp0951* status for PUD significantly increased the risk of a clinical outcome. In contrast, the *jhp0945* or *jhp0949* status significantly decreased the risk for CAG (OR [95 % CI]: 0.214 [0.099 to 0.466]; 0.373 [0.172 to 0.807], respectively). Age significantly decreased the risk of CAG and PUD (OR [95 % CI]: 0.964 [0.937 to 0.992]; 0.963 [0.937 to 0.991], respectively), while it increased the risk for GC (1.098 [1.059 to 1.139]).

Discussion

The plasticity region is a recently identified locus found in the chromosome of *H. pylori* strains J99 and 26695 that displays similar characterics to pathogenicity islands [7, 8]. The majority of the *H. pylori* strain-specific genes that are transferred from other species are located in the plasticity region [9, 12, 13]. The genes present in the plasticity region have been highlighted as potential pathogenic markers and may account for the differences in the *H. pylori* strain virulence, resulting in various clinical outcomes.

The *jhp0940, jhp0945, jhp0947, jhp0949* and *jhp0951* genes, which are specific for strain J99, have recently

Table 5 A multivariate analysis of the risk for CAG, PUD and GC based on age and the status of all five genes

Disease	Parameter	ORd	95 % CIe	p value
CAGa	jhp0945	0.214	0.099–0.466	0.0001
	jhp0949	0.373	0.172–0.807	0.0123
	age	0.964	0.937–0.992	0.0111
PUDb	jhp0951	2.821	1.224–6.499	0.0149
	age	0.963	0.937–0.991	0.0089
GCc	jhp0945	3.460	1.351–8.865	0.0097
	age	1.098	1.059–1.139	<0.0001

[a]CAG chronic active gastritis
[b]PUD peptic ulcer disease
[c]GC gastric carcinoma
[d]OR odds ratio
[e]CI confidence interval

been reported to be associated with *H. pylori*-related diseases and are potential markers for the risk of gastrointestinal diseases [10]. Because of their geographic variation, the relationship between these genes and the severity of certain diseases has been discussed, but the results are often not in agreement. The prevalence of these genes and their relationship with certain diseases in China is currently unknown; therefore, we examined the distribution of these virulence markers and their relationship to the clinical outcomes of patients infected with *H. pylori*.

Previous study found that there were no significant associations between the gastroduodenal diseases and the status of *jhp0940, jhp0945* and *jhp0949* in East Asia strains [10]. Yakoob *et al.* demonstrated that *jhp0940* and *jhp0947* in Pakistan strains were associated with GC and PUD [14]. In our study, there was no association between *jhp0940* and diseases. The positive rates of *jhp0945, jhp0947, jhp0949* and *jhp0951* were much higher in PUD, and there was a significant association between the genes. However, the multivariate analysis showed that only *jhp0951* was independently associated with the development of PUD in our study. *Jhp0951*, which encodes an integrase from the XerCD family, is involved in the response to acidic environments [15]. In DUs, acid secretion increases, causing the mucosa to be continuously exposed to a low pH, which is consistent with our results [9]. As the virulence genes were associated with each other in our study, the strong linkage of *jhp0945, jhp0947* and *jhp0949* with PUD may be due to the significant association between *jhp0951* and PUD. We also speculate that all of these factors act synergistically in causing damage to the host.

It is well known that the development of GC is marked by a slow progression that begins with *H. pylori*-induced chronic superficial gastritis, which then progresses to atrophic gastritis, intestinal metaplasia, dysplasia and eventually GC [16, 17]. In our study, the multivariate analysis showed that the only independent virulence gene that increased the risk of GC was *jhp0945*, indicating a significant association between the two. However, the *jhp0945* status showed a negative association with CAG (Table 5), which conflicts with the process of GC development. In our study, we speculate that the majority of the individuals with CAG do not carry the *jhp0945* gene, while the few *jhp0945*-positive individuals potentially develop GC due to a combination of the bacteria, the host and other environmental factors, which is consistent with the fact that of the *H. pylori*-infected individuals, 80–90 % have clinically asymptomatic gastritis, while only 1–2 % develop GC [18]. *Jhp0945*-positive isolates may be more likely to develop severe diseases, and *jhp0945* status may be a risk indicator for GC development. Additional prospective studies are still necessary to further confirm our speculations.

Conclusions

In conclusion, this was the first study in China to evaluate the relationship between plasticity region genes and clinical disease outcomes. We found that *jhp0951* status is an independent factor for discriminating PUD and may influence the association of other virulence factors with certain diseases. *Jhp0945* may predict the future development of GC in patients with CAG and is considered to be the best candidate disease marker for *H. pylori*-related diseases.

Abbreviations

H. pylori: Helicobacter pylori; CAG: Chronic active gastritis; PUD: Peptic ulcer disease; GC: Gastric carcinoma; HLJ: Heilongjiang; JX: Jiangxi; OR: Odds ratio; CI: Confidence interval.

Competing interests

The authors declare that they have no competing interests.

Authors' contributions

ZJZ designed the research. GYN performed the study and wrote the paper. PXH and LH analyzed the results. HLH and YYH participated in strains recovery. All authors read and approved the final manuscript.

Acknowledgments

This study was supported by the Grant from National Technology R & D Program in the 12th Five-Year Plan of China (No. 2012BAI06B02), the Major Technology Project as part of "Prevention and Control of Major Infectious Diseases including AIDS and Viral Hepatitis" (No. 2013ZX10004216-002) and the grant from National Key Scientific Instrument and Equipment Development Project (No. 2012YQ180117).
We would like to thank all of the participants from the Department of Diagnosis for Communicable Diseases, the National Institute for Communicable Disease Control and Prevention, and the Chinese Center for Disease Control and Prevention.

References

1. Parsonnet J, Friedman GD, Vandersteen DP, Chang Y, Volgeman JH, Orentreich N, et al. *Helicobacter pylori* infection and the risk of gastric carcinoma. N Engl J Med. 1991;325:1127–31.
2. Uemura N, Okamoto S, Yamamoto S, Matsumura N, Yamaguchi S, Yamakido M, et al. *Helicobacter pylori* infection and the development of gastric cancer. N Engl J Med. 2001;345:784–9.
3. Occhialini A, Marais A, Richard A, Garcia F, Sierra R, Mégraud F. Distribution of Open Reading Frames of Plasticity Region of Strain J99 in *Helicobacter pylori* Strains Isolated from Gastric Carcinoma and Gastritis Patients in Costa Rica. Infect Immun. 2000;68:6240–9.
4. Santos A, Queiroz DM, Ménard A, Marais A, Rocha GA, Oliveira CA, et al. New pathogenicity marker found in the plasticity region of the *Helicobacter pylori* genome. J Clin Microbiol. 2003;41:1651–5.
5. Backert S, Schwarz T, Miehlke S, Kirsch C, Sommer C, Kwok T, et al. Functional analysis of the *cag* pathogenicity island in *Helicobacter pylori* isolates from patients with gastritis, peptic ulcer, and gastric cancer. Infect Immun. 2004;72:1043–56.
6. Yamaoka Y. Mechanisms of disease: *Helicobacter pylori* virulence factors. Nat Rev Gastroenterol Hepatol. 2000;7:629–41.
7. Alm RA, Ling LS, Moir DT, King BL, Brown ED, Doig PC, et al. Genomic-sequence comparison of two unrelated isolates of the human gastric pathogen *Helicobacter pylori*. Nature. 1999;397:176–80.
8. Doig P, de Jonge BL, Alm RA, Brown ED, Uria-Nickelsen M, Noonan B, et al. *Helicobacter pylori* physiology predicted from genomic comparison of two strains. Microbiol Mol Biol Rev. 1999;63:675–707.
9. Romo-González C, Salama NR, Burgeño-Ferreira J, Ponce-Castañeda V, Lazcano-Ponce E, Camorlinga-Ponce M, et al. Differences in genome content among *Helicobacter pylori* isolates from patients with gastritis, duodenal ulcer, or gastric cancer reveal novel disease-associated genes. Infect Immun. 2009;77:2201–11.
10. Sugimoto M, Watada M, Jung SW, Graham DY, Yamaoka Y. Role of *Helicobacter pylori* Plasticity Region Genes in development of Gastroduodenal Diseases. J Clin Microbiol. 2012;50:441–8.
11. Proença Módena JL, Lopes Sales AI, Olszanski Acrani G, Russo R, Vilela Ribeiro MA, Fukuhara Y, et al. Association between *Helicobacter pylori* genotypes and gastric disorders in relation to the cag pathogenicity island. Diagn Microbiol Infect Dis. 2007;59:7–16.
12. Rizwan M, Alvi A, Ahmed N. Novel protein antigen (JHP940) from the genomic plasticity region of *Helicobacter pylori* induces tumor necrosis factor alpha and interleukin-8 secretion by human macrophages. J Bacteriol. 2008;190:1146–51.
13. de Jonge R, Kuipers EJ, Langeveld SC, Loffeld RJ, Stoof J, van Vliet AH, et al. The *Helicobacter pylori* plasticity region locus *jhp0947-jhp0949* is associated with duodenal ulcer disease and interleukin-12 production in monocyte cells. FEMS Immunol Med Microbiol. 2004;41:161–7.
14. Yakoob J, Abbas Z, Nas S, Islam M, Abid S, Jafri W. Associations between the plasticity region genes of *Helicobacter pylori* and gastroduodenal diseases in a high-prevalence area. Gut and Liver. 2010;4:345–50.
15. Gancz H, Censini S, Merrell DS. Iron and pH homeostasis intersect at the level of Fur regulation in the gastric pathogen *Helicobacter pylori*. Infect Immun. 2006;74:602–14.
16. Conteduca V, Sansonno D, Lauletta G, Russi S, Ingravallo G, Dammacco F. *H. pylori* infection and gastric cancer: State of the art. Int J Oncol. 2013;42:5–18.
17. Matysiak-Budnik T, Mégraud F. *Helicobacter pylori* infection and gastric cancer. Eur J Cancer. 2006;42:708–16.
18. Wu MS, Chow LP, Lin JT, Chiou SH. Proteomic identification of biomarkers related to *Helicobacter pylori*-associated gastroduodenal disease: Challenges and opportunities. J Gastroenterol Hepatol. 2008;23:1657–61.
19. Watada M, Shiota S, Matsunari O, Suzuki R, Murakami K, Fujioka T, et al. Association between *Helicobacter pylori* cagA-related genes and clinical outcomes in Colombia and Japan. BMC Gastroenterol. 2011;11:141–8.

8

Gastric cancer diagnosed after *Helicobacter pylori* eradication in diabetes mellitus patients

Kosuke Sakitani[1,2*], Yoshihiro Hirata[2], Nobumi Suzuki[1], Satoki Shichijo[2], Ayako Yanai[1], Takako Serizawa[2], Kei Sakamoto[1], Masao Akanuma[1], Shin Maeda[3], Yutaka Yamaji[2], Yasuhiko Iwamoto[1], Shoji Kawazu[1] and Kazuhiko Koike[2]

Abstract

Background: *Helicobacter pylori* infection is the most important risk factor for gastric cancer, for which eradication therapy is commonly performed. However, gastric cancer is sometimes discovered after successful eradication of *H. pylori*. Much evidence indicates that diabetes mellitus (DM) is a risk factor for gastric cancer. The incidence and characteristics of gastric cancer diagnosed after *H. pylori* eradication in DM patients remain to be determined.

Methods: We followed the clinical course of patients who underwent *H. pylori* eradication therapy at our institution. Endoscopy was performed before and after eradication. We compared the incidence and clinical characteristics of gastric cancer arising in DM and non-DM patients.

Results: In total, 965 patients who underwent successful eradication (518 DM and 447 non-DM patients) were followed-up for an average of 4.5 years. During the follow-up period, 21 gastric cancers were diagnosed (12 in DM patients and 9 in non-DM patients). The incidence of gastric cancer after eradication was not significantly different between DM and non-DM patients (0.485 and 0.482 %/year, respectively). There was no significant difference in the pathology, diameter, depth, location, or treatment of gastric cancer between patients with and without DM.

Conclusion: The incidence and characteristics of gastric cancer occurring after *H. pylori* eradication were comparable between DM and non-DM patients.

Keywords: Gastric cancer, *Helicobacter pylori* eradication, Diabetes mellitus

Background

Gastric cancer is a major cause of cancer death worldwide. Infection with *Helicobacter pylori* (*H. pylori*), first isolated by Warren and Marshall [1], together with the subsequent changes in the gastric mucosa, is the most important risk factor for gastric cancer [2–5]. Previous reports have suggested that *H. pylori* eradication reduces the incidence of gastric cancer [6–8]. Therefore, eradication therapy is now commonly performed. However, gastric cancer is occasionally discovered after successful *H. pylori* eradication, and investigations of the risk factors for, and characteristics of, gastric cancer after eradication have been conducted [9, 10].

The infection–inflammation–cancer axis is widely accepted, based in part on epidemiological and basic investigations of *H. pylori* [11]. On the other hand, evidence is accumulating that diseases associated with adult lifestyle factors—*e.g.*, diabetes mellitus (DM)—enhance the risk of malignancies, including gastric cancer [12, 13]. Thus, it is possible that the presence of DM might affect the gastric carcinogenesis such as incidence and histological characteristics of gastric cancer after *H. pylori* eradication.

However, few studies have examined the inhibitory effect of *H. pylori* eradication therapy on gastric cancer in DM patients. In this study, we investigated the incidence and characteristics of gastric cancer diagnosed after *H. pylori* eradication in DM patients.

* Correspondence: sakitani-tky@umin.ac.jp
[1]The Institute for Adult Diseases, Asahi Life Foundation, 2-2-6 Bakuro-cho, Nihon-Bashi, Chuo-ku, Tokyo 113-8655, Japan
[2]Department of Gastroenterology, Graduate School of Medicine, The University of Tokyo, Tokyo, Japan

Methods

Patients

To evaluate the incidence and characteristics of gastric cancer diagnosed after *H. pylori* eradication in DM patients, 991 patients who underwent successful *H. pylori* eradication therapy at our institution between January 1996 and March 2013 and were followed up for over 6 months (the follow-up period was defined as the period from the day of commencement of eradication therapy to the day of the last endoscopy performed at our institution) were analyzed retrospectively. Then, we excluded patients who met the following criteria: i) those in whom endoscopy before eradication was not conducted at our institution ($n = 18$) and ii) those with a previous history of gastrectomy ($n = 8$). Therefore, a total of 965 patients were included in the analysis.

Patients were divided into DM and non-DM groups. DM was diagnosed according to the 2010 Japan Diabetes Society (JDS) criteria [14]. The diagnoses of hypertension (HT), hyperlipidemia (HL), and hyperuricemia (HU) were based on the need for medical treatment. The study design was approved by the Ethics Committee at the Institute for Adult Diseases, Asahi Life Foundation and conformed to the Declaration of Helsinki. The patients' records were anonymized prior to analysis. Written informed consent was obtained from all participants.

H. pylori eradication therapy

H. pylori infection was defined by a positive result for at least one of the following: rapid urease test (Helicocheck, Otsuka Pharmaceuticals, Tokyo, Japan), serological testing for anti-*H. pylori* IgG, ^{13}C-urea urea breath test, or pathological analysis by hematoxylin and eosin or Giemsa staining. Patients in whom *H. pylori* infection was confirmed underwent eradication therapy. Patients in whom eradication therapy had failed received additional treatment: the first-line regimen comprised a proton pump inhibitor (PPI), amoxicillin, and clarithromycin [15]; the second-line regimen comprised a PPI, amoxicillin, and metronidazole; and the third-line regimen comprised a PPI, amoxicillin, and sitafloxacin [16]. The success or failure of eradication therapy was determined by a ^{13}C-urea breath test performed at least 4 weeks after treatment.

Endoscopy

At our institution, patients who receive eradication therapy are recommended to undergo esophagogastroduodenoscopy annually. The upper gastrointestinal endoscopies were performed by experienced endoscopists. Gastric mucosal atrophy was evaluated using the endoscopic scale described by Kimura and Takemoto [17], which has been reported to concord with the histological results [18]. Patients were classified into three groups according to their endoscopic atrophic gastritis grade: the mild (C-I and C-II), moderate (C-III and O-I), and severe atrophic gastritis (O-II and O-III) groups.

Gastric cancer determination

Biopsy specimens were taken from the neoplastic lesion, and the final diagnosis of gastric cancer was based on the pathology results. Gastric cancers were classified pathologically according to Lauren's classification as intestinal or diffuse type [19]. A lesion identified by endoscopy prior to eradication was not counted as gastric cancer after eradication in this study.

Statistical analysis

All statistical analyses were performed using the JMP10 software (SAS Institute, Cary, NC, USA). Welch's t-test was used to compare the means of continuous variables. Comparisons of nominal variables were performed by χ^2 test or Fisher's exact test, as appropriate. The incidence of gastric cancer in patients with and without DM was evaluated using the Kaplan–Meier method, and the statistical significance of the differences was evaluated by log-rank test. The diagnosis of gastric cancer was the primary endpoint, and data were censored at the last endoscopy. The risk of gastric cancer after eradication was assessed using Cox's proportional-hazards model. Since no gastric cancer was detected in the mild atrophic gastritis group, this group served as the control. Odds ratios (OR) with 95 % confidence intervals (CI) were used as a measure of association and were adjusted using unconditional logistic regression models. A two-sided p-value of less than 0.05 was considered to indicate statistical significance.

Results

Baseline characteristics of the patients

The baseline characteristics of the patients are provided in Table 1. In total, 965 patients (729 males and 236 females, mean age 62.9 years, and mean body mass index (BMI) 23.2 kg/m^2) underwent successful *H. pylori* eradication therapy as the first-, second-, and third-line regimens in 782 (81.0 %), 178 (18.4 %), and 5 (0.52 %) patients, respectively. The 965 patients comprised 518 DM patients (13 type 1 DM and 505 type 2 DM patients) and 447 non-DM patients. Patients were followed-up for up to 16.2 years (mean 4.5 years). In terms of the endoscopic atrophic gastritis grade, 173 (17.9 %), 422 (43.7 %), and 370 (38.3 %) patients were categorized as having mild, moderate, and severe atrophic gastritis, respectively.

Non-DM patients who underwent eradication therapy were significantly younger than DM patients (60.7 and 64.8 years, respectively). The mean follow-up period (4.18 years for non-DM patients and 4.78 years for DM patients) and mean endoscopy interval (1.37 years for

Table 1 Characteristics of patients with and without DM who underwent *H. pylori* eradication therapy

Total (*n* = 965)	Non-DM (*n* = 447)	DM (*n* = 518)	*p*
Mean age (range), years	60.7 (27–84)	64.8 (30–86)	<0.0001*
Sex, *n* (%)			<0.0001*
Female	139 (31.1 %)	97 (18.7 %)	
Male	308 (68.9 %)	421 (81.3 %)	
Mean follow-up period (range), years	4.18 (0.54–13.2)	4.78 (0.68–16.2)	0.0006*
Mean endoscopy interval (range), years	1.37 (0.40–8.38)	1.61 (0.34–8.08)	<0.0001*
Mean body mass index (range), kg/m^2	23.1 (14.8–34.9)	23.4 (15.9–32.3)	0.1452
Atrophic gastritis grade, *n* (%)			0.0011*
Mild	95 (21.3 %)	78 (15.1 %)	
Moderate	207 (46.3 %)	215 (41.5 %)	
Severe	145 (32.4 %)	225 (43.4 %)	
Hypertension, *n* (%)	99 (22.1 %)	244 (47.1 %)	<0.0001*
Hyperlipidemia, *n* (%)	89 (19.9 %)	220 (42.5 %)	<0.0001*
Hyperuricemia, *n* (%)	32 (7.16 %)	48 (9.27 %)	0.236

DM diabetes mellitus
*Statistically significant (*p* < 0.05)

non-DM patients and 1.61 years for DM patients) of the non-DM patients were significantly shorter than those of the DM patients. The mean BMI (23.1 kg/m^2 for non-DM patients and 23.4 kg/m^2 for DM patients) was not significantly different between non-DM and DM patients. The proportion of patients who received medications for HT and HL was higher in DM than in non-DM patients.

Incidence and characteristics of gastric cancer after *H. pylori* eradication

During the follow-up period, 21 gastric cancers [9 in non-DM patients (0.482 %/year) and 12 in DM patients (0.485 %/year)] were diagnosed after *H. pylori* eradication (Table 2). No gastric cancer was found in the mild atrophic gastritis group, while 8 (38.1 %) gastric cancers were diagnosed in the moderate atrophic gastritis group and 13 (61.9 %) in the severe atrophic gastritis group. Among these 21 gastric cancers, there were no cardiac cancers. Eleven (52.4 %) gastric cancers had a depth of invasion limited to the mucosa; the remainder [10 (47.6 %)] exhibited submucosal or deeper invasion.

The mean age (69.4 years for non-DM patients and 70.6 years for DM patients), the proportion of males (77.8 % for non-DM patients and 91.7 % for DM patients), mean follow-up duration (4.59 years for non-DM patients and 3.95 years for DM patients), mean endoscopy interval (1.93 years for non-DM patients and 1.62 years for DM patients), mean BMI (23.4 kg/m^2 for non-DM patients and 22.6 kg/m^2 for DM patients) and atrophic gastritis grade were not significantly different between the gastric cancer patients with versus without DM.

In total, 16 (76.2 %) intestinal-type gastric cancer and 5 (23.8 %) diffuse-type gastric cancer cases were diagnosed. Among the non-DM gastric cancer patients, 88.9 % (8/9) were of the intestinal type, compared with 66.7 % (8/12) of the DM gastric cancer patients. Regarding gastric cancer treatment modalities, 11 (52.4 %) patients underwent curative endoscopic treatment. The remaining 10 (47.6 %) patients received curative surgical treatment. There were no significant differences in the pathology, diameter (22.1 mm for non-DM patients and 25.0 mm for DM patients), depth, location, or treatment of the gastric cancers between patients with and without DM.

Kaplan–Meier analysis of the proportions of patients free of gastric cancer after *H. pylori* eradication with and without DM is shown in Fig. 1. No significant difference was found in the incidence of gastric cancer after eradication between non-DM and DM patients by log-rank test (*p* = 0.8754).

Risk factors for gastric cancer after *H. pylori* eradication

We next analyzed the risk factors for gastric cancer after *H. pylori* eradication using Cox's proportional hazards model (Table 3). Age, sex, BMI, DM, HT, HL, and HU were not found to be risk factors for gastric cancer after *H. pylori* eradication in either univariate or multivariate analysis. Severe atrophic gastritis before eradication was identified as a significant risk factor for gastric cancer after *H. pylori* eradication in the multivariate analysis (OR 2.56, 95 % CI 1.03–6.77, *p* = 0.0424), in accordance with a previous report [9].

Table 2 Characteristics of gastric cancer in patients with and without DM after *H. pylori* eradication therapy

Total (n = 21)	Non-DM (n = 9)	DM (n = 12)	p
Mean age (range), years	69.4 (56–80)	70.6 (60–78)	0.7137
Sex, n (%)			0.5533
Female	2 (22.2 %)	1 (8.33 %)	
Male	7 (77.8 %)	11 (91.7 %)	
Mean follow up period (range), years	4.59 (1.03–11.8)	3.95 (0.95–7.15)	0.6990
Mean endoscopy interval (range), years	1.93 (0.99–4.06)	1.62 (0.70–2.95)	0.2527
Mean body mass index (range), kg/m^2	23.4 (19.5–27.5)	22.6 (19.0–30.1)	0.5534
Atrophic gastritis, n (%)			0.2030
Mild	0	0	
Moderate	5 (55.6 %)	3 (25.0 %)	
Severe	4 (44.4 %)	9 (75.0 %)	
Pathology, n (%)			0.3383
Intestinal type	8 (88.9 %)	8 (66.7 %)	
Diffuse type	1 (11.1 %)	4 (33.3 %)	
Diameter, mm	22.1 (3–70)	25.0 (5–60)	0.7543
Depth, n (%)			0.2562
Mucosa	6 (66.7 %)	5 (41.7 %)	
Submucosa and deeper	3 (33.3 %)	7 (58.3 %)	
Location, n (%)			0.7332
Upper third	3 (33.3 %)	2 (16.7 %)	
Middle third	3 (33.3 %)	5 (41.7 %)	
Lower third	3 (33.3 %)	5 (41.7 %)	
Treatment, n (%)			0.3869
Endoscopic	6 (66.7 %)	5 (41.7 %)	
Surgery	3 (33.3 %)	7 (58.3 %)	

DM diabetes mellitus

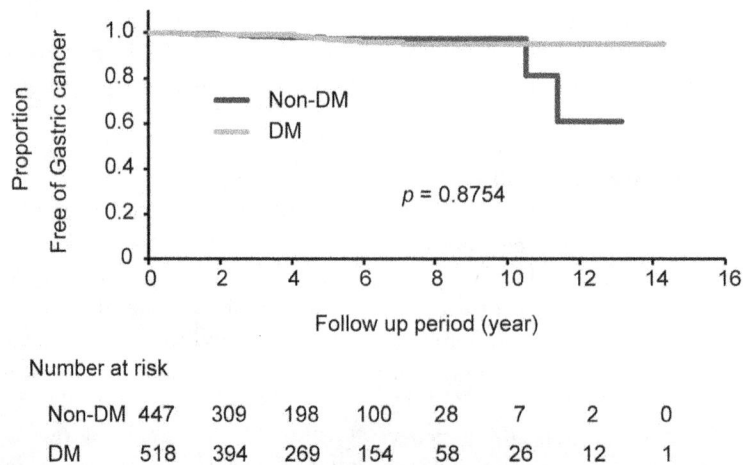

Fig. 1 Kaplan–Meier analysis of the proportion of patients with and without diabetes mellitus (DM) free from gastric cancer after *H. pylori* eradication therapy. Gastric cancer was diagnosed in nine non-DM patients and 12 DM patients during the follow-up period (p =0.8754, log-rank test)

Table 3 Cox's proportional hazards model for factors associated with the incidence of gastric cancer after *H. pylori* eradication

Factor	Univariate OR (95 % CI)	p	Multivariate OR (95 % CI)	p
Age (years)	1.01 (0.96–1.06)	0.6248	1.00 (0.94–1.05)	0.9446
Sex				
Female	1			
Male	1.82 (0.61–7.78)	0.3030	2.13 (0.67–9.46)	0.1914
Body mass index kg/m2) m²)	1.02 (0.83–1.13)	0.7880	1.01 (0.83–1.15)	0.8264
Diabetes mellitus (DM)				
Non-DM	1			
DM	0.93 (0.39–2.30)	0.8756	0.64 (0.25–1.66)	0.3530
Hypertension (HT)				
Non-HT	1			
HT	1.40 (0.57–3.31)	0.4459	1.36 (0.53–3.36)	0.4985
Hyperlipidemia (HL)				
Non-HL	1			
HL	1.15 (0.43–2.83)	0.7600	1.17 (0.42–2.99)	0.7485
Hyperuricemia (HU)				
Non-HU	1			
HU	0.62 (0.03–3.05)	0.6295	0.43 (0.02–2.24)	0.3811
Atrophic gastritis				
Mild-Moderate	1			
Severe	2.63 (1.10–6.67)	0.0280*	2.56 (1.03–6.77)	0.0424*

OR odds ratio; *CI* confidence interval
*Statistically significant ($p < 0.05$)

Discussion

In this study, we aimed to elucidate the incidence and characteristics of gastric cancer after *H. pylori* eradication therapy in DM patients. Our results indicated that the incidence and characteristics of gastric cancer developing after *H. pylori* eradication therapy were not significantly different between DM and non-DM patients. The incidence of gastric cancer after eradication was 0.48 %/year and the mean age of the patients 62 years. The incidence and mean age are in agreement with those reported by Ogura et al. (0.46 %/year and 62 years, respectively) [6]. Kamada et al. reported that severe mucosal atrophy in the corpus is a risk factor for gastric cancer after eradication [9]. This study also showed that severe atrophic gastritis before eradication is the risk for gastric cancer suggesting follow-up endoscopy of patients with severe atrophic gastritis is necessary.

The prevalence of DM is rapidly increasing, and several studies have focused on the interaction of DM with *H. pylori* infection and the gastric cancer axis [20–22]. The prevalence of *H. pylori* infection in DM patients is reportedly higher than that in non-DM patients [23]. Sekikawa et al. reported that open-type atrophic gastritis is found more frequently in DM patients than in non-DM patients (33.4 % (50/148) and 21.1 % (274/1301),

respectively); moreover, the presence of DM increased the risk of development of early gastric cancer. In the present study, the presence of DM did not increase the incidence of gastric cancer after *H. pylori* eradication therapy. It is possible that DM acts synergistically with consistent *H. pylori* infection to increase the risk of gastric cancer, as reported previously [24], and that the presence of DM after *H. pylori* eradication therapy might not enhance the risk of gastric cancer.

Other possible risk factors for gastric cancer (such as smoking and high salt intake) have been reported to increase gastric cancer risk synergistically with *H. pylori* infection [25, 26]. A prospective study conducted in Japan (the Hisayama study) found that the combination of smoking and *H. pylori* infection increased the risk of gastric cancer more than did smoking or *H. pylori* infection alone [25]. The Hisayama study also found a significant association between high salt intake and gastric cancer in a population with atrophic gastritis and *H. pylori* infection [26].

In the present study, the pathological features of gastric cancer after eradication were not significantly different between DM and non-DM patients. This finding is in line with a previous report that there is no significant difference in the histopathological differentiation of gastric cancer in patients with versus without DM [27]. The proportion of those with intestinal-type gastric cancer after eradication (76.2 %, 16/21) in this study is in agreement with that reported by Kamada et al. (75.0 %, 15/20) [9].

There were several limitations to our study. First, it was a retrospective cohort design; therefore, further prospective and longer-term studies are required. Second, several possible risk factors for gastric cancer—such as smoking, alcohol intake, dietary habits, family history and *H. pylori* virulence factors—were not evaluated. Regarding lifestyle factors, a previous report showed that smoking and drinking alcohol were not associated with the development of gastric cancer after *H. pylori* eradication therapy [28].

Conclusion
Our findings indicated that the incidence and characteristics of gastric cancer after *H. pylori* eradication therapy were comparable between DM and non-DM patients.

Abbreviations
DM: Diabetes mellitus.

Competing interests
The authors declare that they have no competing interests.

Authors' contributions
K Sakitani collected and analyzed the data, and drafted the manuscript. YH analyzed the data and revised the manuscript. NS, SS, TS, and YY analyzed the data. AY, K Sakamoto, MA, and SM collected and analyzed the data. YI, SK and KK supervised the study.

Acknowledgements
The authors thank the gastroenterologists who performed the endoscopic procedures and the diabetes specialists who managed the diabetes patients at the Institute for Adult Diseases, Asahi Life Foundation Hospital (Tokyo, Japan). We are grateful to N. Tachibana and Y. ligaya for their arrangement of the database.

Author details
[1]The Institute for Adult Diseases, Asahi Life Foundation, 2-2-6 Bakuro-cho, Nihon-Bashi, Chuo-ku, Tokyo 113-8655, Japan. [2]Department of Gastroenterology, Graduate School of Medicine, The University of Tokyo, Tokyo, Japan. [3]Gastroenterology Division, Yokohama City University Graduate School of Medicine, Yokohama, Japan.

References
1. Warren JR, Marshall BJ. Unidentified curved bacilli on gastric epithelium in active chronic gastritis. Lancet. 1983;1(8336):1273–5.
2. Correa P. Human gastric carcinogenesis - a multistep and multifocul process - 1st American-Cancer-Society Award Lecture on cancer-epidemioplogy and prevention. Cancer Res. 1992;52(24):6735–40.
3. Uemura N, Okamoto S, Yamamoto S, Matsumura N, Yamaguchi S, Yamakido M, et al. Helicobacter pylori infection and the development of gastric cancer. N Engl J Med. 2001;345(11):784–9.
4. Sakitani K, Hirata Y, Watabe H, Yamada A, Sugimoto T, Yamaji Y, et al. Gastric cancer risk according to the distribution of intestinal metaplasia and neutrophil infiltration. J Gastroenterol Hepatol. 2011;26(10):1570–5.
5. Shichijo S, Hirata Y, Sakitani K, Yamamoto S, Serizawa T, Niikura R, et al. The distribution of intestinal metaplasia as a predictor of gastric cancer development. J Gastroenterol Hepatol. 2015;30(8):1260–4.
6. Ogura K, Hirata Y, Yanai A, Shibata W, Ohmae T, Mitsuno Y, et al. The effect of Helicobacter pylori eradication on reducing the incidence of gastric cancer. J Clin Gastroenterol. 2008;42(3):279–83.
7. Fukase K, Kato M, Kikuchi S, Inoue K, Uemura N, Okamoto S, et al. Effect of eradication of Helicobacter pylori on incidence of metachronous gastric carcinoma after endoscopic resection of early gastric cancer: an open-label, randomised controlled trial. Lancet. 2008;372(9636):392–7.
8. Take S, Mizuno M, Ishiki K, Hamada F, Yoshida T, Yokota K, et al. Seventeen-year effects of eradicating Helicobacter pylori on the prevention of gastric cancer in patients with peptic ulcer; a prospective cohort study. J Gastroenterol. 2015;50(6):638–44.
9. Kamada T, Hata J, Sugiu K, Kusunoki H, Ito M, Tanaka S, et al. Clinical features of gastric cancer discovered after successful eradication of Helicobacter pylori: results from a 9-year prospective follow-up study in Japan. Aliment Pharmacol Ther. 2005;21(9):1121–6.
10. Yamamoto K, Kato M, Takahashi M, Haneda M, Shinada K, Nishida U, et al. Clinicopathological analysis of early-stage gastric cancers detected after successful eradication of Helicobacter pylori. Helicobacter. 2011;16(3):210–6.
11. Karin M, Lawrence T, Nizet V. Innate immunity gone awry: linking microbial infections to chronic inflammation and cancer. Cell. 2006;124(4):823–35.
12. Giovannucci E, Harlan DM, Archer MC, Bergenstal RM, Gapstur SM, Habel LA, et al. Diabetes and cancer: a consensus report. Diabetes Care. 2010;33(7):1674–85.
13. Hidaka A, Sasazuki S, Goto A, Sawada N, Shimazu T, Yamaji T, et al. Plasma insulin, C-peptide and blood glucose and the risk of gastric cancer: the Japan Public Health Center-based prospective study. Int J Cancer. 2015;136(6):1402–10.
14. Seino Y, Nanjo K, Tajima N, Kadowaki T, Kashiwagi A, Araki E, et al. Report of the committee on the classification and diagnostic criteria of diabetes mellitus. J Diabetes Investig. 2010;1(5):212–28.
15. Yanai A, Sakamoto K, Akanuma M, Ogura K, Maeda S. Non-bismuth quadruple therapy for first-line Helicobacter pylori eradication: a randomized study in Japan. World J Gastrointest Pharmacol Ther. 2012;3(1):1–6.
16. Hirata Y, Ohmae T, Yanai A, Sakitani K, Hayakawa Y, Yoshida S, et al. Sitafloxacin resistance in Helicobacter pylori isolates and sitafloxacin-based triple therapy as a third-line regimen in Japan. Int J Antimicrob Agents. 2012;39(4):352–5.
17. Kimura K, Takemoto T. an endoscopic recognition of the atrophic border and its significance in chronic gastritis. Endoscopy. 1969;1(3):87–97.
18. Satoh K, Kimura K, Taniguchi Y, Yoshida Y, Kihira K, Takimoto T, et al. Distribution of inflammation and atrophy in the stomach of Helicobacter pylori-positive and -negative patients with chronic gastritis. Am J Gastroenterol. 1996;91(5):963–9.
19. Lauren P. The two histological main types of gastric carcinoma - diffuse and so-called intestinal-type carcinoma - an attempt at a histo-clinical classification. Acta Pathol Et Microbiol Scand. 1965;64(1):31–49.
20. Tseng CH, Tseng FH. Diabetes and gastric cancer: the potential links. World J Gastroenterol. 2014;20(7):1701–11.
21. Tian T, Zhang LQ, Ma XH, Zhou JN, Shen J. Diabetes mellitus and incidence and mortality of gastric cancer: a meta-analysis. Exp Clin Endocrinol Diabetes. 2012;120(4):217–23.
22. Yoon JM, Son KY, Eom CS, Durrance D, Park SM. Pre-existing diabetes mellitus increases the risk of gastric cancer: a meta-analysis. World J Gastroenterol. 2013;19(6):936–45.
23. Zhou X, Zhang C, Wu J, Zhang G. Association between Helicobacter pylori infection and diabetes mellitus: a meta-analysis of observational studies. Diabetes Res Clin Pract. 2013;99(2):200–8.
24. Ikeda F, Doi Y, Yonemoto K, Ninomiya T, Kubo M, Shikata K, et al. Hyperglycemia increases risk of gastric cancer posed by Helicobacter pylori infection: a population-based cohort study. Gastroenterology. 2009;136(4):1234–41.

25. Shikata K, Doi Y, Yonemoto K, Arima H, Ninomiya T, Kubo M, et al. Population-based prospective study of the combined influence of cigarette smoking and Helicobacter pylori infection on gastric cancer incidence: the Hisayama Study. Am J Epidemiol. 2008;168(12):1409–15.

26. Shikata K, Kiyohara Y, Kubo M, Yonemoto K, Ninomiya T, Shirota T, et al. A prospective study of dietary salt intake and gastric cancer incidence in a defined Japanese population: the Hisayama study. Int J Cancer. 2006;119(1):196–201.

27. Wei ZW, Li JL, Wu Y, Xia GK, Schwarz RE, He YL, et al. Impact of pre-existing type-2 diabetes on patient outcomes after radical resection for gastric cancer: a retrospective cohort study. Dig Dis Sci. 2014;59(5):1017–24.

28. Take S, Mizuno M, Ishiki K, Yoshida T, Ohara N, Yokota K, et al. The long-term risk of gastric cancer after the successful eradication of Helicobacter pylori. J Gastroenterol. 2011;46(3):318–24.

9

Comparison of sequential therapy and amoxicillin/tetracycline containing bismuth quadruple therapy for the first-line eradication of *Helicobacter pylori*

Ju Yup Lee[1,2], Nayoung Kim[1*], Kyung Sik Park[2], Hyun Jin Kim[3], Seon Mee Park[4], Gwang Ho Baik[5], Ki-Nam Shim[6], Jung Hwan Oh[7], Suck Chei Choi[8], Sung Eun Kim[9], Won Hee Kim[10], Seon-Young Park[11], Gwang Ha Kim[12], Bong Eun Lee[12], Yunju Jo[13] and Su Jin Hong[14]

Abstract

Background: The <80 % *Helicobacter pylori* eradication rate with sequential therapy is unsatisfactory. Modified bismuth quadruple therapy, replacing metronidazole with amoxicillin, could be promising because *H. pylori* resistance to tetracycline or to amoxicillin is relatively low. A 14-day modified bismuth quadruple protocol as first-line *H. pylori* treatment was compared with 10-day sequential therapy.

Methods: In total, 390 *H. pylori*-infected subjects participated in the randomized clinical trial: 10-day sequential therapy (40 mg pantoprazole plus 1 g amoxicillin twice a day for 5 days, then 40 mg pantoprazole and 500 mg clarithromycin twice a day and 500 mg metronidazole three times a day for 5 days) or 14-day modified bismuth quadruple therapy (40 mg pantoprazole, 600 mg bismuth subcitrate, 1 g tetracycline, and 1 g amoxicillin, twice a day). ^{13}C-urea breath test, rapid urease testing, or histology was performed to check for eradication.

Results: Intention-to-treat (ITT) eradication rates of 10-day sequential and 14-day quadruple therapy were 74.6 % and 68.7 %, respectively, and the per-protocol (PP) rates were 84.2 and 76.5 %, respectively. The eradication rate was higher in the sequential therapy group, but neither the ITT nor the PP analyses had a significant difference ($P = 0.240$ and $P = 0.099$, respectively). However, the adverse events were significantly lower in the modified bismuth quadruple therapy group than the sequential therapy group (36.9 vs. 47.7 %, $P = 0.040$).

Conclusions: Ten-day sequential therapy appears to be more effective despite frequent adverse events. However, both 10-day SQT and 14-day PBAT did not reach the excellent eradication rates that exceed 90 %. Additional trials are needed to identify a more satisfactory first-line eradication therapy.

Keywords: *Helicobacter pylori*, Eradication, Amoxicillin, Tetracycline, Bismuth, Quadruple

* Correspondence: nayoungkim49@empas.com
[1]Department of Internal Medicine, Seoul National University Bundang Hospital, Seongnam, South Korea
Full list of author information is available at the end of the article

Background

Helicobacter pylori is a major cause of gastric diseases such as chronic gastritis, gastroduodenal ulcers, and gastric cancer, and it is well known that the eradication of *H. pylori* is important in preventing and treating these gastric diseases [1, 2]. Recently, the Kyoto Global Consensus Meeting, held in Japan in early February of 2014, presented radical changes in the diagnosis and treatment of *H. pylori* infection, such as recommending eradication treatment for patients with dyspepsia [3]. In addition, eradication therapy was recommended for all *H. pylori*-positive individuals for the purpose of preventing *H. pylori*-related diseases [3]. However, the eradication rates of first-line triple therapy, which consists of a proton pump inhibitor (PPI) and two antibiotics (clarithromycin and amoxicillin), have been continuously decreasing [4]. Only ~18 % of previous studies have reported exceeding 85 % eradication on an intention-to-treat (ITT) analysis, with ~60 % falling short of 80 % [5]. The reason for the decrease in the efficacy of PPI-based triple therapy is mainly due to the increase in *H. pylori* resistance to clarithromycin. As such, in Western countries, standard triple therapy is currently considered a "legacy therapy" [5]. In fact, recent European guidelines recommended triple therapy as the first-line treatment only when the prevalence of clarithromycin resistance is under 20 % [6].

To overcome this unsatisfactory eradication rate, sequential therapy (SQT) is currently recommended as an alternative first-line treatment for *H. pylori* infection. Many European randomized clinical trials (RCTs) and meta-analyses have shown the superiority of SQT over standard PPI-based triple therapy [7–9]. In a Korean meta-analysis based on six RCTs, the eradication rate of SQT was 79.4 % in ITT analysis and 86.4 % in PP analysis; this meta-analysis also proved that SQT is superior to standard PPI-based triple therapy (relative risk [RR] 1.761, 95 % confidence interval [CI]; 1.403–2.209) [10]. However, the eradication rate of SQT in Korea, mostly under 80 % (ITT: 79.4 %, 95 % CI: 76.3–82.2) [10], is not satisfactory and is about 10 % lower than reported in early European studies [10, 11]. This suboptimal eradication rate could be explained by high rates of antibiotic resistance, especially to clarithromycin, metronidazole, or both [12]. Previous studies showed that the rate of resistance to clarithromycin was >20 %, that to metronidazole was >30 %, and that to both was >10 % [13, 14].

The classical bismuth quadruple therapy, which consists of a PPI, bismuth, tetracycline, and metronidazole, is frequently used as a first- or second-line regimen [6, 15–17]. However, it is known that more than 30 % of patients stop taking their medicine due to the complicated regimen and the high rate of adverse events [18]. In view of antibiotic resistance, a modified bismuth quadruple therapy (PBAT), in which metronidazole is replaced with amoxicillin, is very attractive because many studies have

reported that *H. pylori* resistance to amoxicillin and tetracycline is low [19] and furthermore, amoxicillin is easier to take in comparison to metronidazole. Several studies have suggested good eradication rates with this amoxicillin and tetracycline combined quadruple regimen [20–23]; however, the reported efficacies are conflicting. From this background the aim of this study was to evaluate the efficacy of 14-day PBAT as a first-line treatment and compare 10-day SQT to 14-day PBAT in order to establish a more effective first-line regimen for *H. pylori* in terms of eradication rate and adverse effects.

Methods

Study design and participants

A prospective, multi-center, randomized, open-label, parallel design clinical trial was conducted between July 2014 and May 2015 in 14 tertiary hospitals from different regions in Korea. Inclusion criteria were adult Korean men and women (aged ≥ 18 years) who were diagnosed as *H. pylori*-positive by any of the following three methods: 1) a positive rapid urease test (CLOtest [Delta West, Bentley, Australia]), 2) histologic evidence of *H. pylori* by modified Giemsa staining, or a 3) positive ^{13}C-urea breath test. Exclusion criteria were 1) age under 18 years; 2) previous eradication therapy for *H. pylori*; 3) drugs that could influence the study results such as a PPI, H_2 blocker, mucosal protective agent, or antibiotics within the prior 4 weeks; 3) previous gastric surgery; 4) advanced gastric cancer or other malignancy; 5) abnormal liver function or liver cirrhosis; 6) abnormal renal function or chronic kidney disease; 7) other severe concurrent diseases; 8) previous contraindications or allergic reactions to the study drugs; 9) genetic disorders such as galactose intolerance, the Lapp lactase deficiency, or glucose-galactose malabsorption; 10) mental disorders or alcohol or drug addiction; 11) pregnancy or lactation or refusal to use an appropriate method of contraception throughout the course of the study; 12) any condition that might affect the evaluation of the clinical results in the judgment of the principal investigator or sub-investigator; or 13) any specific contraindication to the study drugs.

The study protocol was approved by the Korean Food and Drug Administration (KFDA No. 30157) and by the Institutional Review Board and Ethics Committees of all participating hospitals (Additional file 1). The study was performed according to Good Clinical Practices (GCP) and the Declaration of Helsinki, and written informed consent was obtained from all patients before enrollment. In addition, this study protocol has been registered at ClinicalTrials.gov (NCT02159976) and Clinical Research Information Service (CRIS) (KCT0001176).

Randomization and treatment allocation

An independent statistician at Seoul National University Bundang Hospital (SNUBH) prepared the randomization.

The subjects were randomized in a 1:1 ratio by a block randomization method to receive either 10-day SQT or 14-day PBAT. The 10-day SQT consisted of 40 mg of pantoprazole plus 1 g of amoxicillin twice a day for the initial 5 days, followed by 40 mg of pantoprazole and 500 mg of clarithromycin twice a day and 500 mg of metronidazole three times a day for the subsequent 5 days. The 14-day PBAT consisted of 40 mg of pantoprazole, 600 mg of bismuth subcitrate, 1 g of tetracycline, and 1 g of amoxicillin, twice a day. Four weeks after completing the therapy, successful *H. pylori* eradication was defined by a negative ^{13}C-urea breath test or an invasive test when endoscopic follow-up was needed in cases of benign gastric ulcer. The drug compliance and adverse events were evaluated by a physician via direct questioning. Compliance was considered to be satisfactory when drug intake exceeded 85 %.

Assessment of *H. pylori* infection
Invasive *H. pylori* test (Giemsa histology and CLOtest)
To determine the presence of current *H. pylori* infection, four biopsy specimens (one each from the greater curvature and lesser curvature of the antrum and body) were taken from the gastric mucosa at each endoscopic examination and were fixed in formalin to be used for the evaluation of *H. pylori* infection by Giemsa staining [24]. Two specimens from the lesser curvature of the antrum and body were used for the rapid urease test (CLOtest) [24].

^{13}C-urea breath test
Subjects were fasted for 4 h prior to testing and a pre-dose breath sample was obtained; 100 mg of ^{13}C-urea powder (UBiTkit; Otsuka Pharmaceutical Co. Ltd., Tokyo, Japan) dissolved in 100 mL of water was then administered orally, and a second breath sample was collected 20 min later. The cutoff value was 2.5 %. The collected samples were analyzed using an isotope ratio mass spectrometer (UBiT-IR300; Otsuka Pharmaceutical Co., Ltd.).

Trial outcomes
The primary outcome was comparing the percentage of participants with successful *H. pylori* eradication in the 10-day SQT and 14-day PBAT groups 4–6 weeks after completion of eradication therapy. The secondary outcome was to compare the percentage of patients whose drug compliance was greater than 85 % and the percentage of adverse events in the 10-day SQT and 14-day PBAT groups.

Sample size and statistical analysis
Because the eradication rate of the 10-day SQT was found to be 82.0 % in a previous Korean report [10] the eradication rate of the 14-day PBAT was assumed to be similar to that of the 10-day SQT if the rate difference between the two regimens was less than 10 %. With a power of 80 % at a two-sided type 1 error rate of 5 %, 195 subjects were needed for each treatment arm to allow for 10 % loss to follow-up. The *H. pylori* eradication rate was determined by both an ITT and a per-protocol (PP) analysis. All subjects who received treatment were included in the ITT analysis. For the PP analysis, subjects who were lost to follow-up, had taken less than 85 % of the prescribed drugs, or had dropped out due to severe adverse events were excluded.

Parametric continuous variables were compared using the Student's *t*-test and are presented as mean ± standard deviation (SD). Categorical variables were analyzed using Pearson's chi square test or Fisher's exact test and were presented as numbers (percentages). Univariate and multivariate logistic regression were used for analysis of influencing factors, which were expressed as the odds ratios (OR) and 95 % confidence intervals (CI). A two-sided *P* value of less than 0.05 was considered statistically significant. All statistical analyses were performed using SPSS (version 20.0; SPSS Inc., Chicago, IL, US).

Results
Subjects
A total of 390 *H. pylori*-infected treatment-naïve subjects were randomly assigned to the 10-day SQT group (n = 195) or the 14-day PBAT group (n = 195) (Fig. 1). Nineteen subjects in the SQT group and 18 subjects in the PBAT group did not complete the study due to adverse events, loss of follow-up, or withdrawal of consent. Therefore, 176 subjects in the SQT group and 175 subjects in the PBAT group completed the follow-up. After exclusion of 11 and 7 noncompliant subjects who consumed <85 % of the prescribed medications, 165 and 170 subjects in the SQT and PBAT groups, respectively, became the objects of the PP analysis (Fig. 1). There were no significant differences in the baseline characteristics or endoscopic findings between the two groups (Table 1).

Eradication rates
ITT eradication rates of the 10-day SQT and 14-day PBAT groups were 74.6 % (146/195) and 68.7 % (134/195) and the PP eradication rates were 84.2 % (139/165) and 76.5 % (130/170), respectively. The eradication rate was higher in the SQT than the PBAT group, but there was no statistical significance on either ITT or PP analysis (*P* = 0.240 and *P* = 0.099, respectively) (Fig. 2). There also was no statistical significance in the ITT analysis conducted independently at each institution (Fig. 3).

Compliance and adverse events
The complete follow-up rate was 90.3 % (176/195) in the 10-day SQT and 90.8 % in the 14-day PBAT group. The numbers of subjects who took more than 85 % of the prescribed medicine were 93.8 % (165/176) in the

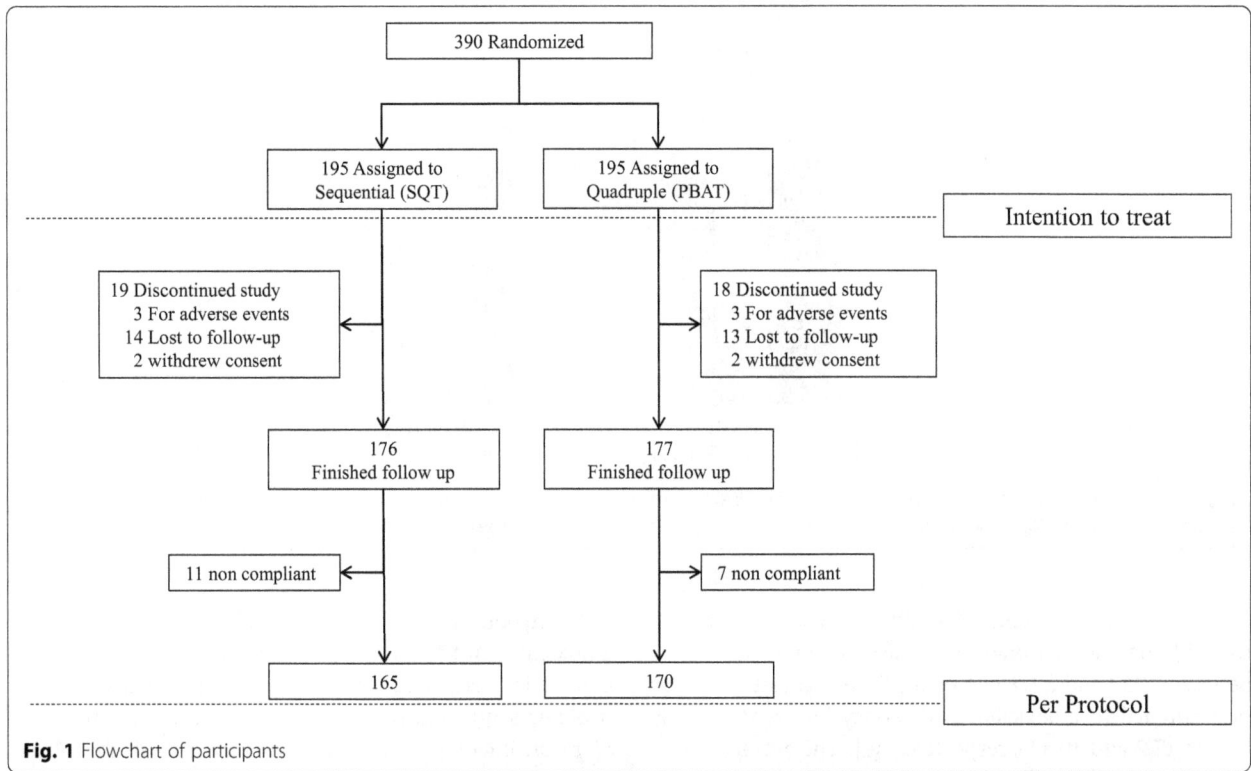

Fig. 1 Flowchart of participants

Table 1 Baseline characteristics of the subjects

	SQT ($n = 195$)	PBAT ($n = 195$)	p-value
Gender, n (%)			0.184
Male	103 (52.8)	117 (60.0)	
Female	92 (47.2)	78 (40.0)	
Age (mean ± SD), year	53.1 ± 12.6	53.6 ± 13.2	0.697
BMI, kg/m^2	23.5 ± 3.1	23.9 ± 3.4	0.328
Smoking, n (%)	38 (19.5)	36 (18.5)	0.897
Alcohol, n (%)	75 (38.5)	72 (36.9)	0.835
Endoscopic finding, n (%)			
Normal	10 (5.1)	11 (5.6)	1.000
Atrophic gastritis with or without intestinal metaplasia	43 (22.1)	31 (15.9)	0.155
Other gastritis	12 (6.2)	16 (8.2)	0.556
Gastric ulcer	47 (24.1)	43 (22.1)	0.718
Duodenal ulcer	15 (7.7)	20 (10.3)	0.479
Gastric ulcer + Duodenal ulcer	4 (2.1)	7 (3.6)	0.541
EMR, ESD for dysplasia or EGC	16 (8.2)	18 (9.2)	0.858
MALToma	1 (0.5)	0 (0.0)	1.000
Reflux esophagitis	1 (0.5)	3 (1.5)	0.615
Others	10 (5.1)	7 (3.6)	0.620

SQT sequential therapy, *PBAT* quadruple therapy consist of pantoprazole, bismuth, amoxicillin, and tetracycline, *BMI* body mass index, *EMR* endoscopic mucosal resection, *ESD* endoscopic submucosal dissection, *EGC* early gastric cancer, *MALToma* mucosal associated lymphoid tissue lymphoma

10-day SQT group and 96.1 % (170/177) in the 14-day PBAT group. There was also no significant difference between the two groups ($P = 0.460$). Ninety-three patients (47.7 %) who took the sequential regimen and 72 patients (36.9 %) who took the quadruple regimen experienced at least one adverse event. The adverse event rate was significantly lower in the PBAT group than in the SQT group ($P = 0.040$). In the 10-day SQT group, the most frequent adverse events were taste distortion (25.8 %) and abdominal bloating (22.6 %). In the 14-day PBAT group, the most frequent adverse events were epigastric discomfort (23.6 %) and diarrhea (16.7 %). Taste distortion was more frequently reported in the 10-day SQT group ($P < 0.001$) and diarrhea was more frequently reported in the 14-day PBAT group ($P = 0.014$) (Table 2).

Factors associated with eradication failure in PBAT

On univariate analysis, male sex (OR, 0.38; 95 % CI, 0.31–1.30) and BMI ≥ 25 kg/m^2 (OR, 2.28; 95 % CI, 1.12–4.63) were associated with treatment failure in the 14-day PBAT group. The multivariate analysis confirmed that both male sex (OR, 0.27; 95 % CI, 0.34–1.51) and BMI (OR, 2.16; 95 % CI, 1.05–4.43) were associated with treatment failure in the 14-day PBAT group (Table 3).

Discussion

Antibiotic resistance is one of the main causes of treatment failure in *H. pylori* eradication. The rates of clarithromycin

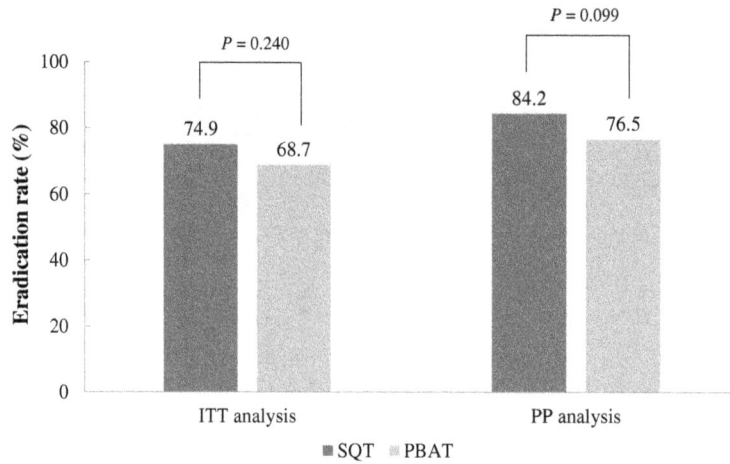

Fig. 2 *H. pylori* eradication rate of 10-day SQT and 14-day PBAT according to the ITT and PP analyses. SQT, sequential therapy; PBAT, quadruple therapy consists of pantoprazole, bismuth, amoxicillin, and tetracycline; ITT, intention-to-treat; PP, per-protocol

resistance increased rapidly from 23.2 to 37.3 % from 2003 to 2012 and the metronidazole resistance rate was 35.8 % between 2009 and 2012 in Korea [4]. In contrast, the rates of resistance to amoxicillin and tetracycline are relatively low, at 17.2 and 10.8 %, respectively [4]. The average resistance rate to amoxicillin in Europe is reported to be lower than 2 %, and the resistance rate to tetracycline is reported to be below 5 % in most countries [25–27].

We hypothesized that a quadruple regimen containing amoxicillin and tetracycline would demonstrate a superior eradication rate and could be a suitable substitute for triple or sequential regimens in the first-line treatment of *H. pylori* infection. The ITT eradication rate of the 14-day PBAT was 68.7 % and that of 10-day SQT was 74.6 %. There was no statistically significance difference between these two treatment groups (*P* = 0.240), suggesting that

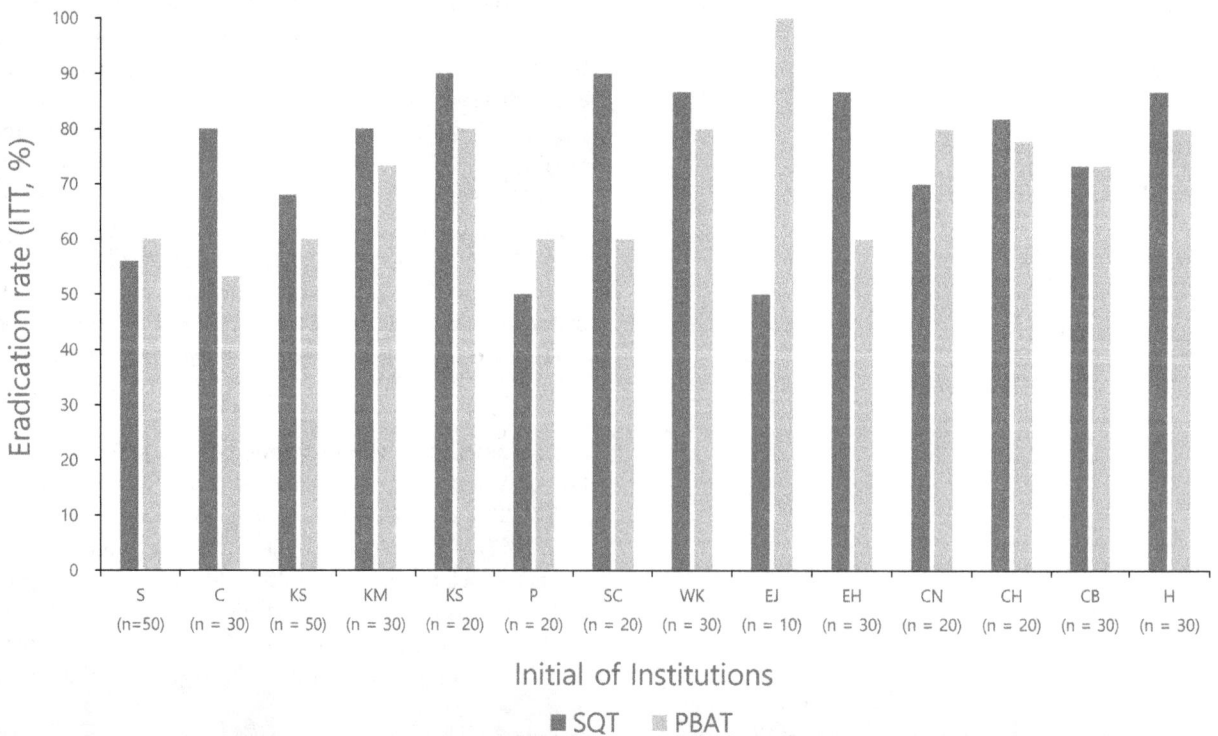

Fig. 3 *H. pylori* eradication rate of 10-day SQT and 14-day PBAT according to each institution. SQT, sequential therapy; PBAT, quadruple therapy consists of pantoprazole, bismuth, amoxicillin, and tetracycline; ITT, intention-to-treat

Table 2 Adverse events of the subjects

	SQT (n = 195)	PBAT (n = 195)	p-value
	n (%)	n (%)	
Bloating	21 (22.6)	11 (15.3)	0.097
Epigastric soreness	15 (16.1)	17 (23.6)	0.854
Anorexia	2 (2.2)	1 (1.4)	1.000
Taste distortions	24 (25.8)	4 (5.6)	**<0.001**
Nausea	14 (15.1)	6 (8.3)	0.108
Vomiting	0	2 (2.8)	0.478
Abdominal pain	4 (4.3)	4 (5.6)	0.721
Headache	1 (1.1)	2 (2.8)	1.000
Dyspepsia	4 (4.3)	4 (5.6)	0.721
Diarrhea	2 (2.2)	12 (16.7)	**0.014**
Constipation	2 (2.2)	3 (4.2)	1.000
Reflux	1 (1.1)	1 (1.4)	0.478
Rash and itching	2 (2.2)	5 (2.8)	0.446
Dizziness	1 (1.1)	0	1.000
Stool color change	0	3 (4.2)	0.246
Total	93 (47.7)	72 (36.9)	**0.040**

Bold style, means statistical significance

SQT sequential therapy, *PBAT* quadruple therapy consist of pantoprazole, bismuth, amoxicillin, and tetracycline

14-day PBAT was not inferior to 10-day SQT and therefore 14-day PBAT could be another treatment option.

However, some controversies in the results and large heterogeneity in the duration or the first- or second-line regimen exists in previous studies of amoxicillin- and tetracycline-containing quadruple regimens. For instance, in a study of the 14-day quadruple regimen, the eradication rate was 33.3 % in amoxicillin-susceptible *H. pylori*-infected patients [28]. In contrast, a Chinese study showed that the eradication rate of 14-day LBAT (lansoprazole, bismuth, amoxicillin, and tetracycline) was 83.8 % (95 % CI: 76.8–90.9 %) [20]. Furthermore, an RCT performed in Turkey reported the eradication rate of 14-day EBAT (esomeprazole, bismuth, amoxicillin, and tetracycline) as 79.0 % (95 % CI: 71–87 %) [21]. Chi et al. [23] reported that quadruple therapy containing

amoxicillin and tetracycline is an effective regimen to rescue patients after a failed triple therapy by overcoming the antimicrobial resistance of *H. pylori* with an eradication rate of 78 % in ITT and 89 % in PP.

Since *H. pylori* resistance to amoxicillin and tetracycline is uncommon, the explanation for the heterogeneous results could be that both amoxicillin and tetracycline are weak against *H. pylori* or possibly there is an antagonistic effect. However, any possible antagonistic effect between these two antibiotics is unclear and it is difficult to elucidate because data on the gastric bioavailability of tetracycline is lacking [29]. Furthermore, several studies showed a good eradication rate (78.0–83.8 %), which was not inferior to other regimens, and this positive tendency was also proven in a recent meta-analysis. Published in 2015, the meta-analysis, which included 9 RCTs, showed that the total eradication rate of a quadruple regimen containing amoxicillin and tetracycline was 78.1 % in ITT and 84.5 % in PP, which was not inferior to other quadruple regimens (pooled odds ratio [OR]: 0.9, 95 % CI: 0.42–1.78) [30]. In subgroup analysis, the eradication rates of 7-day, 10-day, and 14-day amoxicillin/tetracycline quadruple regimens were 67.4, 84.6, and 82.3 %, respectively, and the pooled OR of an amoxicillin/tetracycline quadruple regimen used as first-line therapy was 2.34 (95 % CI: 0.74–7.42) [30].

In our study, we used different doses and intervals of PBAT compared with those of previous studies to maximize subject compliance. In previous studies, bismuth was administered at 300 mg and tetracycline at 500 mg, both four times a day [21, 31]. The mixture of twice a day and four times a day can influence drug compliance. A recently developed three-in-one capsule containing bismuth, tetracycline, and metronidazole improved the eradication rate of bismuth quadruple therapy over 90 % by reducing the number of medicines and therefore improving patient compliance [32]. In the present clinical trial bismuth 600 mg twice a day and tetracycline 1000 mg twice a day were chosen to increase compliance.

Tetracycline is a time-dependent (half-life 8–10 h) antibiotic agent and has a long post-antibiotic effect (PAE) [33]. Even though a high blood concentration of

Table 3 Factors associated with eradication failure in amoxicillin- and tetracycline containing quadruple therapy

Factors	Crude	Univariated	Adjusted	Multivariated
	OR (95 % CI)	p-value[a]	OR (95 % CI)[b]	p-value[c]
Age ≥ 50 (y)	1.12 (0.54–2.32)	0.763		
Female	0.38 (0.31–1.30)	<0.0001	0.27 (0.34–1.51)	<0.0001
Cigarette smoking	1.35 (0.57–3.20)	0.499		
Alcohol drinking	1.42 (0.70–2.88)	0.325		
BMI ≥ 25 (kg/m²)	2.28 (1.12–4.63)	0.023	2.16 (1.05–4.43)	0.037

OR odds ratio, *CI* confidence intervals, *BMI* body mass index
[a]Univariate logistic regression
[b]Adjusted for gender and BMI
[c]Multivariate logistic regression

tetracycline does not increase its sterilizing power, it can inhibit bacterial regrowth for a longer period of time [34, 35]. From these pharmacokinetic considerations, a twice-a-day regimen is also appropriate and is likely to promote patient compliance. The drug compliance in the present study was 96.1 % in the PBAT group, which is comparable to that in the SQT group (93.8 %). In addition, this rate is higher than the 88.6 % [20] and 92.0 % [31] reported by other studies.

This clinical trial had some limitations. First, *H. pylori* culture was not routinely performed and we could not evaluate the eradication rate of amoxicillin- and/or tetracycline-susceptible *H. pylori* strains. However, one center (SNUBH) performed *H. pylori* cultures and antibiotic susceptibility testing by the agar dilution method in a small number of patients. The first-line or second-line eradication rate of PBAT was 57.1 % (8/14) in amoxicillin- and tetracycline-susceptible subjects (data not shown). More antibiotic susceptibility data are needed in a future study to confirm the eradication effect of amoxicillin and tetracycline-containing regimens both in vitro and in vivo. Second, the limited accuracy of ^{13}C-UBT at 4–6 weeks after the completion of a bismuth-based treatment that makes possible, at least in part, a false negative diagnosis of *H. pylori* eradication leading to an overestimation of success rates with the bismuth-based regimen (PBAT). However, ^{13}C-UBT is a convenient non-invasive method for *H. pylori* diagnosis and popularly used for eradication success. It is very difficult to perform invasive *H. pylori* test such as histology or CLOtest via upper endoscopy to all patients in real clinical setting who did not need follow-up endoscopy and medical cost is also a problem. Third, we cannot elucidate the reason why PBAT showed a lower eradication rate than expected. However, there is a fairly large eradication rate gap between positive and negative studies. Further study is needed in the future.

Conclusions

In conclusion, this prospective, multi-center, randomized, open-label, parallel design clinical trial demonstrated that SQT for 10 days appears more effective than PBAT in spite of frequent adverse events. However, both 10-day SQT and 14-day PBAT did not achieve excellent eradication rates (>90 %). Thus, additional trials are necessary to identify a more satisfactory first-line eradication therapy for *H. pylori*.

Abbreviations

EGC, early gastric cancer; EMR, endoscopic mucosal resection; ESD, endoscopic submucosal dissection; *H. pylori*, *Helicobacter pylori*; MALToma, mucosal associated lymphoid tissue lymphoma; PBAT, quadruple therapy consist of pantoprazole, bismuth, amoxicillin, and tetracycline; SQT, sequential therapy

Acknowledgements

This work was supported by grant no 06-2014-074 from the Seoul National University Bundang Hospital Research. The authors thank Division of Statistics in Medical Research Collaborating Center at Seoul National University Bundang Hospital for providing statistical consultation.

Authors' contributions

JYL reviewed the literature and drafted the manuscript; NK designed and supervised research; KSP reviewed draft and performed research; HJK and GHK advised and performed research; SMP, GHB, KNS, JHO, SCC, SEK, WHK, SYP, BEL, JYJ, SJH performed clinical procedures including endoscopies, patient enroll, and data collection. JYL and SEK analyzed data. All authors read and approved the final manuscript.

Competing interests

The authors declare that they have no competing interests.

Consent for publication

Not applicable.

Author details

[1]Department of Internal Medicine, Seoul National University Bundang Hospital, Seongnam, South Korea. [2]Department of Internal Medicine, Keimyung University School of Medicine, Daegu, South Korea. [3]Department of Internal Medicine and Institute of Health Science, Gyeongsang National University School of Medicine, Jinju, Gyeongsangnam-do, South Korea. [4]Department of Internal Medicine, College of Medicine, Chungbuk National University, Cheongju, South Korea. [5]Department of Internal Medicine, Hallym University College of Medicine, Chuncheon Sacred Heart Hospital, Chuncheon, South Korea. [6]Department of Internal Medicine, Ewha Womans University School of Medicine, Seoul, South Korea. [7]Departments of Internal Medicine, College of Medicine, The Catholic University of Korea, Seoul, Republic of Korea. [8]Department of Internal Medicine, Wonkwang University School of Medicine, Iksan, South Korea. [9]Department of Internal Medicine, Kosin University College of Medicine, Busan, South Korea. [10]Digestive Disease Center, CHA Bundang Medical Center, CHA University, Seongnam, South Korea. [11]Department of Internal Medicine, Chonnam National University Medical School, Gwangju, South Korea. [12]Department of Internal Medicine, Pusan National University School of Medicine and Biomedical Research Institute, Pusan National University Hospital, Busan, South Korea. [13]Department of Internal Medicine, Eulji General Hospital, Eulji University School of Medicine, Seoul, South Korea. [14]Department of Internal Medicine and Research Institute, Soonchunhyang University College of Medicine, Bucheon, South Korea.

References

1. McColl KE. Clinical practice. *Helicobacter pylori* infection. New Engl J Med. 2010;362:1597–604.
2. Graham DY, Lu H, Yamaoka Y. A report card to grade *Helicobacter pylori* therapy. Helicobacter. 2007;12:275–8.
3. Sugano K, Tack J, Kuipers EJ, Graham DY, El-Omar EM, Miura S, Haruma K, Asaka M, Uemura N, Malfertheiner P, et al. Kyoto global consensus report on *Helicobacter pylori* gastritis. Gut. 2015;64:1353–67.
4. Lee JY, Kim N, Kim MS, Choi YJ, Lee JW, Yoon H, Shin CM, Park YS, Lee DH, Jung HC. Factors affecting first-line triple therapy of *Helicobacter pylori* including CYP2C19 genotype and antibiotic resistance. Dig Dis Sci. 2014;59:1235–43.
5. Graham DY, Fischbach L. *Helicobacter pylori* treatment in the era of increasing antibiotic resistance. Gut. 2010;59:1143–53.
6. Malfertheiner P, Megraud F, O'Morain CA, Atherton J, Axon AT, Bazzoli F, Gensini GF, Gisbert JP, Graham DY, Rokkas T, et al. Management of *Helicobacter pylori* infection–the Maastricht IV/Florence Consensus Report. Gut. 2012;61:646–64.

7. Jafri NS, Hornung CA, Howden CW. Meta-analysis: sequential therapy appears superior to standard therapy for *Helicobacter pylori* infection in patients naive to treatment. Annals Intern Med. 2008;148:923–31.

8. Gatta L, Vakil N, Leandro G, Di Mario F, Vaira D. Sequential therapy or triple therapy for *Helicobacter pylori* infection: systematic review and meta-analysis of randomized controlled trials in adults and children. Am J Gastroenterol. 2009;104:3069–79.

9. Tong JL, Ran ZH, Shen J, Xiao SD. Sequential therapy vs. standard triple therapies for *Helicobacter pylori* infection: a meta-analysis. J Clin Pharm Ther. 2009;34:41–53.

10. Kim JS, Kim BW, Ham JH, Park HW, Kim YK, Lee MY, Ji JS, Lee BI, Choi H. Sequential Therapy for *Helicobacter pylori* Infection in Korea: Systematic Review and Meta-Analysis. Gut Liver. 2013;7:546–51.

11. Zullo A, Rinaldi V, Winn S, Meddi P, Lionetti R, Hassan C, Ripani C, Tomaselli G, Attili AF. A new highly effective short-term therapy schedule for *Helicobacter pylori* eradication. Aliment Pharmacol Tther. 2000;14:715–8.

12. Yoon H, Lee DH, Kim N, Park YS, Shin CM, Kang KK, Oh DH, Jang DK, Chung JW. Meta-analysis: Is sequential therapy superior to standard triple therapy for *Helicobacter pylori* infection in Asian adults? J Gastroenterol Hepatol. 2013;28:1801–9.

13. Chung JW, Jung YK, Kim YJ, Kwon KA, Kim JH, Lee JJ, Lee SM, Hahm KB, Lee SM, Jeong JY, et al. Ten-day sequential versus triple therapy for *Helicobacter pylori* eradication: a prospective, open-label, randomized trial. J Gastroenterol Hepatol. 2012;27:1675–80.

14. Lee JY, Kim N. Future trends of *Helicobacter pylori* eradication therapy in Korea. Korean J Gastroenterol. 2014;63:158–70.

15. Kim SG, Jung HK, Lee HL, Jang JY, Lee H, Kim CG, Shin WG, Shin ES, Lee YC. Guidelines for the diagnosis and treatment of *Helicobacter pylori* infection in Korea, 2013 revised edition. J Gastroenterol Hepatol. 2014;29:1371–86.

16. Marin AC, McNicholl AG, Gisbert JP. A review of rescue regimens after clarithromycin-containing triple therapy failure (for *Helicobacter pylori* eradication). Exp opin Pharmacotherapy. 2013;14:843–61.

17. Venerito M, Krieger T, Ecker T, Leandro G, Malfertheiner P. Meta-analysis of bismuth quadruple therapy versus clarithromycin triple therapy for empiric primary treatment of *Helicobacter pylori* infection. Digestion. 2013;88:33–45.

18. Lee BH, Kim N, Hwang TJ, Lee SH, Park YS, Hwang JH, Kim JW, Jeong SH, Lee DH, Jung HC, et al. Bismuth-containing quadruple therapy as second-line treatment for Helicobacter pylori infection: effect of treatment duration and antibiotic resistance on the eradication rate in Korea. Helicobacter. 2010;15:38–45.

19. Lee JW, Kim N, Kim JM, Nam RH, Chang H, Kim JY, Shin CM, Park YS, Lee DH, Jung HC. Prevalence of primary and secondary antimicrobial resistance of *Helicobacter pylori* in Korea from 2003 through 2012. Helicobacter. 2013;18:206–14.

20. Liang X, Xu X, Zheng Q, Zhang W, Sun Q, Liu W, Xiao S, Lu H. Efficacy of bismuth-containing quadruple therapies for clarithromycin-, metronidazole-, and fluoroquinolone-resistant *Helicobacter pylori* infections in a prospective study. Clin Gastroenterol Hepatol. 2013;11:802–807.e801.

21. Kadayifci A, Uygun A, Polat Z, Kantarcioglu M, Kilciler G, Baser O, Ozcan A, Emer O. Comparison of bismuth-containing quadruple and concomitant therapies as a first-line treatment option for *Helicobacter pylori*. Turkish J Gastroenterol. 2012;23:8–13.

22. Cetinkaya ZA, Sezikli M, Guzelbulut F, Cosgun S, Duzgun S, Kurdas OO. Comparison of the efficacy of the two tetracycline-containing sequential therapy regimens for the eradication of *Helicobacter pylori*: 5 days versus 14 days amoxicillin. Helicobacter. 2010;15:143–7.

23. Chi CH, Lin CY, Sheu BS, Yang HB, Huang AH, Wu JJ. Quadruple therapy containing amoxicillin and tetracycline is an effective regimen to rescue failed triple therapy by overcoming the antimicrobial resistance of *Helicobacter pylori*. Aliment Pharmacol Ther. 2003;18:347–53.

24. Kim SE, Park YS, Kim N, Kim MS, Jo HJ, Shin CM, Lee SH, Hwang JH, Kim JW, Jeong SH, et al. Effect of *Helicobacter pylori* Eradication on Functional Dyspepsia. J Neurogastroenterol Motility. 2013;19:233–43.

25. Megraud F, Coenen S, Versporten A, Kist M, Lopez-Brea M, Hirschl AM, Andersen LP, Goossens H, Glupczynski Y. *Helicobacter pylori* resistance to antibiotics in Europe and its relationship to antibiotic consumption. Gut. 2013;62:34–42.

26. Boyanova L, Mitov I. Geographic map and evolution of primary *Helicobacter pylori* resistance to antibacterial agents. Exp Rev Anti-infect Ther. 2010;8:59–70.

27. Vakil N, Vaira D. Treatment for *H. pylori* infection: new challenges with antimicrobial resistance. J Clin Gastroenterol. 2013;47:383 8.

28. Gomollon F, Sicilia B, Ducons JA, Sierra E, Revillo MJ, Ferrero M. Third line treatment for *Helicobacter pylori*: a prospective, culture-guided study in peptic ulcer patients. Aliment Pharmacol Ther. 2000;14:1335–8.

29. Perri F, Festa V, Merla A, Quitadamo M, Clemente R, Andriulli A. Amoxicillin/ tetracycline combinations are inadequate as alternative therapies for *Helicobacter pylori* infection. Helicobacter. 2002;7:99–104.

30. Lv ZF, Wang FC, Zheng HL, Wang B, Xie Y, Zhou XJ, Lv NH. Meta-analysis: is combination of tetracycline and amoxicillin suitable for *Helicobacter pylori* infection? World J Gastroenterol. 2015;21:2522–33.

31. Uygun A, Ozel AM, Yildiz O, Aslan M, Yesilova Z, Erdil A, Bagci S, Gunhan O. Comparison of three different second-line quadruple therapies including bismuth subcitrate in Turkish patients with non-ulcer dyspepsia who failed to eradicate *Helicobacter pylori* with a 14-day standard first-line therapy. J Gastroenterol Hepatol. 2008;23:42–5.

32. Malfertheiner P, Bazzoli F, Delchier JC, Celinski K, Giguere M, Riviere M, Megraud F. Helicobacter pylori eradication with a capsule containing bismuth subcitrate potassium, metronidazole, and tetracycline given with omeprazole versus clarithromycin-based triple therapy: a randomised, open-label, non-inferiority, phase 3 trial. Lancet. 2011;377(9769):905–13.

33. Levison ME. Pharmacodynamics of antimicrobial agents. Bactericidal and postantibiotic effects. Infect Dis Clin North Am. 1995;9:483–95.

34. Adir J, Barr WH. Dose-dependent bioavailability of tetracycline in man. J Pharmacokinet Biopharm. 1978;6:99–110.

35. Liu P, Muller M, Derendorf H. Rational dosing of antibiotics: the use of plasma concentrations versus tissue concentrations. Intern J Antimicrob Agents. 2002;19:285–90.

10

Changes in plasma ghrelin and leptin levels in patients with peptic ulcer and gastritis following eradication of *Helicobacter pylori* infection

Chika Kasai[1], Kazushi Sugimoto[2,3*], Isao Moritani[1], Junichiro Tanaka[1], Yumi Oya[1], Hidekazu Inoue[1], Masahiko Tameda[2,3], Katsuya Shiraki[1], Masaaki Ito[4], Yoshiyuki Takei[3] and Kojiro Takase[1]

Abstract

Background: *Helicobacter pylori* (*H. pylori*) infection and eradication therapy have been known to influence gastric ghrelin and leptin secretion, which may lead to weight gain. However, the exact relationship between plasma ghrelin/leptin levels and *H. pylori* infection has remained controversial. The aim of this study was to investigate plasma ghrelin and leptin levels in *H. pylori*-positive and -negative patients, to compare the two levels of the hormones before and after *H. pylori* eradication, and to examine the correlation between body mass index (BMI) and active ghrelin or leptin levels, as well as that between atrophic pattern and active ghrelin or leptin levels.

Methods: Seventy-two *H. pylori*-positive patients who underwent upper gastrointestinal endoscopy, 46 diagnosed as having peptic ulcer and 26 as atrophic gastritis, were enrolled. Control samples were obtained from 15 healthy *H. pylori*-negative volunteers. The extent of atrophic change of the gastric mucosa was assessed endoscopically. Body weight was measured and blood was collected before and 12 weeks after *H. pylori* eradication therapy. Blood samples were taken between 8 and 10 AM after an overnight fast.

Results: Plasma ghrelin levels were significantly lower in *H. pylori*-positive patients than in *H. pylori*-negative patients. In particular, plasma active ghrelin levels were significantly lower in patients with gastritis compared with patients with peptic ulcer. Plasma ghrelin levels decreased after *H. pylori* eradication in both peptic ulcer and gastritis patients, while plasma leptin levels increased only in peptic ulcer patients. Plasma leptin levels and BMI were positively correlated, and active ghrelin levels and atrophic pattern were weakly negatively correlated in peptic ulcer patients.

Conclusion: *H. pylori* infection and eradication therapy may affect circulating ghrelin/leptin levels. This finding suggests a relationship between gastric mucosal injury induced by *H. pylori* infection and changes in plasma ghrelin and leptin levels.

Keywords: Plasma Ghrelin and Leptin, *Helicobacter pylori*, Eradication

* Correspondence: kazushi@clin.medic.mie-u.ac.jp
[2]Department of Molecular and Laboratory Medicine, Mie University School of Medicine, 2-174 Edobashi, Tsu, Mie 514-8507, Japan
[3]Department of Gastroenterology and Hepatology, Mie University School of Medicine, Tsu, Japan

Background

Helicobacter pylori (*H. pylori*), a Gram-negative, spiral-shaped bacterium that colonizes the stomach, is a major cause of atrophic and chronic gastritis, peptic ulcers, and gastric malignant lesions such as mucosa-associated lymphoid tissue lymphoma and adenocarcinoma [1–3]. Eradication of *H. pylori* reduces the relapse rate of peptic ulcer [4] and the incidence of gastric cancer [5]. However, much attention has recently been paid to the inverse relationship of *H. pylori* infection and obesity [6, 7].

Appetite and energy expenditure are regulated mainly by two hormones, ghrelin and leptin, produced in the gastric mucosa, which may be modified by *H. pylori* colonization [8]. Ghrelin, a 28-amino acid, novel appetite-stimulating peptide produced predominantly by the stomach, is thought to be a strong growth hormone releaser [9]. Ghrelin exists in two different forms: acylated ghrelin, octanoylated, in serine3 (active ghrelin), and desacyl-ghrelin, without the octanoyl group [10]. Active ghrelin has a short half-life, and once released, it will be subsequently converted to desacyl-ghrelin [11]. Activation of ghrelin occurs via the enzyme ghrelin O-acyltransferase (GOAT) which is responsible for adding an N-octanoylated serine in potion 3 to the proghrelin peptide [12]. Desacyl-ghrelin is notably less potent on the GHS-receptor than active ghrelin [13]. It is generally known that these two forms of ghrelin have differential effects in the tissues. While active ghrelin has been implicated in the control of food intake and shown to evoke weight gain by actions in the hypothalamus [14, 15], desacyl-ghrelin is thought to be also involved in energy balance in some way, but its exact role is unknown. On the other hand, leptin is a 16-kDa protein, a product of the Ob gene, secreted primarily from adipose tissue cells [16]. It has recently been found that leptin is also present in gastric mucosa [17–19]. This hormone plays a role of mediator in the long-term regulation of energy balance, suppressing food intake, and thereby inducing weight loss [8, 20].

A number of studies have reported the relationship between plasma ghrelin/leptin levels and the effects of *H. pylori* infection and eradication. A study by Nwokolo et al., first reporting on the possible relationship between ghrelin and the effect of *H. pylori* eradication, showed that cure of *H. pylori* increased plasma ghrelin levels in healthy asymptomatic subjects, which in turn may lead to increased appetite and weight gain [21]. In contrast, some studies reported that plasma ghrelin levels decreased following *H. pylori* eradication [22, 23]. Nonetheless, a number of other studies showed that *H. pylori* infection and/or eradication therapy had no effect on ghrelin levels [24, 25] and leptin levels [26]. In addition, Azuma et al. reported that gastric leptin expression was significantly increased by *H. pylori* infection, and gastric leptin expression was reduced after *H. pylori* eradication,

but serum leptin levels did not change significantly after cure of *H. pylori* infection [27]. It has been thought that the relationships between *H. pylori* and production of these hormones are regulated by the *H. pylori* strain [28], the extent of atrophic gastritis induced by *H. pylori* infection [29], the duration of follow-up, and other unexplained factors. However, the exact mechanism by which *H. pylori* eradication may interface with plasma ghrelin and leptin to affect body weight has remained unknown.

Therefore, in the present study, plasma ghrelin and leptin levels were measured in *H. pylori*-positive and -negative patients, and the levels of the two hormones were compared before and after *H. pylori* eradication. Furthermore, the correlations between body mass index (BMI) and active ghrelin or leptin levels and between atrophic pattern and active ghrelin or leptin levels were also examined.

Methods

Human subjects

The study subjects were 72 *H. pylori*-positive patients referred for upper gastrointestinal endoscopy at Mie Prefectural General Medical Center, Yokkaichi, Japan, between November 2011 and October 2014. The subjects' diagnoses were duodenal and gastric ulcer in 46 and atrophic gastritis in 26. Control samples were obtained from 15 healthy *H. pylori*-negative volunteers. All patients and controls received an explanation of the procedures and possible risks associated with the study and gave their written, informed consent to participate. This study was performed in conformity with the Declaration of Helsinki and was approved by our institutional ethics committee (authorization number 2011-4, Mie Prefectural General Medical Center, Yokkaichi, Japan). The exclusion criteria were pregnancy, BMI >30 kg/m^2, diabetes mellitus, cachectic state including advanced cancer, systemic infection, thyroid and liver disease, renal impairment, use of medications effective against *H. pylori* during the preceding 3 months, history of eradication therapy before the study, and history of previous gastric surgery.

Eradication therapy and data collection

H. pylori-positive patients received triple therapy with lansoprazole 30 mg, amoxicillin 750 mg, and clarithromycin 200 mg twice per day for 7 days after the endoscopic examination. Body weight was measured and blood was collected before and 12 weeks after the treatment. Blood samples were taken between 8 and 10 AM after an overnight fast, transferred into BD™ P800 tubes (Becton-Dickinson, Franklin Lakes, NJ) containing spray-dried K$_2$EDTA anticoagulant and a proprietary cocktail of protease, esterase, and dipeptidyl peptidase 4 (DPP-4) inhibitors. The collected samples were centrifuged at

1100–1300 × g for 10 min, and plasma was separated and stored at -80 °C until assay.

Endoscopic diagnosis of atrophic gastritis

Endoscopic diagnosis of gastric mucosal atrophy was performed using the Kimura-Takemoto classification of atrophic pattern [30]. According to this classification, gastric mucosal atrophy is classified as closed-type if an atrophic boundary exists between the fundic mucosa and the pyloric mucosa in the antrum or lesser curvature of the gastric body. In the C-0 type, there are no atrophic changes. In the C-1 type, there are atrophic changes visible only in the antrum. In the C-2 type, the atrophic borders exist on the lesser curvature of the lower portion of the stomach body. In the C-3 type, atrophic borders are found on the lesser curvature of the upper portion of the stomach body. On the other hand, atrophy is classified as open type if an atrophic border lies in the lateral wall or greater curvature of the gastric body. In the O-1 type, atrophic borders are found between the lesser curvature and the lateral wall of the gastric body. In the O-2 type, atrophic changes are spread along the lateral wall. In the O-3 type, a border exists between the lateral wall and the greater curvature.

Schedule of examinations for H. pylori infection

Endoscopic examination and determination of *H. pylori* infection were performed by RUT (Pyloritek, Serim Laboratories, Elkhart, IN) before treatment. The success of the *H. pylori* eradication therapy was assessed by ImmunoCard STAT!®HpSA®Stool antigen test (Meridian Bioscience Inc., Cincinnati, OH) 12 weeks after the cessation of therapy.

Hormone assays

ELISA kits were used for the measurement of active serum ghrelin (SCETI K.K., Tokyo, Japan), des-acyl serum ghrelin (SCETI K.K.), and leptin (Cosmic Corporation, Tokyo, Japan). Serum levels of both ghrelin and leptin were measured and calculated according to the manufacturer instructions. Ghrelin levels are expressed as fmol/mL and leptin levels as ng/ml.

Statistical analysis

Continuous variables were compared using the Kruskal-Wallis test or the Mann-Whitney test (two-sided), and categorical variables were compared using Fisher's exact test. Paired measures of plasma ghrelin and leptin levels were analyzed using the Wilcoxon signed-rank test. Ghrelin/leptin levels and BMI or atrophic pattern were assessed for correlations with Pearson correlation coefficients. All statistical analyses were performed with IBM SPSS software Ver. 22. Data are expressed as mean ± SD. *P* values less than 0.05 were considered significant.

Results

Baseline characteristics

The characteristics of the subjects are shown in Table 1. A total of 72 *H. pylori*-positive patients (46 peptic ulcer and 26 atrophic gastritis) and 15 healthy *H. pylori*-negative volunteers were studied. There were no significant differences in BMI between each pair of groups. They included 20 current smokers and 31 alcohol drinkers. There were no differences in laboratory data (data not shown). *H. pylori* eradication was successful in 39 of 46 peptic ulcer patients and 18 of 26 atrophic gastritis patients who received eradication therapy.

Ghrelin and leptin levels at the initial assessment

Plasma active ghrelin levels were significantly lower in patients with gastritis than in patients with peptic ulcer (Fig. 1a). Notably, plasma desacyl-ghrelin levels were significantly higher in *H. pylori*-negative control patients than in *H. pylori*-positive patients (both peptic ulcer and gastritis) (Fig. 1b). With regard to plasma leptin levels, no significant differences were found between each pair of three groups (Fig. 1c). Since plasma ghrelin levels were affected by the presence or absence of *H. pylori*, whether *H. pylori* eradication affects BMI and circulating ghrelin/leptin levels, as well as whether the treatment regulates the levels of these two hormones to those of *H. pylori*-negative patients, was evaluated.

Changes in BMI after H. pylori eradication

There were no significant changes in BMI in after *H. pylori* eradication in both peptic ulcer and gastritis groups, regardless of its success (data not shown).

Ghrelin and leptin levels at the initial and 12th week assessment

Whereas significant changes in BMI were not found in patients after successful *H. pylori* eradication, altered levels of circulating ghrelin and leptin were observed. In peptic ulcer patients, although not significant in all cases, ghrelin levels decreased after *H. pylori* eradication (Fig. 2a and b). There was a significant increase in leptin levels in both successfully and unsuccessfully eradicated patients (Fig. 2c). In the case of gastritis patients, there

Table 1 Demographic and clinical characteristics of the study groups

	Control	Peptic Ulcer	Chronic Gastritis	P value
	N = 15	N = 46	N = 26	
Age	45.9 ± 9.3	53.0 ± 15.6	60.8 ± 11.7	0.001
Gender, M: n (%)	6 (40 %)	32 (69.5 %)	10 (38.5 %)	0.017
BMI (kg/m²)	21.7 ± 2.2	23.0 ± 3.4	22.1 ± 2.9	0.260

P values are based on Kruskal-Wallis test or the Mann-Whitney test (two-sided) for continuous variables and Fisher' exact test for categorical variable
BMI body mass index

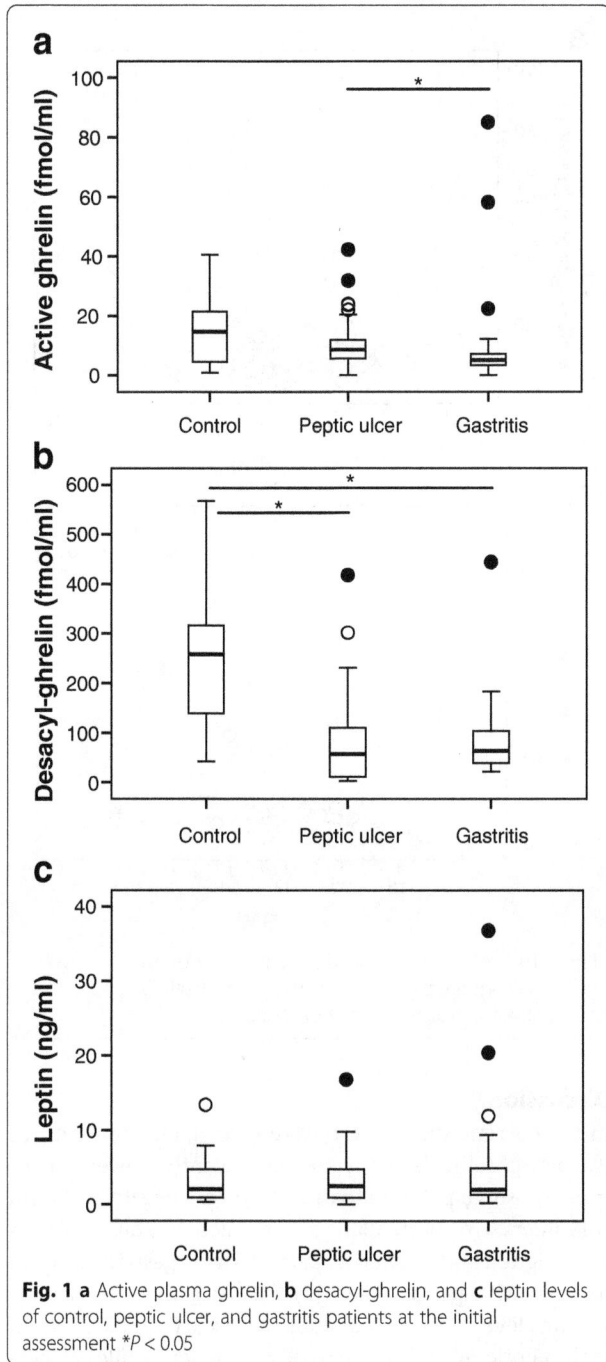

Fig. 1 a Active plasma ghrelin, **b** desacyl-ghrelin, and **c** leptin levels of control, peptic ulcer, and gastritis patients at the initial assessment *P < 0.05

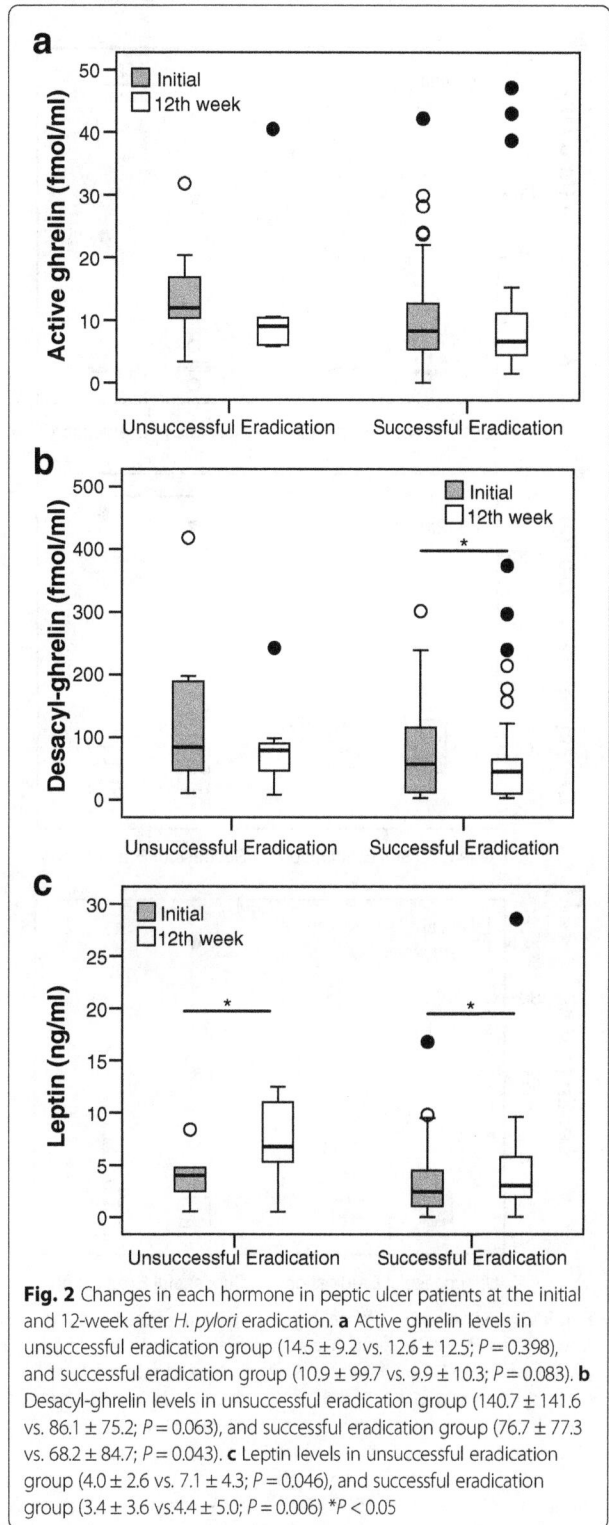

Fig. 2 Changes in each hormone in peptic ulcer patients at the initial and 12-week after *H. pylori* eradication. **a** Active ghrelin levels in unsuccessful eradication group (14.5 ± 9.2 vs. 12.6 ± 12.5; *P* = 0.398), and successful eradication group (10.9 ± 99.7 vs. 9.9 ± 10.3; *P* = 0.083). **b** Desacyl-ghrelin levels in unsuccessful eradication group (140.7 ± 141.6 vs. 86.1 ± 75.2; *P* = 0.063), and successful eradication group (76.7 ± 77.3 vs. 68.2 ± 84.7; *P* = 0.043). **c** Leptin levels in unsuccessful eradication group (4.0 ± 2.6 vs. 7.1 ± 4.3; *P* = 0.046), and successful eradication group (3.4 ± 3.6 vs.4.4 ± 5.0; *P* = 0.006) *P < 0.05

was a significant decrease in ghrelin levels in eradicated patients (Fig. 3a and b), while no changes were found in leptin levels (Fig. 3c).

Relationships between BMI and active ghrelin or leptin levels

Although the initial active ghrelin levels and BMI were not correlated, the initial plasma leptin levels and BMI were positively correlated ($r = 0.420$, $P < 0.001$) (Fig. 4). This correlation might be attributed to the fact that leptin is secreted primarily from adipose tissue cells.

Relationships between atrophic pattern and active ghrelin or leptin levels

Although not significant, the initial active ghrelin levels showed a weak negative correlation with atrophic pattern in peptic ulcer patients, but no correlation

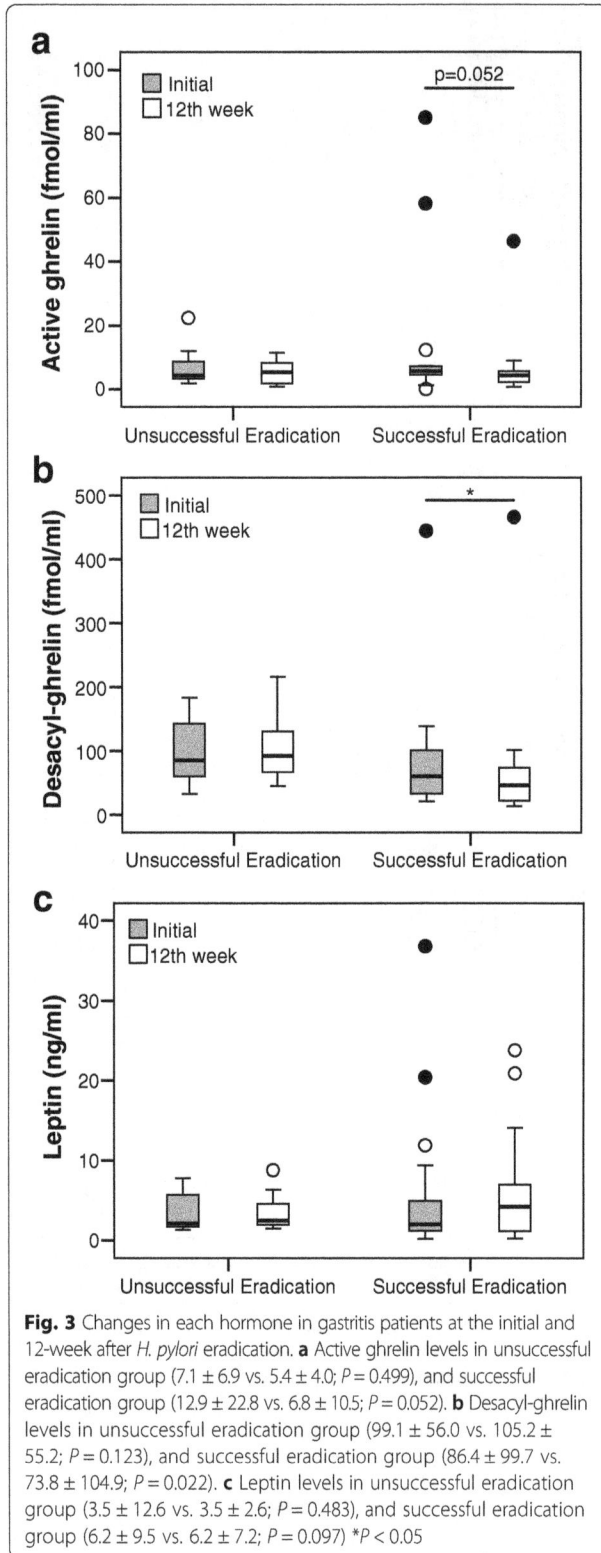

Fig. 3 Changes in each hormone in gastritis patients at the initial and 12-week after *H. pylori* eradication. **a** Active ghrelin levels in unsuccessful eradication group (7.1 ± 6.9 vs. 5.4 ± 4.0; $P = 0.499$), and successful eradication group (12.9 ± 22.8 vs. 6.8 ± 10.5; $P = 0.052$). **b** Desacyl-ghrelin levels in unsuccessful eradication group (99.1 ± 56.0 vs. 105.2 ± 55.2; $P = 0.123$), and successful eradication group (86.4 ± 99.7 vs. 73.8 ± 104.9; $P = 0.022$). **c** Leptin levels in unsuccessful eradication group (3.5 ± 12.6 vs. 3.5 ± 2.6; $P = 0.483$), and successful eradication group (6.2 ± 9.5 vs. 6.2 ± 7.2; $P = 0.097$) *$P < 0.05$

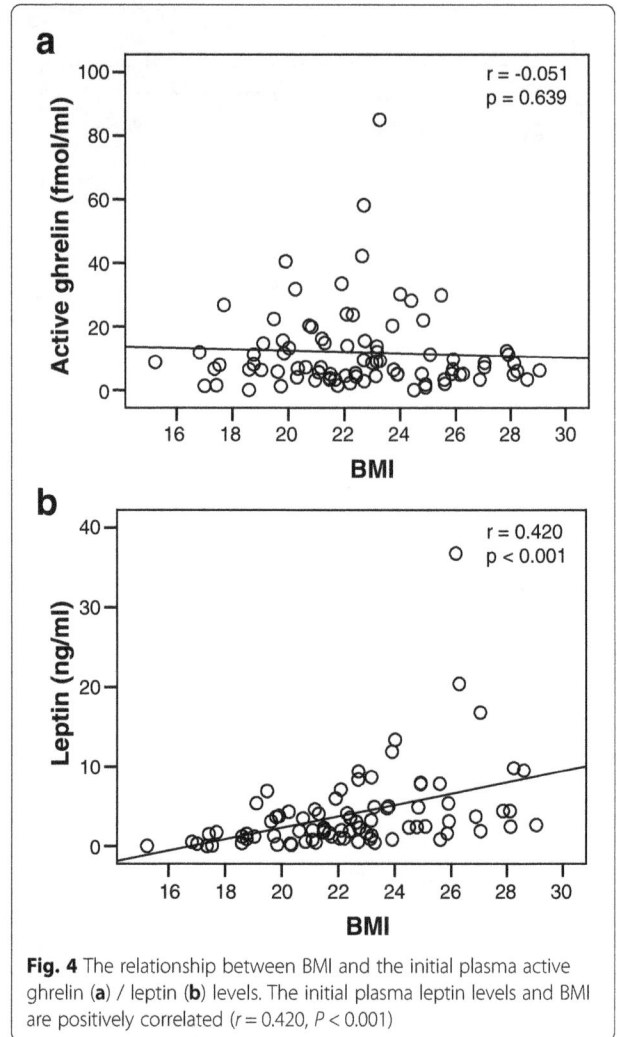

Fig. 4 The relationship between BMI and the initial plasma active ghrelin (**a**) / leptin (**b**) levels. The initial plasma leptin levels and BMI are positively correlated ($r = 0.420$, $P < 0.001$)

Discussion

In the current study, there were three major findings. (i) Plasma ghrelin levels were significantly lower in *H. pylori*-positive patients than in *H. pylori*-negative control volunteers. In particular, plasma active ghrelin levels were significantly lower in patients with gastritis than in patients with peptic ulcer. (ii) Plasma active and desacyl ghrelin levels decreased after *H. pylori* eradication in both peptic ulcer and gastritis patients, while plasma leptin levels increased only in peptic ulcer patients. (iii) Plasma leptin levels and BMI were positively correlated, and the active ghrelin levels and atrophic pattern were weakly negatively correlated in peptic ulcer patients.

In common with previous studies [29, 31–33], plasma ghrelin levels were significantly lower in *H. pylori*-positive patients than in *H. pylori*-negative control volunteers. It seems logical that *H. pylori*-positive patients with atrophic gastric mucosa have low plasma ghrelin levels, considering the negative correlation between active ghrelin levels and atrophic pattern, as also proposed by Kawashima et al

in gastritis patients (Fig. 5a and b). The initial leptin levels showed no correlation with atrophic pattern in peptic ulcer and gastritis patients (Fig. 5c).

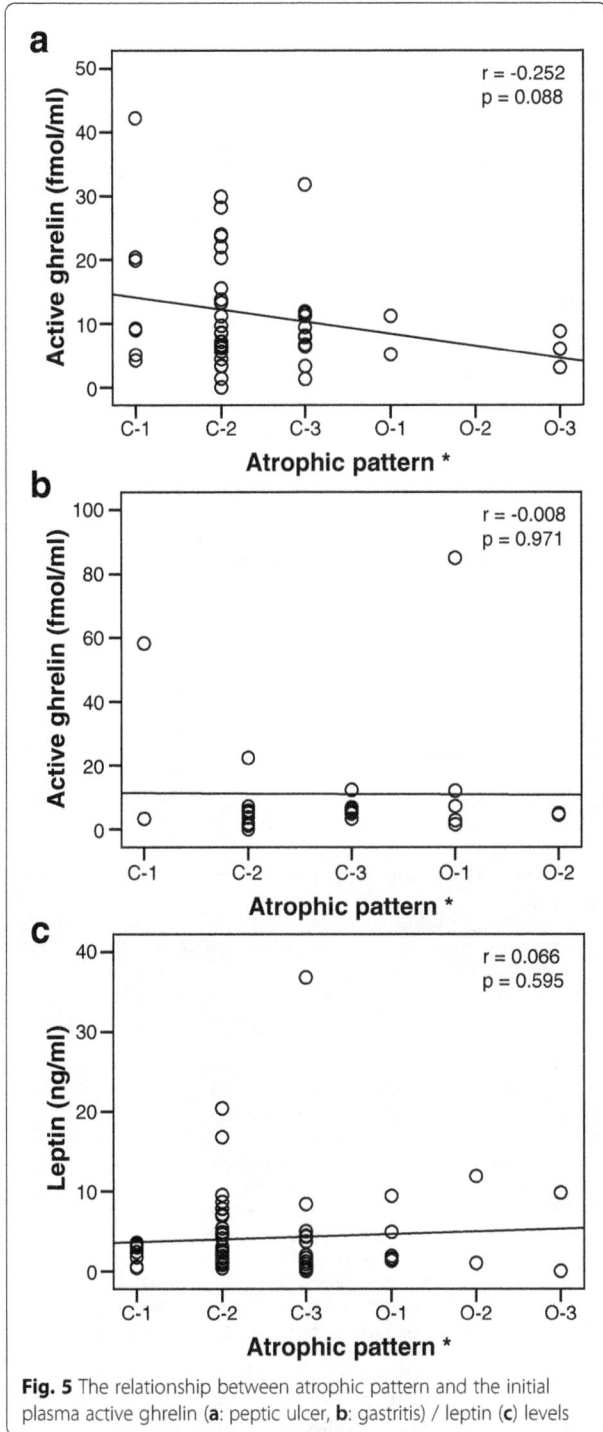

Fig. 5 The relationship between atrophic pattern and the initial plasma active ghrelin (**a**: peptic ulcer, **b**: gastritis) / leptin (**c**) levels

cancer) [34], hence the lower plasma ghrelin levels in *H. pylori*-positive patients than in *H. pylori*-negative patients.

Furthermore, consistent with Suzuki et al.[35] and Isomoto et al.[36], plasma ghrelin levels were significantly lower in patients with gastritis than in those with peptic ulcer. A recent study suggested that plasma ghrelin levels increase in response to severe gastric mucosal oxidative stress induced by acute gastritis and peptic ulcer [37]. These results suggested that long duration of *H. pylori* infection reduced circulating ghrelin levels, presumably by destroying ghrelin-producing cells, and that acute gastric mucosal injury such as peptic ulcer increased circulating ghrelin levels because of stress related to ghrelin secretion.

The effect of *H. pylori* eradication on circulating ghrelin/leptin levels has remained controversial. Nweneka et al. reviewed previous studies on circulating ghrelin levels before and after *H. pylori* eradication in a meta-analysis [38]. Some studies reported that there was no significant difference in circulating ghrelin levels after *H. pylori* eradication [24, 31, 39], while others reported an increase [21, 29, 40] or a decrease [22, 23]. They concluded that *H. pylori* eradication did not have any significant effect on circulating ghrelin levels. On the other hand, Bocian et al. showed that *H. pylori* eradication was associated with increased circulating leptin levels and decreased ghrelin levels, thereby resulting in an increased BMI in many studies [7]. Consistent with Bocian et al. [7], the present results showed that plasma ghrelin levels decreased after *H. pylori* eradication in both peptic ulcer and gastritis patients, and plasma leptin levels increased in peptic ulcer patients. A possible mechanism for decreased levels of plasma ghrelin after *H. pylori* eradication is as follows: before eradication, plasma ghrelin is released transiently into blood due to gastric mucosal oxidative stress and injury induced by *H. pylori* infection, and after eradication, the release of plasma ghrelin decreases in accordance with improvement of gastric mucosal injury. The decreased ghrelin levels in the present study are possibly attributed to the relatively short term of observation and it can be further assumed that the ghrelin levels would return to normal or even higher in a longer-term follow-up observation.

The increase of plasma leptin levels after eradication in peptic ulcer patients needs explanation. Plasma leptin levels and BMI were positively correlated, while there were no significant changes in BMI after eradication in the present study. Previous studies suggested that short-term fasting caused a decline in circulating leptin concentration much greater than the change in adipose mass [41, 42]. Regardless of the success or failure of *H. pylori* eradication, presumably, the suppressed appetite of peptic ulcer patients improved with the healing of the ulcer, which led to increased food intake and increased

[29]. In addition, Isomoto et al. reported that *H. pylori*-positive patients with type I strain (expressing the virulence factors of cytotoxin-associated gene-A and Vacuolating cytotoxin A) have lower circulating ghrelin levels than those with the less virulent type II strain (expressing no virulence factors) [28]. The population analyzed in the present study was a Japanese population with Type I strain (a known contributor to a higher incidence of gastric

plasma leptin levels as a consequence. In contrast, gastritis patients did not show a reduced appetite in the first place. That is probably the reason they exhibited changes neither in dietary behavior, nor in the concomitant plasma leptin levels. We suspect that there is a complex relationship among leptin secretion, adipose tissue mass, and gastric mucosal injury.

Remarkably, in the present study, both ghrelin and leptin levels before/after *H.pylori* eradication were measured in relation to peptic ulcer and gastritis. The most important findings are that our study showed the levels of the hormones changed independently and that the changes differed in peptic ulcer and gastritis patients.

The present study had certain limitations: lack of histological evaluation such as ghrelin/leptin expression in the stomach, small sample size, and short-duration of follow-up. Therefore, we believe further research including histological evaluation will definitely improve our understanding in a future long-term study.

Conclusion

In conclusion, the results of the current study showed that plasma ghrelin levels were significantly lower in *H. pylori*-positive patients than in *H. pylori*-negative patients. Furthermore, plasma active and desacyl ghrelin levels decreased and plasma leptin levels increased after *H. pylori* eradication. However, the precise mechanism remains an open question for research. Further study will be necessary to elucidate the exact effect of *H. pylori* eradication on plasma ghrelin/leptin levels, which may lead to body weight gain and the ultimate development of lifestyle-related diseases.

Abbreviations
BMI: Body mass index; *H. pylori*: Helicobacter pylori

Acknowledgements
The authors would like to thank Mina Tenpaku for her technical assistance.

Funding
Not applicable.

Authors' contributions
Conceived and designed the study: CK KS1 KT. Recruited the subjects: CK IM JT YO HI KT. Wrote the paper CK KS1 MT. Supervised the study; KS2 MI YT KT. KS1 is corresponding to Kazushi Sugimoto, KS2 is corresponding to KS. All authors read and approved the final manuscript.

Competing interests
The authors declare that they have no competing interests.

Consent for publication
Not applicable.

Author details
[1]Department of Gastroenterology, Mie Prefectural General Medical Center, Yokkaichi, Japan. [2]Department of Molecular and Laboratory Medicine, Mie University School of Medicine, 2-174 Edobashi, Tsu, Mie 514-8507, Japan. [3]Department of Gastroenterology and Hepatology, Mie University School of Medicine, Tsu, Japan. [4]Department of Cardiology and Nephrology, Mie University School of Medicine, Tsu, Japan.

References
1. Parsonnet J, Hansen S, Rodriguez L, Gelb AB, Warnke RA, Jellum E, Orentreich N, Vogelman JH, Friedman GD. Helicobacter pylori infection and gastric lymphoma. N Engl J Med. 1994;330(18):1267–71.
2. Uemura N, Okamoto S, Yamamoto S, Matsumura N, Yamaguchi S, Yamakido M, Taniyama K, Sasaki N, Schlemper RJ. Helicobacter pylori infection and the development of gastric cancer. N Engl J Med. 2001;345(11):784–9.
3. Forman D, Newell DG, Fullerton F, Yarnell JW, Stacey AR, Wald N, Sitas F. Association between infection with Helicobacter pylori and risk of gastric cancer: evidence from a prospective investigation. BMJ. 1991;302(6788):1302–5.
4. Gisbert JP, Khorrami S, Carballo F, Calvet X, Gene E, Dominguez-Munoz JE: H. pylori eradication therapy vs. antisecretory non-eradication therapy (with or without long-term maintenance antisecretory therapy) for the prevention of recurrent bleeding from peptic ulcer. Cochrane Database Syst Rev. 2004(2):CD004062. doi:10.1002/14651858.CD004062.pub2.
5. Ford AC, Forman D, Hunt R, Yuan Y, Moayyedi P. Helicobacter pylori eradication for the prevention of gastric neoplasia. Cochrane Database Syst Rev. 2015;7:CD005583.
6. Lender N, Talley NJ, Enck P, Haag S, Zipfel S, Morrison M, Holtmann GJ. Review article: Associations between Helicobacter pylori and obesity–an ecological study. Aliment Pharmacol Ther. 2014;40(1):24–31.
7. Bocian KM, Jagusztyn-Krynicka EK. The controversy over anti-Helicobacter pylori therapy. Pol J Microbiol. 2012;61(4):239–46.
8. Klok MD, Jakobsdottir S, Drent ML. The role of leptin and ghrelin in the regulation of food intake and body weight in humans: a review. Obes Rev. 2007;8(1):21–34.
9. Kojima M, Hosoda H, Date Y, Nakazato M, Matsuo H, Kangawa K. Ghrelin is a growth-hormone-releasing acylated peptide from stomach. Nature. 1999; 402(6762):656–60.
10. Hosoda H, Kojima M, Matsuo H, Kangawa K. Ghrelin and des-acyl ghrelin: two major forms of rat ghrelin peptide in gastrointestinal tissue. Biochem Biophys Res Commun. 2000;279(3):909–13.
11. De Vriese C, Gregoire F, Lema-Kisoka R, Waelbroeck M, Robberecht P, Delporte C. Ghrelin degradation by serum and tissue homogenates: identification of the cleavage sites. Endocrinology. 2004;145(11):4997–5005.
12. Gutierrez JA, Solenberg PJ, Perkins DR, Willency JA, Knierman MD, Jin Z, Witcher DR, Luo S, Onyia JE, Hale JE. Ghrelin octanoylation mediated by an orphan lipid transferase. Proc Natl Acad Sci U S A. 2008;105(17):6320–5.
13. Thompson NM, Gill DA, Davies R, Loveridge N, Houston PA, Robinson IC, Wells T. Ghrelin and des-octanoyl ghrelin promote adipogenesis directly in vivo by a mechanism independent of the type 1a growth hormone secretagogue receptor. Endocrinology. 2004;145(1):234–42.
14. Nakazato M, Murakami N, Date Y, Kojima M, Matsuo H, Kangawa K, Matsukura S. A role for ghrelin in the central regulation of feeding. Nature. 2001;409(6817):194–8.
15. Wren AM, Seal LJ, Cohen MA, Brynes AE, Frost GS, Murphy KG, Dhillo WS, Ghatei MA, Bloom SR. Ghrelin enhances appetite and increases food intake in humans. J Clin Endocrinol Metab. 2001;86(12):5992.
16. Zhang Y, Proenca R, Maffei M, Barone M, Leopold L, Friedman JM. Positional cloning of the mouse obese gene and its human homologue. Nature. 1994; 372(6505):425–32.
17. Bado A, Levasseur S, Attoub S, Kermorgant S, Laigneau JP, Bortoluzzi MN, Moizo L, Lehy T, Guerre-Millo M, Le Marchand-Brustel Y, et al. The stomach is a source of leptin. Nature. 1998;394(6695):790–3.
18. Sobhani I, Bado A, Vissuzaine C, Buyse M, Kermorgant S, Laigneau JP, Attoub S, Lehy T, Henin D, Mignon M, et al. Leptin secretion and leptin receptor in the human stomach. Gut. 2000;47(2):178–83.

19. Guilmeau S, Buyse M, Bado A. Gastric leptin: a new manager of gastrointestinal function. Curr Opin Pharmacol. 2004;4(6):561–6.

20. Trayhurn P, Hoggard N, Mercer JG, Rayner DV. Leptin: fundamental aspects. Int J Obes Relat Metab Disord. 1999;23 Suppl 1:22–8.

21. Nwokolo CU, Freshwater DA, O'Hare P, Randeva HS. Plasma ghrelin following cure of Helicobacter pylori. Gut. 2003;52(5):637–40.

22. Osawa H, Kita H, Ohnishi H, Nakazato M, Date Y, Bowlus CL, Ishino Y, Watanabe E, Shiiya T, Ueno H, et al. Changes in plasma ghrelin levels, gastric ghrelin production, and body weight after Helicobacter pylori cure. J Gastroenterol. 2006;41(10):954–61.

23. Pacifico L, Anania C, Osborn JF, Ferrara E, Schiavo E, Bonamico M, Chiesa C. Long-term effects of Helicobacter pylori eradication on circulating ghrelin and leptin concentrations and body composition in prepubertal children. Eur J Endocrinol. 2008;158(3):323–32.

24. Choe YH, Lee JH, Lee HJ, Paik KH, Jin DK, Song SY, Lee JH. Ghrelin Levels in Gastric Mucosa before and after Eradication of Helicobacter pylori. Gut Liver. 2007;1(2):132–7.

25. Gokcel A, Gumurdulu Y, Kayaselcuk F, Serin E, Ozer B, Ozsahin AK, Guvener N. Helicobacter pylori has no effect on plasma ghrelin levels. Eur J Endocrinol. 2003;148(4):423–6.

26. Chuang CH, Sheu BS, Yang HB, Lee SC, Kao AW, Cheng HC, Chang WL, Yao WJ. Gender difference of circulating ghrelin and leptin concentrations in chronic Helicobacter pylori infection. Helicobacter. 2009;14(1):54–60.

27. Azuma T, Suto H, Ito Y, Ohtani M, Dojo M, Kuriyama M, Kato T. Gastric leptin and Helicobacter pylori infection. Gut. 2001;49(3):324–9.

28. Isomoto H, Nishi Y, Ohnita K, Mizuta Y, Kohno S, Ueno H, Nakazato M. The Relationship between Plasma and Gastric Ghrelin Levels and Strain Diversity in Helicobacter pylori Virulence. Am J Gastroenterol. 2005;100(6):1425–7.

29. Kawashima J, Ohno S, Sakurada T, Takabayashi H, Kudo M, Ro S, Kato S, Yakabi K. Circulating acylated ghrelin level decreases in accordance with the extent of atrophic gastritis. J Gastroenterol. 2009;44(10):1046–54.

30. Kimura K, Takemoto T. An endoscopic recognition of the atrophic border and its significance in chronic gastritis. Endoscopy. 1969;1(03):87–97.

31. Isomoto H, Ueno H, Saenko VA, Mondal MS, Nishi Y, Kawano N, Ohnita K, Mizuta Y, Ohtsuru A, Yamashita S, et al. Impact of Helicobacter pylori infection on gastric and plasma ghrelin dynamics in humans. Am J Gastroenterol. 2005;100(8):1711–20.

32. Osawa H, Nakazato M, Date Y, Kita H, Ohnishi H, Ueno H, Shiiya T, Satoh K, Ishino Y, Sugano K. Impaired production of gastric ghrelin in chronic gastritis associated with Helicobacter pylori. J Clin Endocrinol Metab. 2005;90(1):10–6.

33. Plonka M, Bielanski W, Konturek SJ, Targosz A, Sliwowski Z, Dobrzanska M, Kaminska A, Sito E, Konturek PC, Brzozowski T. Helicobacter pylori infection and serum gastrin, ghrelin and leptin in children of Polish shepherds. Dig Liver Dis. 2006;38(2):91–7.

34. Yamaoka Y, Kodama T, Gutierrez O, Kim JG, Kashima K, Graham DY. Relationship between Helicobacter pylori iceA, cagA, and vacA status and clinical outcome: studies in four different countries. J Clin Microbiol. 1999; 37(7):2274–9.

35. Suzuki H, Masaoka T, Nomoto Y, Hosoda H, Mori M, Nishizawa T, Minegishi Y, Kangawa K, Hibi T. Increased levels of plasma ghrelin in peptic ulcer disease. Aliment Pharmacol Ther. 2006;24(s4):120–6.

36. Isomoto H, Ueno H, Nishi Y, Yasutake T, Tanaka K, Kawano N, Ohnita K, Mizuta Y, Inoue K, Nakazato M, et al. Circulating ghrelin levels in patients with various upper gastrointestinal diseases. Dig Dis Sci. 2005;50(5):833–8.

37. Suzuki H, Matsuzaki J, Hibi T. Ghrelin and oxidative stress in gastrointestinal tract. J Clin Biochem Nutr. 2011;48(2):122–5.

38. Nweneka CV, Prentice AM. Helicobacter pylori infection and circulating ghrelin levels - a systematic review. BMC Gastroenterol. 2011;11:7.

39. Lee ES, Yoon YS, Park CY, Kim HS, Um TH, Baik HW, Jang EJ, Lee S, Park HS, Oh SW. Eradication of Helicobacter pylori increases ghrelin mRNA expression in the gastric mucosa. J Korean Med Sci. 2010;25(2):265–71.

40. Czesnikiewicz-Guzik M, Loster B, Bielanski W, Guzik TJ, Konturek PC, Zapala J, Konturek SJ. Implications of oral Helicobacter pylori for the outcome of its gastric eradication therapy. J Clin Gastroenterol. 2007;41(2):145–51.

41. Weigle DS, Duell PB, Connor WE, Steiner RA, Soules MR, Kuijper JL. Effect of fasting, refeeding, and dietary fat restriction on plasma leptin levels. J Clin Endocrinol Metab. 1997;82(2):561–5.

42. Kolaczynski JW, Considine RV, Ohannesian J, Marco C, Opentanova I, Nyce MR, Myint M, Caro JF. Responses of leptin to short-term fasting and refeeding in humans: a link with ketogenesis but not ketones themselves. Diabetes. 1996;45(11):1511–5.

11

Analyzing the influence of gastric intestinal metaplasia on gastric ulcer healing in *Helicobacter pylori*–infected patients without atrophic gastritis

Li-Wei Chen[1], Liang-Che Chang[2], Chung-Ching Hua[3], Bor-Jen Hsieh[1], Shuo-Wei Chen[1] and Rong-Nan Chien[1*]

Abstract

Background: Gastric epithelial hyper-proliferation was reported in patients with *Helicobacter pylori* (*H. pylori*)–infected gastric mucosa with intestinal metaplasia (IM) changes. In patients with gastric ulcer (GU) and IM, the GU may have a different healing rate in comparison to patients without IM. This study aimed to compare the difference in GU healing between *H. pylori*–infected patients with IM and those without IM.

Methods: We retrospectively analyzed patients at the Keelung Chung Gung Memorial Hospital during the period from March 2005 to January 2011. The inclusion criteria were: 1) endoscopic findings of GU and biopsy histological examination plus rapid urease test indicating *H. pylori* infection; 2) gastric IM adjacent to a GU but with no atrophic gastritis changes; 3) patients receiving *H. pylori* eradication triple therapy and 8 weeks of maintenance therapy with a proton pump inhibitor; and 4) patients receiving follow-up endoscopy within the 3rd and the 4th months after treatment.

Results: In total, 327 patients with GU and *H. pylori* infection (136 with IM and 191 without IM) were included. Patients with IM had a higher GU healing rate than those without IM (91.9% vs. 84.3%, $P = 0.040$). Multivariate logistical regression analysis revealed that failure of *H. pylori* eradication (Odds = 4.013, 95% CI: 1.840–8.951, $P < 0.001$) and gastric IM (Odds = 0.369, 95% CI: 0.168–0.812, $P = 0.013$) were the predictors of non-healing GU following treatment.

Conclusions: Patient with gastric IM change may have a higher GU healing rate than those without gastric IM. However, successful *H. pylori* eradication is a more important factor for GU healing than gastric IM.

Keywords: *Helicobacter pylori*, Intestinal metaplasia, Peptic ulcer

Background

Intestinal metaplasia (IM) is a common finding in patients with *Helicobacter pylori* (*H. pylori*) infection. The prevalence of IM in patients with *H. pylori* infection is 30–40% in patients approximately 50 years old [1, 2]. Some studies revealed that the Wingless-Int (Wnt)/β catenin pathway plays an important role in the progression of *H. pylori*-related IM [3–6]. The Wnt signal transduction pathway is also important in intestinal epithelial homeostasis, wound repair and epithelial proliferation [7]. Gastric epithelial hyperproliferation has been observed in patients with gastritis and IM caused by *H. pylori* infection [8–11]. Epithelial cell proliferation is one of the mechanisms governing the repair of a gastric ulcer (GU) [12–14]. Patients with a condition of IM near the GU might have a different outcome of GU healing due to gastric mucosal hyperproliferation. To the best of our knowledge, no study has analyzed whether IM influences GU healing or *H. pylori* eradication. This study aimed to compare the difference in GU healing between *H. pylori*–infected patients with and those without IM adjacent to the GU.

---

* Correspondence: ronald@cgmh.org.tw
[1]Departments of Gastroenterology and Hepatology, Chang-Gung Memorial Hospital and University, 12F, No 222, Mai-Jin Road, Keelung, Taiwan

Methods

We retrospectively analyzed the clinical presentations, endoscopic findings and pathologic records of all patients treated for peptic ulcers at Keelung Chang Gung Memorial Hospital from March 2005 to January 2011. The inclusion criteria in the study were: patients with esophagogastroduodenoscopy (EGD) evidence of active GU in the gastric antrum or body; patients with histological findings by GU biopsy and rapid urease tests indicating *H. pylori* infection with or without IM change; patients who received standard triple therapy (including proton pump inhibitor (PPI), lansoprazole 30 mg or esomerpazole 40 mg, 1 g amoxicillin, and 500 mg clarithromycin twice daily for 7 days) and 8 weeks of maintenance PPI therapy; and patients receiving follow-up EGD and undergoing a rapid urease test and a histological study within the 3rd and the 4th month following treatment. The exclusion criteria were patients receiving PPI or antibiotics two weeks before any of the follow-up EGD studies, and patients taking non-steroid anti-inflammatory drugs (NSAIDs) or aspirin during the healing phase.

If a patient had several EGD studies, only the findings of the 1st and 2nd (follow-up) EGD studies were included in the analysis. The exclusion criteria included patients with underlying malignancy, gastric malignancy revealed by GU biopsy or dysplasia change detected via GU biopsy. In some patients, long-term *H. pylori* infection will induce a progressive gastric atrophy including loss of acid-producing parietal cells. Gastric atrophy leads to lowered gastric acid output which might influence GU healing [15]. Moreover, this study aimed to elucidate the influence of IM adjacent to GU on GU healing and the data of intra-gastric pH could not be available in this retrospective study. Patients with gastric mucosal atrophy according to the results of GU biopsy were also excluded to avoid low gastric acid interfering with GU healing in this study.

Endoscopic study

Patients who experienced epigastric pain, dyspepsia or acid reflux symptoms received EGD. Wide base ulcer was defined as GU base more than 1.5 cm in size. During the EGD study, GU biopsies (4 specimens from each GU margin mucosa, another specimen from the gastric antrum and one from the incisura angularis of corpus) were obtained except in patients with active ulcer bleeding or NSAID-related shallow ulcers. The rapid urease test (RUT) was administered to confirm the presence of *H. pylori* infection. Patients with positive results from both the histological examination and RUT test were included. In patients who had completed standard triple therapy for *H. pylori* eradication and maintenance PPI therapy, EGD was performed between the 3rd and the

4th month after treatment to evaluate the status of gastric ulcer healing and *H. pylori* eradication success. Therefore, biopsies were repeated for histological analysis and RUT, likewise to the initial EGD. Three stages of GU were defined by endoscopy, based on the cycle of ulcer formation and resolution. Gastric healed ulcer in this study was defined as the regeneration of epithelium that completely covered the floor of the ulcer (scarring status), replacing the white coating ulcer base. Patients with partially healing GU (not scarring status) or active GU detected in the following EGD were recognized as persistent GU in this study.

Histology and immunohistochemical (IHC) stain for *H. pylori* detection

All patients received GU biopsy for histology (hematoxylin and eosin) and IHC staining (polyclone, Zytomed Systems GmbH, Berlin, Germany) to evaluate *H. pylori* infection status. Histological sections of all biopsies were routinely examined to determine *H. pylori* infection, IM, atrophic gastritis and malignancy. Atrophy of the gastric mucosa was defined as loss of glandular tissue and mucosal thinning changes. IM was detected on the basis of the morphological features in the stomach observed by performing H & E and Alcian blue staining [16–18]. This study applied the most widely used classification, in which there are two types of IM:

1) Complete type IM: presence of small intestinal-type mucosa with goblet cells, a brush border and eosinophilic enterocytes.
2) Incomplete type IM: presence of colonic epithelium with multiple, irregular mucin droplets of variable size in the cytoplasm and absence of a brush border.

IM was scored according to the visual analog scale of the updated Sydney classification [16]. The results of the histological analyses were reviewed by a single experienced pathologist (Dr. Chang LC).

Rapid urease test (RUT)

RUT (Pronto dry test; Medical Instruments Corporation, Switzerland) was performed. The sensitivity and specificity of RUT for detecting *H. pylori* infection were 99 and 96%, respectively [19].

Antigen Ki-67 stain for epithelial cell proliferation

For patients with adequate residual biopsy specimens from GU margin after staining with an *H. pylori* antibody, an additional Ki-67 IHC stain was applied to assess cell proliferation. Antigen Ki-67 IHC staining was performed using DAKO autostain agent (Cytomation, Carpinteria, CA). REAL EnVision Detection System,

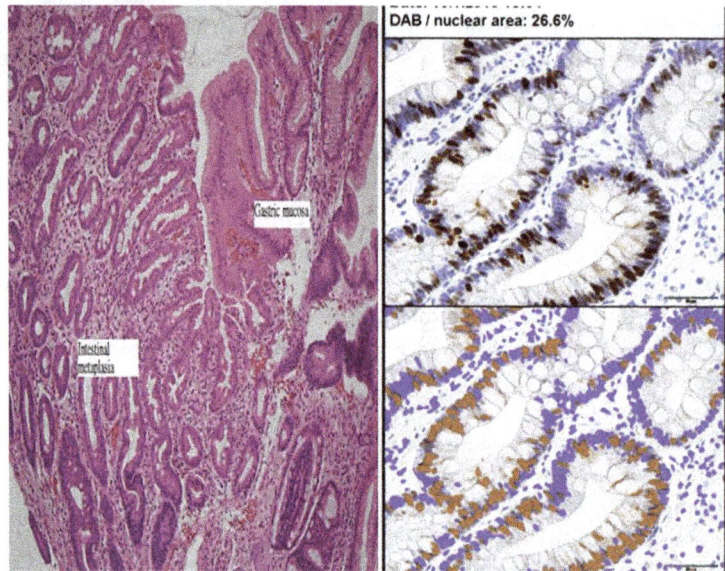

Fig. 1 *Left* side: Photomicrographs of gastric intestinal metaplasia. Gastric mucosa on the left show intestinal metaplasia with histological features similar to the small bowel epithelium. Gastric mucosa lined by foveolar cells at the right upper portion. (Hematoxylin and eosin stain; 100×). *Right* side: ImmunoRatio was applied to calculate the percentage of positively stained nuclear area (labeling index, DAB: diaminobenzidine area) among the background hematoxylin stain area (Ki-67 index: DAB/nuclear area = 26.6% in this slide)

Peroxidase/diaminobenzidine (DAB) (K5007, DAKO) was used to visualize the staining.

Digital data analysis

Digital data analysis was performed with computer software to prevent manual or inter-observer bias for the Ki-67 index score counting. The digital data analysis was processed with ImageJ (1.45i) [20]. The color deconvolution plug-in was used to separate the stains into two 8-bit component images: the DAB image and the hematoxylin image. The DAB image was used for density measurement. We calculated the percentage of positively stained nuclei (labeling index) by using a color deconvolution algorithm to separate the staining

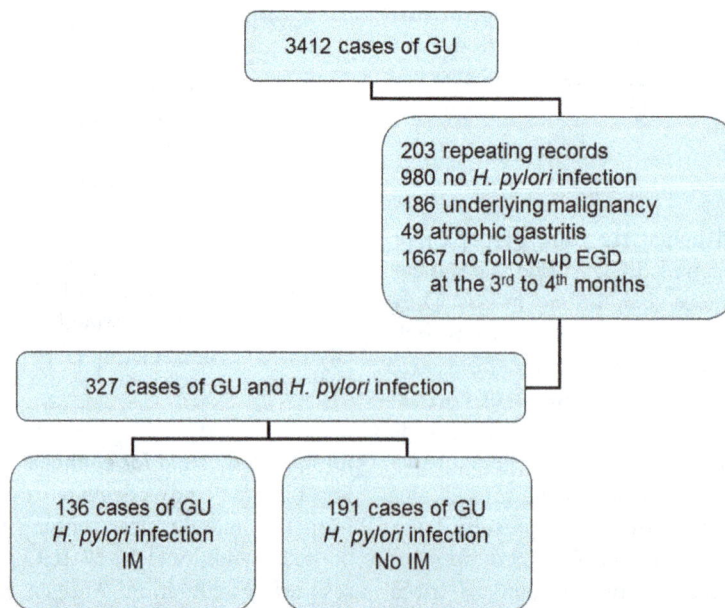

Fig. 2 Case selection flow chart. GU: gastric ulcer; EGD: esophagogastroduodenoscopy; IM: intestinal metaplasia

components and an adaptive threshold for nuclear area segmentation (Fig. 1, right side) [21]. Five pictures from the targeted gastric epithelium adjacent to GU were applied for digital data analysis. The result was recorded as a mean Ki-67 labeling index (%).

Statistical methods

To the best of our knowledge, there are no previous reports on peptic ulcer-healing rate or *H. pylori* eradication rate following PPI administration in patients with GU and IM. Because GU patients with *H. pylori* infection and IM exhibit gastric epithelial hyperproliferation, the null hypothesis was that patients with IM had a higher rate of GU scarring (prediction: 95%) than patients without IM (80% in our previous study) following standard triple eradication and PPI therapy [18]. To obtain a power of 0.8 at the significant level of 0.05, the minimal required number of patients was 70 for each

Table 1 Demographics and other characteristics of patients with gastric ulcer and *H. pylori* infections

Characteristic	IM	No IM	P value
Number	136	191	
Age (years)*	63.3 ± 12.1	59. 3 ± 13.4	0.006
Gender (F/M)	58/78	74/117	0.478
Symptoms			
Abdominal pain	100 (73.5%)	149 (78.0%)	0.349
Abdominal fullness	54 (39.7%)	82 (42.9%)	0.560
GERD	14 (10.3%)	17 (8.9%)	0.672
Personal history			
Smoking	32 (23.5%)	49 (25.7%)	0.661
Alcohol	24 (17.6%)	32 (16.8%)	0.833
Co morbidity			
Cirrhosis	6 (4.4%)	11 (5.8%)	0.589
Uremia	5 (3.7%)	7 (3.7%)	0.996
Diabetic mellitus	28 (20.6%)	34 (17.8%)	0.526
IM type			
Complete type	14 (10.3%)		
Incomplete type	122 (89.7%)		
Gastric ulcer			
Wide base (>1.5 cm)	23 (16.9%)	21 (11.0%)	0.122
Location			
antrum	62 (45.6%)	101 (52.9%)	0.194
body	74 (54.4%)	90 (47.1%)	0.194
GU-scarring rate	125 (91.9%)	161 (84.3%)	0.040
H. pylori eradication rate	111 (81.6%)	163 (85.3%)	0.368

*Data presented as the mean ± standard deviation; number (%)
IM Intestinal metaplasia, *GERD* Gastro-esophageal reflux disease, *GU-scaring rate* Healed (scarred) gastric ulcer rate (%) following treatment, *H. pylori eradication rate H. pylori* eradication success rate following treatment

Table 2 A correlation analysis among factors of non-healing gastric ulcer, persistent *H. pylori* infection and other factors, data are presented as correlation coefficients (Spearmen's rho)

Variables	NHGU	Persistent Hp
Gender	0.010	0.024
Age	0.126*	0.069
Smoking	−0.025	−0.002
Alcohol	−0.025	−0.046
Cirrhosis	0.078	0.084
Uremia	0.073	−0.042
DM	0.029	0.020
Wide base ulcer	0.013	0.118*
Persistent Hp	0.209*	1.000
IM	−0.113*	0.050
NHGU	1.000	0.209*

DM diabetic mellitus, *Wide base ulcer* gastric ulcer base more than 1.5 cm, *IM* intestinal metaplasia besides the gastric ulcer, *Persistent Hp* persistent *H. pylori* infection after treatment (eradication failure), *NHGU* non-healing gastric ulcer after treatment
*P-value < 0.05

group. Hence, it was reasonable to enroll at least 140 patients in this study.

Continuous data were expressed as the mean ± standard deviation (SD). Continuous data were evaluated using the paired-*t* test if the sample size was more than 30 in each group and the Mann–Whitney test was applied if the sample size was less than 30. The chi-square test was used for nominal data. Categorical data were analyzed with the chi-square test or Fisher's exact test, where appropriate. All statistical tests were 2-tailed. A *P*-value of <0.05 was considered statistically significant. The correlation coefficients such as Pearson's correlation coefficient, Point bi-serial correlation coefficient and Spearman's co-efficiency rho were appropriately chosen based on the data types including numerical, nominal or ordinal data. A multivariate logistic regression analysis was applied for the predictors' evaluation for non-healing GU and persistent *H. pylori* infection after treatment.

Statistical analyses were performed using the Statistical Package for the Social Science software version 16.0 for Windows (SPSS, Chicago, IL, USA).

Table 3 Predictors for non-healing gastric ulcer after treatment according to logistic regression analysis

Variables	Odds ratio (95% CI)	P-value
Age	1.035 (1.007–1.064)	0.015
Persistent Hp	3.924 (1.857–8.294)	<0.001
IM	0.366 (0.170–0.792)	0.011

CI confidence interval

Table 4 Predictors for persistent *H. pylori* infection after treatment according to logistic regression analysis

Variables	Odds ratio (95% CI)	P-value
Wide base ulcer	2.256 (1.053–4.836)	0.036
NHGU	3.808 (1.836–7.896)	<0.001

This research was approved by the Institutional Review Board of the Chang-Gung Memorial Hospital (IRB No: 99-2661B). Written informed consent was obtained from all enrolled subjects in this study.

Results

We initially included 3412 cases of GU, which were diagnosed by EGD and pathologic studies. In total, 136 cases of GU with IM (IM group), and 191 cases of GU without IM (no IM group) were enrolled in the final analysis (Fig. 2). Most patients with gastric IM were of the incomplete type (122/136, 89.7%). Because patients with atrophic mucosa in histological findings were excluded in this study, the majority of patients had minimal foci of IM and were scored as 0 (absent) or 1 (mild) (107/136, 78.7%) by using the Sydney system visual analog scale. Only 29 patients with incomplete IM were scored as 2 (moderate). No patient was scored as 3 (marked).

Demographic and other characteristics of the patients are listed in Table 1. No significant inter-group differences were observed in the distribution of gender, symptoms, personal history, co-morbidities, GU size and location. Patients in the IM group were older than those in the no IM group (mean age, 63.5 ± 12.3 years vs. 59.4 ± 13.4 years, $P = 0.004$). Patients with IM had higher GU-healing rate than those without IM (92.1% vs. 84.3%, $P = 0.036$). However, there were no significant differences in the *H. pylori* eradication rates between the two groups [81.6% (IM group) vs. 85.3% (no IM group), $P = 0.405$]. A subgroup analysis from 274 patients with successful *H. pylori* eradication was performed and the result revealed no significant difference in GU healing rate between patients with IM (104/111, 93.7%) and those without IM (144/163, 88.3%) ($P = 0.125$).

The bivariate correlation test revealed that non-healing GU (NHGU) was positively correlated with age and persistent *H. pylori* infection (failure of *H. pylori* eradication), but negatively correlated with IM (Table 2). Because patients with IM were older than those without IM in this study, multivariate logistical regression analysis was performed to determine the predictor of GU healing by adjusting the factor of age (Table 3). As positive predictors for NHGU, the analysis revealed age [odds ratio (OR) =1.035, 95% confidence interval (CI) = 1.007–1.064; $P = 0.015$] and persistent *H. pylori* infection [OR = 3.924, 95% CI = 1.857–8.294, $P < 0.001$]. A negative predictor was IM [OR = 0.366, 95% CI = 0.170–0.792, $P = 0.011$].

For failure of *H. pylori* eradication, only the factor of NHGU was a predictor. IM was not a predictor and was not correlated with failure of *H. pylori* eradication (Table 4).

Because this was a retrospective analysis, only adequate GU biopsy specimens from patients before and after *H. pylori* eradication therapy were used for the IHC stain study. A total of 64 GU biopsy specimens (30 from patients with non-IM, 34 patients with IM) underwent Ki-67 staining (Table 5). There was no significant difference in Ki-67 index between patients with IM and those without IM. The mean Ki-67 index change before or after treatment was only marginally different between patients with IM and those without IM (0.5 ± 1.7 vs. 0.6 ± 1.9, $P = 0.06$).

Discussion

IM is a common pathologic finding in patients with endoscopy-proven GU [22–24]. Previous studies focused on the precancerous condition of IM; however, few studies have investigated the influence of IM on gastric ulcer healing and *H. pylori* eradication. Factors such as age, smoking and *H. pylori* eradication were reported as important factors for GU healing [25–27]. In our study, although patients with gastric mucosal IM had a higher GU healing rate than those without IM, the GU healing rates were not significantly different when the focus was on the patients with successful *H. pylori* eradication. Multivariate logistic regression analyses revealed that failure of *H. pylori* eradication was a positive predictor (OR = 4.013) and IM was a negative predictor (OR = 0.369) for non-healing GU. Hence, successful *H. pylori* eradication is a more important predictor than IM for GU healing in this study.

Table 5 Mean Ki-67 stain index in patients before and after *H. pylori* eradication and maintenance of proton pump inhibitor therapy for 8 weeks

Ki-67 index	No Intestinal metaplasia (n = 30)			Intestinal metaplasia (n = 34)		
	Before	After	P value	Before	After	P value
Mean index (%)	19.1 ± 15.0	17.3 ± 15.6	0.20	19.8 ± 13.4	17.8 ± 12.2	0.34
Change (%)*	0.6 ± 1.9			0.5 ± 1.7		0.06

*Index change (%) calculated as the mean Ki-67 index (before-after)/before × 100%

The mechanisms associated with GU healing and repair include epithelial cell proliferation, growth control, epidermal growth factors, angiogenesis and inhibition of acid secretion [12, 13, 28, 29]. Although our original hypothesis was that cell hyperproliferation in IM might influence GU healing, we found that there was no significant difference in cell proliferation Ki-67 stain index between the IM group and the no IM group. Antigen Ki-67 is a nuclear protein that is associated with cellular proliferation and ribosomal RNA transcription. The Ki-67 protein is present during all active phases of the cell cycle (G1, S, G2 and mitosis), but is absent from resting cells (G0). In previous studies, patients with H. pylori infection and chronic gastritis exhibited significantly increased rates of epithelial cell proliferation. Cell proliferation decreases after successful H. pylori eradication [30, 31]. Although the mean Ki-67 index was decreased (decreased cell proliferation) following H. pylori eradication in our study, there was no significant difference in mean Ki-67 index between patients with IM and those without IM. The condition of gastric mucosal cell proliferation might be due to the status of H. pylori infection and chronic gastritis, but not the status of IM [30, 31].

There were two limitations in the present study. First, this study only included patients with GU and IM adjacent to GU, but patients with atrophic gastritis were excluded. It is common to detect atrophic gastritis and IM coexistence in patients with an H. pylori infection [16–18]. Although the intra-gastric juice pH value and serum pepsinogen value are important for the evaluation of atrophic gastritis and GU healing, these data were not available in this retrospective study. It would be difficult to elucidate whether atrophic gastritis or IM has an influence on GU healing when a patient has both pathologic findings of atrophic gastritis and IM in the stomach. Hence, we excluded the patients with atrophic gastritis detected via histological examination in this study. Second, most of the IM types in this study were mild according to the Sydney system. We could not compare differences in GU healing between patients with mild forms of IM and those with marked forms of IM.

Conclusions

Patients with gastric IM may have a higher GU healing rate than those without gastric IM. Age, successful H. pylori eradication and gastric IM were the predictors for GU healing. However, successful H. pylori eradication was a more important factor for GU healing than gastric IM.

Abbreviations

H. pylori: Helicobacter pylori; GU: Gastric ulcer; IM: Intestinal metaplasia; EGD: Esophagogastroduodenoscopy; PPI: Proton pump inhibitor; RUT: Rapid urease test; DAB: Diaminobenzidine; IHC: Immunohistochemical; SD: Standard deviation

Acknowledgments
We acknowledge Miss Chia-Wen Hsieh for help in collecting and analyzing data.

Funding
This study was not supported by any grant.

Authors' contributions
CLW, HBJ, CSW analyzed and interpreted the patient data regarding the gastric ulcers, H. pylori infection and pathologic findings. CLC performed the histological examination of GU and HCC performed the immunohistochemical study. CLW and CRN were the major contributors in writing the manuscript. All authors read and approved the final manuscript.

Competing interests
The authors declare that they have no competing interests.

Consent for publication
Not applicable.

Personal interest
None.

Author details
[1]Departments of Gastroenterology and Hepatology, Chang-Gung Memorial Hospital and University, 12F, No 222, Mai-Jin Road, Keelung, Taiwan. [2]Departments of Pathology, Chang-Gung Memorial Hospital and University, 12F, No 222, Mai-Jin Road, Keelung, Taiwan. [3]Departments of Internal Medicine, Chang-Gung Memorial Hospital and University, 12F, No 222, Mai-Jin Road, Keelung, Taiwan.

References
1. Wong BC, Lam SK, Wong WM, Chen JS, Zheng TT, Feng RE, et al. Helicobacter pylori eradication to prevent gastric cancer in a high-risk region of China: a randomized controlled trial. JAMA. 2004;291:187–94.
2. Asaka M, Sugiyama T, Nobuta A, Kato M, Takeda H, Graham DY. Atrophic gastritis and intestinal metaplasia in Japan: results of a large multicenter study. Helicobacter. 2001;6:294–9.
3. Franco AT, Israel DA, Washington MK, Krishna U, Fox JG, Rogers AB, et al. Activation of β-catenin by carcinogenic Helicobacter pylori. Proc Natl Acad Sci U S A. 2005;102:10646–51.
4. Murata-Kamiya N, Kurashima Y, Teishikata Y, Yamahashi Y, Saito Y, Higashi H, et al. Helicobacter pylori CagA interacts with Ecadherin and deregulates the β-catenin signal that promotes intestinal transdifferentiation in gastric epithelial cells. Oncogene. 2007;26:4617–26.
5. Clevers H. Wnt/β-catenis signaling in development and disease. Cell. 2006; 127:469–80.
6. Hung KH, Wu JJ, Yang HB, Su LJ, Sheu BS. Host Wnt/β-catenin pathway triggered by Helicobacter pylori correlates with regression of gastric intestinal metaplasia after H. pylori eradication. J Med Microbiol. 2009;58:567–76.
7. Koch S, Nava P, Addis C, Kim W, Denning TL, Li L, et al. The Wnt antagonist Dkk1 regulates intestinal epithelial homeostasis and wound repair. Gastroenterology. 2011;141:259–68.
8. Bechi P, Balzi M, Becciolini A, Maugeri A, Raggi CC, Amorosi A, et al. Helicobacter pylori and cell proliferation of the gastric mucosa: possible implications for gastric carcinogenesis. Am J Gastroenterol. 1996;91:271–6.
9. Ierardi E, Francavilla R, Panella C. Effect of Helicobacter pylori eradication on intestinal metaplasia and gastric epithelium proliferation. Ital J Gastroenterol Hepatol. 1997;29:470–5.
10. Peek Jr RM, Moss SF, Tham KT, Pérez-Pérez GI, Wang S, Miller GG, et al. Helicobacter pylori cagA+ strains and dissociation of gastric epithelial cell proliferation from apoptosis. J Natl Cancer Inst. 1997;89:863–8.

11. Xia HH, Talley NJ. Apoptosis in gastric epithelium induced by *Helicobacter pylori* infection: implications in gastric carcinogenesis. Am J Gastroenterol. 2001;96:16–26.

12. Levi S, Goodlad RA, Lee CY, Walport MJ, Wright NA, Hodgson HJ. Inhibitory effect of non-steroidal anti-inflammatory drugs on mucosal cell proliferation associated with gastric ulcer healing. Lancet. 1990;336:840–3.

13. Tibble J, Sigthorsson G, Caldwell C, Palmer RH, Bjarnason I. Effects of NSAIDs on cryoprobe-injeced gastric ulcer healing in rats. Aliment Pharmacol Ther. 2001;15:2001–8.

14. Zhang C, Yamada N, Wu YL, Wen M, Matsuhisa T, Matsukura N. *Helicobacter pylori* infection, glandular atrophy and intestinal metaplasia in superficial gastritis, gastric erosion, erosive gastritis, gastric ulcer and early gastric cancer. World J Gastroenterol. 2005;11:791–6.

15. Blaser MJ, Atherton JC. *Helicobacter pylori* persistence: biology and disease. J Clin Invest. 2004;113:321–33.

16. Dixon MF, Genta RM, Yardley JH, Correa P. Classification and grading of gastritis. The updated Sydney System. International Workshop on the Histopathology of Gastritis, Houston 1994. Am J Surg Pathol. 1996;20:1161–81.

17. Capelle LG, de Vries AC, Haringsma J, Ter Borg F, de Vries RA, Bruno MJ, van Dekken H, Meijer J, van Grieken NC, Kuipers EJ. The staging of gastritis with the OLGA system by using intestinal metaplasia as an accurate alternative for atrophic gastritis. Gastrointest Endosc. 2010;71:1150–8.

18. Rugge M, Correa P, Dixon MF, Fiocca R, Hattori T, Lechago J, Leandro G, Price AB, Sipponen P, Solcia E, Watanabe H, Genta RM. Gastric mucosal atrophy: interobserver consistency using new criteria for classification and grading. Aliment Pharmacol Ther. 2002;16:1249–59.

19. Chen LW, Chien RN, Fang KM, Yen CL, Chang JJ, Lee TS, et al. A comparative study on *Helicobacter pylori* infection in peptic ulcer disease patients with or without previous eradication therapy. Hepatogastroenterology. 2007;54:2209–11.

20. Schneider CA, Rasband WS, Eliceiri KW. NIH Image to ImageJ: 25 years of image analysis. Nat Methods. 2012;9:671–5.

21. Tuominen VJ, Ruotoistenmäki S, Viitanen A, Jumppanen M, Isola J. ImmunoRatio: a publicly available web application for quantitative image analysis of estrogen receptor (ER), progresterone receptor (PR), and Ki-67. Breast Cancer Res. 2012;12:R56. doi:10.1186/bcr2615.

22. Craanen ME, Dekker W, Blok P, Ferwerda J, Tytgat GN. Intestinal metaplasia and *Helicobacter pylori*: an endoscopic bioptic study of the gastric antrum. Gut. 1992;33:16–20.

23. Filipe MI, Muñoz N, Matko I, Kato I, Pompe-Kirn V, Jutersek A, et al. Intestinal metaplasia types and the risk of gastric cancer: a cohort study in Solvenia. Int J Cancer. 1994;57:24–9.

24. Correa P, Piazuelo B, Wilson KT. Pathology of gastric intestinal metaplasia: clinical implications. Am J Gastroenterol. 2010;105:493–8.

25. Arkkila PE, Kokkola A, Seppälä K, Sipponen P. Size of the peptic ulcer in *Helicobacter pylori*-positive patients: association with the clinical and histological characteristics. Scand J Gastroenterol. 2007;42:695–701.

26. Graham DY, Lew GM, Klein PD, Evans DG, Evans Jr DJ, Saeed ZA. Effect of treatment of *Helicobacter pylori* infection on the long-term recurrence of gastric or duodenal ulcer: a randomized, controlled study. Ann Intern Med. 1992;116:705–8.

27. Labenz J, Borsch G. Evidence for the essential role of *Helicobacter pylori* in gastric ulcer disease. Gut. 1994;35:19–22.

28. Konturek PC, Konturek SJ, Brzozowski T, Ernst H. Epidermal growth factor and transforming growth factor-α: Role in protection and healing of gastric mucosal lesions. Eur J Gastroenterol Hepatol. 1995;7:933–7.

29. Kamada T, Kawano S, Sato N, Fukuda M, Fusamoto H, Abe H. Gastric mucosal blood distribution and its changes in the healing process of gastric ulcer. Gastroenterology. 1983;84:1541–6.

30. Unger Z, Molnar B, Szaleczky E, Torgyekes E, Muller F, Zagoni T, et al. Effect of *Helicobacter pylori* infection and eradication on gastric epithelial cell proliferation and apoptosis. J Physiol Paris. 2001;95:355–60.

31. Szaleczky E, Prónai L, Molnár B, Berczi L, Fehér J, Tulassay Z. Increased cell proliferation in chronic *Helicobacter pylori* positive gastritis and gastric carcinoma–correlation between immuno-histochemistry and Tv image cytometry. Anal Cell Pathol. 2000;20(2–3):131–9.

12

Levofloxacin or Clarithromycin-based quadruple regimens: what is the best alternative as first-line treatment for *Helicobacter pylori* eradication in a country with high resistance rates for both antibiotics?

Diogo Branquinho[1,2]* (iD), Nuno Almeida[1,2], Carlos Gregório[1], José Eduardo Pina Cabral[1], Adriano Casela[1], Maria Manuel Donato[2] and Luís Tomé[1,2]

Abstract

Background: *Helicobacter pylori* eradication rates in Portugal are declining, due to increased resistance of this bacterium to antimicrobial agents, especially Clarithromycin. Quadruple Levofloxacin-containing regimens could be an option for first-line treatment, but its efficacy should be evaluated as fluoroquinolone resistance is rapidly increasing.

Our aim was to compare the efficacy of Clarithromycin and Levofloxacin-based sequential quadruple therapies as first-line treatment options and determine factors associated with treatment failure.

Methods: A total of 200 *Helicobacter pylori* infected patients were retrospectively included (female 57.5%; average age: 53.2 ± 15.7) and received either 10-day sequential therapy (Proton-Pump Inhibitor + Amoxicillin 1 g bid for 5 days and Proton-Pump Inhibitor + Clarithromycin 500 mg + Metronidazole/Tinidazole 500 mg bid/tid in the following 5 days; group A) or a 10-day modified sequential therapy with Levofloxacin 500 mg id instead of Clarithromycin (group B). Eradication was confirmed with urea breath test. Variables that could influence success rate were analyzed.

Results: There were no differences between groups in terms of gender, age, smoking habits and indications for treatment. The eradication rate obtained with Clarithromycin-based sequential treatment was significantly higher than with Levofloxacin-based therapy (90%, CI95%: 84–96% vs. 79%, CI95%: 71–87%, $p = 0.001$). Using full-dose proton-pump inhibitor and high-dose Metronidazole in group A, and full-dose proton-pump inhibitor and prescription from a Gastroenterologist in group B were associated with eradication success.

Conclusions: Ten-day Levofloxacin-based sequential treatment achieved inadequate efficacy rate (<80%) and should not be adopted as first-line therapy. Standard sequential therapy showed significantly better results in this *naïve* population. Using full-dose proton-pump inhibitor and higher doses of Metronidazole is essential to achieve such results.

Keywords: Eradication, First-line, *Helicobacter pylori*, Levofloxacin, Sequential therapy

* Correspondence: diogofbranquinho@yahoo.com
[1]Gastroenterology Department, Coimbra University Hospital, Praceta Prof. Mota Pinto, 3000-075 Coimbra, Portugal
[2]Gastroenterology Centre, Faculty of Medicine, Coimbra University, R. Larga, 3004-504 Coimbra, Portugal

Background

Helicobacter pylori (H. pylori) is a Gram negative, micro-aerophilic bacterium that is presumed to infect from one-third to over half of the world's population [1]. It is known to be a major responsible for a significant number of gastric pathologies, but its role in extra-gastric diseases is also becoming well documented. *H. pylori* leads to an inflammatory state, induces molecular mimicry and alters the absorbance of several nutrients [2]. These discoveries are increasing physicians' awareness to the need to eradicate this bacterium.

Initially, the adopted treatment to eradicate *H. pylori*, the so-called 'legacy' triple therapy with a proton-pump inhibitor (PPI), Clarithromycin and Amoxicillin was quite effective. However, in the last 10 years, its' efficacy has decreased to unacceptable levels in many countries, especially due to increasing levels of bacterial resistance [3]. Excessive and misjudged use of antibiotics contributed to this decreased susceptibility, leading to 50% resistance rates to Clarithromycin in the central region of Portugal (primary 21.4%; secondary 88.3%) [4]. Accordingly, current guidelines recommend bismuth-containing quadruple therapies or, alternatively, sequential or non-bismuth quadruple therapy, if Clarithromycin resistance is above the 15–20% threshold [5]. Unfortunately, *H. pylori* antibiotic resistance has reached alarming levels not only for macrolides but also to other drugs. Metronidazole resistance has been stable in Europe, reaching 34.9% of *H. pylori* isolates. Fortunately, its impact on the success of eradication regimens is limited, as it can be overcome by prolonging duration of treatment or increasing the dosage of Metronidazole [6]. Despite obtaining adequate eradication rates, standard sequential treatment should not be prescribed if the combined Clarithromycin and Metronidazole resistance is over 5% (which is the case in several European countries) [6]. To overcome these problems, some physicians prefer prescribing an adapted sequential treatment with Levofloxacin instead of Clarithromycin, as quinolones have been suggested as an alternative in both first- and second-line regimens [7]. Patients with reported history of penicillin allergy were also often prescribed with such regimens. Regrettably, resistance rates to quinolones also reached worrisome figures in Portugal and in Europe, reflecting its ubiquitous use for minor respiratory and urinary infections. According to Almeida *et al* [4], overall resistance to Levofloxacin in the center of Portugal is currently 33.9% (primary: 26.2%; secondary: 44.2%). Facing such adverse ecological scenario, our aim was to compare the efficacy of Clarithromycin and Levofloxacin-based sequential quadruple therapies as first-line treatment options and determine factors associated with treatment failure.

Methods

Study design

This retrospective study was conducted at the Coimbra University Hospital from January 2014 to December 2015. Adult patients with infection by *H. pylori* defined by histology or ^{13}C-urea breath test (UBT) and treated with either standard sequential treatment (SST; group A) or Levofloxacin-based sequential treatment (LST; group B) were considered for inclusion. The treatment regimen was chosen according to their physicians' preference. Other inclusion criteria were: (1) age over 18 years-old, (2) absence of known allergies for antibiotics used in either regimen, (3) signed informed consent. A total of 358 patients treated with one of these regimens were interviewed after treatment completion (group A – 250 patients; group B – 108 patients). Collected data included age, gender, smoking and alcohol consumption, indication for treatment, side effects and adherence. In order to obtain two groups with similar dimension, and therefore avoid statistical bias, we opted to include 100 patients in each group. The selection of patients was performed randomly, using SPSS software (as detailed below). Eradication therapy was prescribed by Gastroenterologists or other physicians working in our hospital.

The exclusion criteria were: (1) patients with previous *H. pylori* eradication attempts; (2) patients treated with proton-pump inhibitor (PPI), H_2 receptor antagonist or antibiotics in the 4 to 6 weeks previous to UBT; (3) patients that interrupted the treatment before completion for any reason; (4) non-adherence to treatment. The stricter definition of non-adherence was used, and patients that failed at least one dose of medication were excluded.

All patients were submitted to UBT at least 2 months after completing treatment. The primary outcome of the study was the eradication rate of *H. pylori* infection with SST and LST. Finding factors associated with treatment failure was the secondary outcome.

Therapeutic regimens

Patients in group A were treated with standard sequential therapy (SST) for 10 days: PPI twice daily + Amoxicillin 1 g twice daily for 5 days; followed by PPI twice daily + Clarithromycin 500 mg twice daily + Metronidazole 500 mg twice / thrice daily or Tinidazole 500 mg twice daily for five more days. Group B patients were treated with Levofloxacin-containing sequential therapy (LST) for 10 days: PPI twice daily + Amoxicillin 1 g twice daily for 5 days followed by PPI twice daily + Levofloxacin 250 mg twice daily + Metronidazole 500 mg twice / thrice or Tinidazole 500 mg twice daily for five more days. The choice between different PPI's, Metronidazole or Tinidazole and its dosage was made by the prescribing physician.

Statistical analysis

Statistical analysis of the results was performed using chi-square test, Student's t-test and Fisher's exact test as well as binomial logistic regression for multivariate analysis. For all analysis, P values <0.05 were considered significant. The 95% confidence intervals (CIs) were calculated by normal approximation. The analysis was performed using SPSS for Windows (version 21; SPSS Inc.).

Results

Study population

These groups were compared regarding demographic and clinical characteristics, as described in Table 1. There was no significant age or gender difference between both groups. The same can be said for smoking habits and alcohol consumption (defined as more than 10 cigars/day and >20 g alcohol each day). The main indication for prescribing eradication therapy was non-ulcer dyspepsia in both groups. First-generation and full-dose PPI were preferred in both the SST and the LST regimens. There were

significant differences in the choice of the nitroimidazole antibiotics: Tinidazole was prescribed more often in both groups, but especially in group B ($p = 0.001$). The most used dosage for Metronidazole was 500 mg three times a day in both groups. The majority of the prescribing physicians were Gastroenterologists, especially in group B ($p = 0.002$).

Efficacy of eradication therapy

The overall eradication rate was 84.5% (169/200). The eradication rates were 90% (90/100) for group A and 79% (79/100) for group B. Standard sequential therapy was more effective than Levofloxacin-based modified sequential therapy ($p = 0.03$; OR = 2.39; IC95% = 1.06–5.38).

Factors associated with eradication failure

In group A, the use of Metronidazole instead of Tinidazole ($p = 0.006$; OR = 10.15; IC95%:1.34–77.15), a lower dose of Metronidazole ($p = 0.001$; OR = 8.25; IC95% = 1.95–34.81) and not using an adequate dosage of PPI ($p = 0.001$;

Table 1 Patients' demographic and clinical characteristics

	Group A (SST) n = 100	Group B (LST) n = 100	p
Mean age (years)	52.4 ± 16.2 (range 18–89)	54 ± 15.3 (range 18–81)	0.458
Gender			
- Female	55%	60%	0.567
- Male	45%	40%	
Smoking habits	8%	8%	1
Alcohol consumption	19%	10%	0.107
Indication(s) for *H. pylori* eradication			
- Non-ulcer dyspepsia	63%	72%	0.307
- Peptic ulcer	14%	10%	0.452
- GERD/chronic use of PPI	11%	11%	1
- Before bariatric surgery	9%	—	—
- Anemia or thrombocytopenia	2%	7%	0.229
- Familial history of gastric cancer	1%	—	—
Nitroimidazole antibiotic			
- Tinidazole	53%	81%	0.001
- Metronidazole	47%	19%	
Metronidazole dosage			
- 500 mg 12–12 h (1000 mg)	29,8%	21,1%	0.554
- 500 mg 8–8 h (1500 mg)	70,2%	79,9%	
PPI 1st or 2nd generation			
- Omeprazole / Pantoprazole / Lansoprazole	81%	89%	0.165
- Esomeprazole / Rabeprazole	19%	11%	
PPI dosage			
- Full-dose	91%	88%	0.645
- Half-dose	9%	12%	
Prescribing Physician			
- Gastroenterologist	79%	94%	0.002
- Non-Gastroenterologist	21%	6%	

SST standard sequential treatment, *LST* levofloxacin-based sequential treatment, *GERD* gastroesophageal reflux disease, *PPI* proton-pump inhibitor

OR = 10.11; IC95% = 3.60–28.41) were risk factors for eradication failure – as described in Table 2. Multivariate analysis confirmed that half-dose PPI ($p = 0.001$; OR = 16.25; IC95% = 2.91–89.21) and a lower dose of Metronidazole ($p = 0.007$; OR = 13.58; IC95% = 2.07–89.04) were associated with unsuccessful eradication (Table 2). In group B, half-dose PPI and prescription from non-Gastroenterologists were the two factors associated with unsuccessful eradication ($p = 0.001$; OR = 3.67; IC95% = 1.86–7.22 and $p = 0.017$; OR = 3.68; IC95% = 1.81–7.50, respectively). Only the use of half-dose PPI was associated with unsuccessful eradication in multivariate analysis ($p = 0.011$; OR = 5.69; IC95% = 1.48–21.90).

Discussion

In southern European countries, such as Portugal, with alarming resistance rates to most commonly used antibiotics, recommending an effective first-line treatment for *H. pylori* eradication is becoming increasingly difficult. Taking into account resistance rates to Clarithromycin of over 30%, an alternative quadruple regimen with Levofloxacin could be an effective option. However, with a resistance rate to Levofloxacin over 25%, its utility may be compromised. But if the resistance rates to Clarithromycin and Levofloxacin are similar, why did the two therapies showed such different results? Probably this is due to the interaction between Amoxicillin and Clarithromycin. Amoxicillin acts on the bacterial wall, destroying a transmembrane efflux system that allows elimination of Clarithromycin in resistant bacterium.

Therefore there is a higher intracellular concentration of Clarithromycin which can overcome other resistance mechanisms [8]. The first 5 days of Amoxicillin act as an inductor for the following 5 days of Clarithromycin. This is probably the reason behind the ability of the sequential regimen to eradicate a significant percentage of Clarithromycin-resistant strains (as high as 82% according to Zullo *et al* [9]). Interestingly, our results are quite different from those obtained in a randomized trial conducted in Italy, where Levofloxacin-based sequential regimens obtained >95% eradication rates, while a Clarithromycin-based sequential regimen obtained only an 80.8% success rate [10]. Other studies showed the same superiority for Levofloxacin-based triple and sequential regimens [11–14]. A recently published meta-analysis compared Levofloxacin-based sequential therapy and Clarithromycin-based triple and sequential treatment, and revealed superiority for the regimens that included fluoroquinolones (87.8% vs. 71.1%, respectively) [15]. This is probably due to the very low resistance to Levofloxacin reported in such studies (as low as 3.7% in the Italian study by Romano *et al* [10]).

The patients included in our study were treated with Metronidazole 500 mg in an 8–8 h or 12–12 h or with Tinidazole 500 mg 12–12 h. Tinidazole was chosen more often in both groups, but this preference was only significant in the LST group. When comparing both antibiotics, Metronidazole was inferior to Tinidazole in the SST group. This difference is probably due to the use of lower doses of Metronidazole (1000 mg) in almost

Table 2 Potential risk factors associated with eradication failure

	Group A (n = 100) Standard Sequential Therapy			Group B (n = 100) Levofloxacin-based Sequential		
	Success (n = 90)	Failure (n = 10)	p/OR (95%CI)	Success (n = 79)	Failure (n = 21)	p/OR (95%CI)
Age	52.1 ± 1.8	55,5 ± 3,8	0.528	55.7 ± 1.6	47.7 ± 3.9	0.068
>65 years	23 (25.6%)	2 (20%)	0.720	23 (29.1%)	7 (33.3%)	0.708
Female	50 (55.6%)	5 (50%)	0.738	49 (62%)	11 (52.4%)	0.423
Smoking habits	6 (6.7%)	2 (20%)	0.182	5 (6.3%)	3 (14.3%)	0.359
Alcohol consumption	16 (17.8%)	3 (30%)	0.350	8 (10.1%)	2 (9.5%)	0.952
Non-ulcer dyspepsia	14 (17.9%)	0	0.353	63 (83.3%)	20 (95.2%)	0.112
Metronidazole (vs. Tinidazole)	38 (42.2%)	9 (90%)	0.006/10.15 (1.34–77.15)	16 (20.3%)	3 (14.3%)	0.756
Metronidazole 1000 mg (vs. 1500 mg)	7 (7.8%)	7 (70%)	0.001/ 8.25 (1.95–34.89)	4 (25%)	0	0.964
1st Generation PPI (vs. 2nd Generation)	74 (82.2%)	7 (70%)	0.396	69 (87.3%)	20 (95.2%)	0.450
Half-dose PPI (vs. full-dose)	4 (4.4%)	5 (50%)	0.001/ 10.11 (3.60–28.41)	5 (6.3%)	7 (33.3%)	0.001/3.67 (1.86–7.22)
Prescription by non-Gastroenterologist	20 (22.2%)	1 (10%)	0.684	2 (2.5%)	4 (19%)	0.017/3.68 (1.81–7.50)

CI95% 95% confidence interval, *OR* odds ratio, *PPI* proton-pump inhibitor

a quarter of the patients. It is known that resistance to Metronidazole in southern European countries is over 30% [4, 16], but can be overcome by using longer treatments or higher doses of the drug. This hypothesis is supported by the fact that high-dose Metronidazole (1500 mg) obtained similar results to Tinidazole. This difference in efficacy when using different Metronidazole dosages was not observed in the LST group, probably due to the low number of patients treated with Metronidazole (19%), not allowing for statistically significant differences to be noted.

When facing high resistance levels to Metronidazole, it has been suggested that the optimum duration of quadruple therapies should be 14 days, combined with high doses of the drug (up to 1500–1600 mg in divided dosages) [17]. Despite being recommended to avoid 10-day sequential treatment if Metronidazole resistance is over 20%, in our population a 90% eradication rate was obtained nevertheless.

Besides antibiotic resistance, there are other factors that may contribute to treatment failure. Smoking is often associated with unsuccessful eradication [18, 19], but this was not the case in our study, probably due to the low number of smokers included in our sample population. Non-ulcer dyspepsia patients also tend to respond worse to eradication treatment, when compared to those with peptic ulcers [20], but this tendency was not observed in our study groups. There was also no difference in eradication rates for patients submitted to treatment for hematologic conditions such as anemia or thrombocytopenia. In fact, the most consistent factor that influenced eradication success for both groups was the proton-pump inhibitor (PPI) dose. The crucial role of acid inhibition in optimizing the action of antibiotics such as Amoxicillin led to the recommendation of twice-daily full-dose PPI regimen [5, 21]. While the use of full-dose PPI is widely recommended, the need to use more recent PPI's instead of first-generation drugs is more controversial. A meta-analysis by McNicholl *et al* [22], revealed superiority of esomeprazole and rabeprazole, but other studies failed to show the same benefit [23]. Using new-generation PPI's may be more beneficial in populations where CYP2C19 extensive metabolizer phenotype is prevalent [24]. In our population the use of new-generation PPI's was not associated with a higher eradication rate. Another interesting finding was the difference in the eradication rates obtained by Gastroenterologists and non-Gastroenterologists in the LST group. While there is no obvious explanation for this difference, it has been suggested that providing the patient with a written plan with prescription details and warning about expected adverse effects may improve adherence and therefore may contribute to eradication success [25, 26].

Our study has some limitations. The strict non-adherence definition used in our study led to the exclusion of a significant number of patients. Furthermore, to obtain two groups with similar dimension, a randomized sampling of patients was performed. Despite these constraints, our study groups' size is within range when compared to other published studies [4, 12, 16, 25]. Its' retrospective nature does not allow comparison in intention-to-treat and per-protocol analysis and *H. pylori* antibiotic resistance was not determined for each included patient.

Conclusions

We can conclude that standard sequential treatment was quite effective and achieved an eradication rate that reached the threshold of 90%, despite Metronidazole resistance over 20% and simultaneous resistance to Clarithromycin and Metronidazole over 5% in our country. Full-dose PPI and a higher dose of Metronidazole should be adopted to insure positive outcomes. Levofloxacin-based sequential regimen achieved an eradication rate under 80% and should not be considered as first-line therapy.

To achieve such results with standard sequential therapy, a full-dose of PPI and high doses of Metronidazole or Tinidazole should be used. Despite adequate success rate demonstrated by Clarithromycin-based sequential therapy, a prospective study comparing different non-bismuth quadruple therapies (sequential, hybrid and concomitant) should be conducted in the near future to find out which is the most effective in a country with high Clarithromycin and Levofloxacin resistance such as Portugal.

Abbreviations

BID/TID: Two/three times a day; CI95%: 95% confidence interval; GERD: Gastroesophageal reflux disease; LST: Levofloxacin-based sequential treatment; OR: Odds ratio; PPI: Proton-pump inhibitor; SST: Standard sequential treatment; UBT: Urea breath test

Acknowledgements

The authors would like to thank Dr. Carlos Alberto Calhau for his work during data collection.

Funding

All authors certify that no funding was received.

Authors' contributions

The involvement of each author was as follows: DB (1–8); NA (1–8); CG (1,2,4,5); JEPC (1,2,4,5); AC (1,2,4,5); MMD (1,5,6,7,8); LT (1,4,5,8). Key: (1) Study concept and design; (2) Acquisition of data; (3) Analysis and interpretation of data; (4) Drafting of the manuscript; (5) Critical revision of the manuscript for important intellectual content; (6) Statistical analysis; (7) Administrative, technical, or material support; (8) Study supervision. All authors read the final version of this manuscript, approve its' content and submission for publication. All authors agreed to be accountable for all aspects of the work in ensuring that questions related to the accuracy or integrity of any part of the work are appropriately investigated and resolved.

Competing interests
The authors declare that they have no competing interest.

Consent for publication
Not applicable. No details, images, or videos relating to individual participants are included in the manuscript.

References

1. Eusebi LH, Zagari RM, Bazzoli F. Epidemiology of Helicobacter pylori infection. Helicobacter. 2014;19.s1:1–5.
2. Roubaud Baudron C, Franceschi F, Salles N, Gasbarrini A. Extragastric diseases and Helicobacter pylori. Helicobacter. 2013;18(s1):44–51.
3. Graham DY, Fischbach L. Helicobacter pylori treatment in the era of increasing antibiotic resistance. Gut. 2010;59:1143–53.
4. Almeida N, Romãozinho JM, Donato MM, Luxo C, Cardoso O, Cipriano MA, et al. Helicobacter pylori antimicrobial resistance rates in the central region of Portugal. Clin Microbiol Infect. 2014;11:1127–33.
5. Malfertheiner P, Megraud F, O'Morain CA, Atherton J, Axon AT, Bazzoli F, et al. Management of Helicobacter pylori infection — the Maastricht IV / Florence consensus report. Gut. 2012;61(5):646–64.
6. Megraud F, Coenen S, Versporten A, Kist M, Lopez-Brea M, Hirschl AM, et al. Helicobacter pylori resistance to antibiotics in Europe and its relationship to antibiotic consumption. Gut. 2013;62(1):34–42.
7. Gisbert JP, Morena F. Systematic review and meta-analysis: levofloxacin-based rescue regimens after Helicobacter pylori treatment failure. Aliment Pharmacol Ther. 2006;23(1):35–44.
8. De Francesco V, Margiotta M, Zullo A, Hassan C, Troiani L, Burattini O, et al. Clarithromycin-resistant genotypes and eradication of Helicobacter pylori. Ann Intern Med. 2006;144(2):94–100.
9. Zullo A, De Francesco V, Hassan C, Morini S, Vaira D. The sequential therapy regimen for Helicobacter pylori eradication: a pooled-data analysis. Gut. 2007;56(10):1353–7.
10. Romano M, Cuomo A, Gravina AG, Miranda A, Lovene MR, Tiso A, et al. Empirical Levofloxacin-containing versus Clarithromycin-containing sequential therapy for Helicobacter pylori eradication: a randomised trial. Gut. 2010;59(11):1465–70.
11. Molina-Infante J, Perez-Gallardo B, Fernandez-Bermejo M, Hernandez-Alonso M, Vinagre G, Duenas C, et al. Clinical trial: clarithromycin vs. levofloxacin in first-line triple and sequential regimens for Helicobacter pylori eradication. Aliment Pharmacol Ther. 2010;31:1077–84.
12. Polat Z, Kadayifci A, Kantarcioglu M, Ozcan A, Emer O, Uygun A. Comparison of Levofloxacin-containing sequential and standard triple therapies for the eradication of Helicobacter pylori. Eur J Intern Med. 2012;23:165–8.
13. Qian J, Ye F, Zhang J, Yang YM, Tu HM, Jiang Q, et al. Levofloxacin-containing Triple and Sequential Therapy or Standard Sequential Therapy as the First Line Treatment for Helicobacter pylori Eradication in China. Helicobacter. 2012;17:478–85.
14. Lee H, Hong SN, Min BH, Lee JH, Rhee PL, Lee YC, et al. Comparison of efficacy and safety of Levofloxacin-containing versus standard sequential therapy in eradication of Helicobacter pylori infection in Korea. Dig Liver Dis. 2015;47:114–8.
15. Kale-Pradhan PB, Mihaescu A, Wilhelm SM. Fluoroquinolone sequential therapy for helicobacter pylori: a meta-analysis. Pharmacotherapy. 2015;35(8):719–30.
16. Georgopoulos SD, Xirouchakis E, Martinez-Gonzalez B, Sgouras DN, Spiliadi C, Mentis AF, et al. Clinical evaluation of a ten-day regimen with esomeprazole, metronidazole, amoxicillin, and clarithromycin for the eradication of helicobacter pylori in a high clarithromycin resistance area. Helicobacter. 2013;18(6):459–67.
17. Graham DY, Lee SY. How to effectively use bismuth quadruple therapy: the good, the bad, and the ugly, Gastroenterology clinics of North America. 2015. p. 537–63.
18. Kim SE, Park MI, Park SJ, Moon W, Choi YJ, Cheon JH, et al. Trends in Helicobacter pylori eradication rates by first-line triple therapy and related factors in eradication therapy. Korean J Intern Med. 2015;30(6):801–7.
19. Pan KF, Zhang L, Gerhard M, Ma JL, Liu WD, Ulm K, et al. A large randomised controlled intervention trial to prevent gastric cancer by eradication of Helicobacter pylori in Linqu County, China: baseline results and factors affecting the eradication. Gut. 2015; Gutjnl.
20. Wolle K, Malfertheiner P. Treatment of Helicobacter pylori. Best Pract Res Clin Gastroenterol. 2007;21(2):315–24.
21. Villoria A, Garcia P, Calvet X, Gisbert JP, Vergara M. Meta-analysis: high-dose proton pump inhibitors vs. standard dose in triple therapy for Helicobacter pylori eradication. Aliment Pharmacol Ther. 2008;28(7):868–77.
22. McNicholl AG, Linares PM, Nyssen OP, Calvet X, Gisbert JP. Meta-analysis: esomeprazole or rabeprazole vs. first-generation pump inhibitors in the treatment of Helicobacter pylori infection. Aliment Pharmacol Ther. 2012;36(5):414–25.
23. Choi HS, Park DI, Hwang SJ, Park JS, Kim HJ, Cho YK, et al. Double-dose, new-generation proton pump inhibitors do not improve Helicobacter pylori eradication rate. Helicobacter. 2007;12(6):638–42.
24. Georgopoulos SD, Papastergiou V, Karatapanis S. Treatment of Helicobacter Pylori infection: optimization strategies in a high resistance era. Expert Opin Pharmacother. 2015;16(15):2307–17.
25. Lee M, Kemp JA, Canning A, Egan C, Tataronis G, Farraye FA. A randomized controlled trial of an enhanced patient compliance program for helicobacter pylori therapy. Arch Intern Med. 1999;159(19):2312–6.
26. Al-Eidan FA, McElnay JC, Scott MG, McConnell JB. Management of Helicobacter pylori eradication–the influence of structured counselling and follow-up. Br J Clin Pharmacol. 2002;53(2):163–71.

13

Systematic review of the relationship of *Helicobacter pylori* infection with geographical latitude, average annual temperature and average daily sunshine

Chao Lu[1†], Ye Yu[2†], Lan Li[1], Chaohui Yu[1] and Ping Xu[1*]

Abstract

Background: *Helicobacter pylori* (*H. pylori*) infection is a worldwide threat to human health with high prevalence. In this study, we analyzed the relationship between latitude, average annual temperature, average daily sunshine time and *H. pylori* infection.

Methods: The PubMed, ClinicalTrials.gov, EBSCO and Web of Science databases were searched to identify studies reporting *H. pylori* infection. Latitude 30° was the cut-off level for low and mid-latitude areas. We obtained information for latitude, average annual temperature, average daily sunshine, and Human Development Index (HDI) from reports of studies of the relationships with *H. pylori* infection.

Results: Of the 51 studies included, there was significant difference in *H. pylori* infection between the low- and mid-latitude areas ($P = 0.05$). There was no significant difference in the prevalence of *H. pylori* infection in each 15°-latitude zone analyzed ($P = 0.061$). Subgroup analysis revealed the highest and lowest *H. pylori* infection rates in the developing regions at > 30° latitude subgroup and the developed regions at < 30° latitude subgroup, respectively ($P < 0.001$). Multivariate analysis showed that average annual temperature, average daily sunshine time and HDI were significantly correlated with *H. pylori* infection ($P = 0.009$, $P < 0.001$, $P < 0.001$), while there was no correlation between *H. pylori* infection and latitude.

Conclusions: Our analysis showed that higher average annual temperature was associated with lower *H. pylori* infection rates, while average daily sunshine time correlated positively with *H. pylori* infection. HDI was also found to be a significant factor, with higher HDI associated with lower infection rates. These findings provide evidence that can be used to devise strategies for the prevention and control of *H. pylori*.

Keywords: Latitude, Temperature, Sunshine, *Helicobacter pylori*

Background

Helicobacter pylori (*H. pylori*) is a Gram-negative micro-aerophilic bacterium that dwells in human gastric mucosa, causing stomach injury. *H. pylori* infection is commonly associated with gastroduodenal diseases in humans, such as chronic gastritis and peptic ulcers [1], gastric mucosa-associated lymphoid tissue lymphoma [2], and even gastric cancer [3, 4]. Almost 50% of the human population worldwide is infected, with a higher rate in people living in developing countries [5]. A large number of studies have provided evidence of *H. pylori* in dental plaques, houseflies, human and animal feces, and natural environmental waters [6]. Therefore, water supplies contaminated by sewage containing fluids or feces from infected people have been considered to be a potential route of *H. pylori* transmission [6]. Several factors may contribute to *H. pylori* infection, such as socioeconomic status and living conditions [7], metabolic syndrome [8], sex [9], education and smoking [10].

* Correspondence: ymsego@zju.edu.cn
†Equal contributors
[1]Department of Gastroenterology, the First Affiliated Hospital, College of Medicine, Zhejiang University, No. 79 Qingchun Road, Hangzhou 310003, China

Among these factors, socioeconomic conditions play an important role in *H. pylori* infection. Our previous analysis of the Human Development Index (HDI) confirmed that high *H. pylori* recurrence rates are more likely in less-developed areas [7]. Thus, prevention and therapy of *H. pylori* have become a public health challenge.

There is clear geographic variation in the prevalence of *H. pylori* infection [11, 12]. Furthermore, vitamin D and vitamin D receptor (VDR) play an important protective role in *H. pylori* infection [13]. Vitamin D is an immunoregulatory agent widely known to mediate bone metabolism and plays a key role in target tissues, such as the kidney, thyroid, intestine, skin, immune cells, nonparenchymal hepatocytes, and biliary epithelial cells [14, 15]. Vitamin D synthesis depends on exposure to sunlight and solar ultraviolet radiation, which is affected by latitude, season, temperature and duration of daily sunshine [16]. Therefore, we hypothesized that the prevalence of *H. pylori* infection varies with changes in geographic areas (different latitudes, temperature and average daily sunshine time) that are associated with differences in the rates of vitamin D synthesis.

The purpose of this study was to determine the influence of different latitudes, temperature, HDI and average daily sunshine time on *H. pylori* infection rates. This information will highlight a novel epidemiologic and global perspective of *H. pylori* infection.

Methods

Search strategy and study selection

We searched articles published from January 1, 2000 to December 1, 2016 in the PubMed, ClinicalTrials.gov, EMBASE and Web of Science databases using the following search terms: (*Helicobacter pylori* OR *H. pylori* OR *Helicobacter infection* OR *Helicobacter** OR *HP* OR *Helicobacter pylori (MeSH)*), *and* (*infection* OR *infectious (MeSH)*). Our study was limited to humans only and studies involving participants undergoing physical examination were included. People with digestive disease, such as gastritis, peptic ulcer, and stomach cancer, were excluded if they underwent physical examination. In addition, we focused on studies with participants aged over 18 years. Age, sex, smoking, HDI and other confounding factors were also considered. Eligibility was evaluated by two investigators independently. The quality of papers was assessed using the Strengthening the Reporting of Observational studies in Epidemiology (STROBE) checklist [17]. Any study-related disagreements were resolved by a third reviewer.

Definitions

Diagnostic methods for H. pylori infection

Combining the guidelines [18] and previous meta-analysis [19], a diagnosis of *H. pylori* infection was confirmed on the basis of at least one positive result from the following tests: (1) $^{13}C/^{14}C$ urea breath test (UBT); (2) rapid urease test (RUT); (3) *H. pylori* culture; (4) stool antigen test; or (5) histology of biopsy staining. Because many medical centers used a serologic test for physical examination, serologic tests were also used to confirm diagnosis.

Average daily sunshine time, latitude, temperature and HDI

After identification of the geographical location of the city or area participating in the study, we used the Hong Kong Observatory (http://gb.weather.gov.hk/contentc.htm) to obtain information for calculation of the average daily sunshine time and the average daily temperature of every city included in this study. The average daily sunshine time was calculated according to the following equation:

Average daily sunshine time = annual average sunshine time/365; Annual average temperature was used in the analysis.

HDI was chosen to assess the socioeconomic status at the national level. This index is a measure of three basic dimensions of human development: health index (according to life expectancy at birth), education index (according to mean and expected years of schooling), and decent standard of living (gross national income per capita) [7]. The HDI data (1990–2012) is available on the United Nations Development Programme website (http://hdr.undp.org/en/reports/). Countries with a high HDI score (0.788 or higher) are regarded as developed, while others are defined as developing according to the United Nations [20].

Data abstraction

Data were extracted to Microsoft Excel (2007 edition; Microsoft, Redmond, WA, USA) for effective organization. The following data were obtained from included studies: the study area, latitude, average annual temperature and average daily sunshine duration (according to study area or country), year of study, participant number, diagnostic method used for *H. pylori* infection, HDI levels (according to study country in the relevant years), age, sex, and smoking.

We excluded papers without information for latitude, average annual temperature or average daily sunshine time. All data were double-checked by two authors.

Statistical analysis

The data obtained in this study exhibited normal distribution; therefore, Student's *t*-test was used to compare numerical variables for each latitude zone and different HDI zones. One-way analysis of variance (ANOVA) was performed to compare multiple groups and analysis of covariance (ANCOVA) was performed to analyze influence effects. Pair-wise comparisons of multiple groups were performed with Bonferroni Correction [21] if necessary. In the multivariate analysis, stepwise linear regression analysis was used to correlate *H. pylori* infection with HDI, latitude, average annual temperature and average daily sunshine time. Adjustment and discretization of different variables were conducted if necessary. Moreover, the potential of sex, age and smoking as influencing factors was analyzed in a randomized controlled model ($I^2 > 50\%$) or a fixed controlled model ($I^2 \leq 50\%$) to compare differences between infected and non-infected individuals. In the multivariate analysis, $P \leq 0.05$ was considered to indicate a significant correlation and $0.1 > P > 0.05$ was considered to indicate a suggestive correlation. For other statistical methods, $P \leq 0.05$ was considered to indicate statistical significance. All statistical analysis was performed using SPSS 17.0 (IBM, Chicago, IL, USA). Associated data were calculated and plotted using GraphPad Prism 5 (Graph Pad, San Diego, CA, USA). The randomized controlled model was performed using Stata 12.0 (StataCorp, College Station, TX, USA).

Results

Study selection

Fifty-one studies originating from 58 regions were included in our final analysis (Fig. 1). Primary data and results for author, study area, HDI, latitude, average annual temperature, and average daily sunshine time are listed in Table 1. Geographically, studies originated mainly from Asia (25/58), Europe (19/58), America (11/58), Africa (2/58) and Oceania (1/58). In addition, according to the dichotomy of HDI, additional studies were included

from developed countries (32/58) and developing countries (26/58). The cut-off level between the low and mid-latitude was set at 30° latitude. Based on latitude, 13 studies originated from low latitude zones, and 45 from zones 30° latitude and higher. Statistically significant heterogeneity was observed among all studies in this analysis.

Prevalence of *H. pylori* infection

The overall prevalence of *H. pylori* infection was 49.73% ± 20.68%, with a significant difference in the prevalence of *H. pylori* infection between the latitude zones < 30° and ≥ 30° (39.92% ± 21.15% vs. 52.56% ± 19.88%, $P = 0.05$) (Fig. 2a). We further analyzed the prevalence of *H. pylori* infection in every 15°-latitude zone. The *H. pylori* infection rate was 35.43% ± 24.68% (0–15°), 43.77% ± 18.71% (15–30°), 56.29% ± 17.24% (30–45°), and 45.10% ± 23.18% (≥ 45°), respectively. ANOVA did not show a significant difference in the prevalence of *H. pylori* infection for each latitude zone ($P = 0.061$). However, we observed a rising trend in the prevalence of *H. pylori* infection from latitude 0° to 45° (Fig. 2b). Most of the regions in the latitude ≥45° zones are developed areas; therefore, we used ANCOVA to assess the existence of confounding effects caused by the HDI. The results showed a linear relationship between HDI and latitude (F = 22.328, $P < 0.001$) and HDI affected the result of latitude as a confounding factor ($P = 0.001$). We then conducted a subgroup analysis. In the developing and developed regions, we also observed a similar rising trend in the prevalence of *H. pylori* infection from latitude 0 to

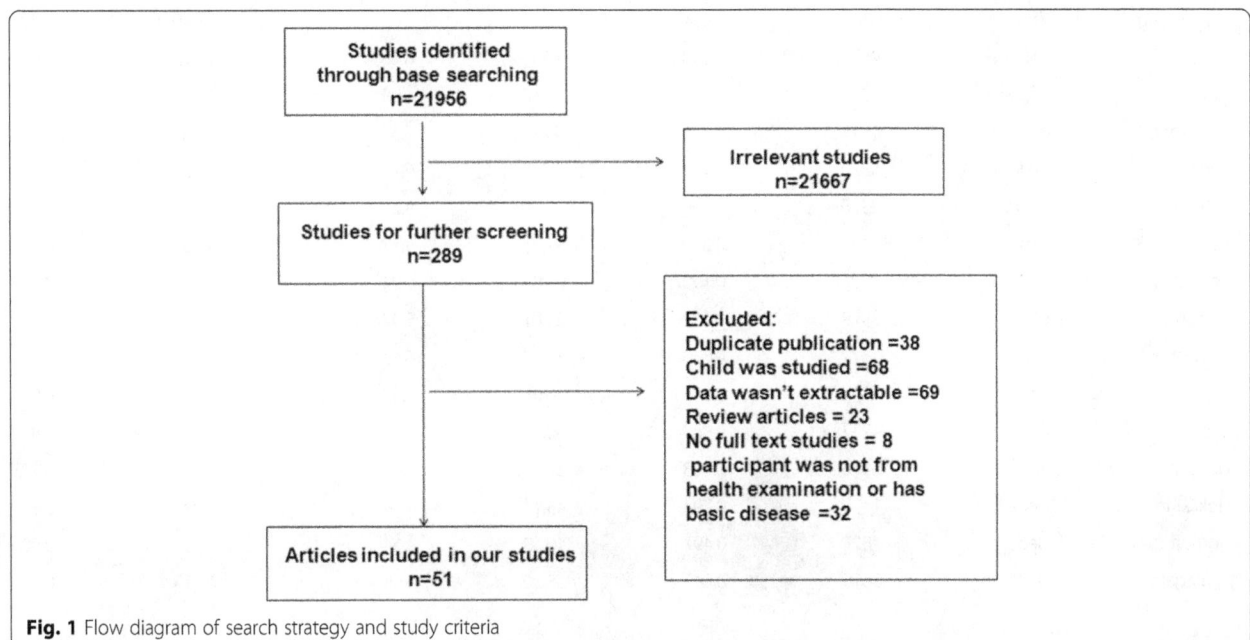

Fig. 1 Flow diagram of search strategy and study criteria

Table 1 The basic characteristics of included papers

Region	Author	Number (n)	Positive rate	Latitude (°)	Temperature (°C)	Sunshine (h)	HDI
Europe							
Israel	Niv	2128	0.328	31.00	9.31	16.45	0.872
Nottingham	Jackson	2437	0.264	52.56	3.77	9.80	0.768
Lebanon	Naja	308	0.520	33.45	8.05	20.87	0.761
Berlin	Berg	1806	0.392	52.30	4.45	8.88	0.801
Rome	Gasbarrini	655	0.400	41.80	6.77	15.20	0.825
Leeds	Moayyedi	8429	0.276	53.48	3.36	8.76	0.818
Magdeburg	Wex	2318	0.444	52.80	4.45	8.75	0.906
Novosibirsk	Reshetnikov	438	0.884	55.20	6.03	1.73	0.723
Prague	Bures	1406	0.292	50.05	4.57	7.85	0.867
Loiano	Bazzoli	1533	0.679	44.16	5.59	8.60	0.803
Stockholm	Sorberg	3502	0.177	59.19	4.99	6.63	0.855
Wroclaw	Iwanczak	3307	0.842	51.10	4.10	8.32	0.794
Tbilisi	Kretsinger	125	0.719	41.70	5.63	13.00	0.690
Heidelberg	Michel	1797	0.481	49.25	4.49	11.50	0.916
Bratislava	Kuzela	1838	0.351	48.08	5.58	10.50	0.836
Tirana	Monno	1088	0.707	41.19	6.97	15.20	0.682
Reykjavik	Thjodleifsson	447	0.363	64.08	3.48	4.30	0.859
Uppsala	Thjodleifsson	359	0.112	59.51	4.86	6.50	0.897
Tartu	Thjodleifsson	240	0.692	58.23	4.59	4.84	0.780
Asia							
Beijing	Zhang	2006	0.833	40.15	7.52	11.80	0.645
Ankara	Akin	1089	0.774	39.52	6.71	11.71	0.653
Korea	Yim	13,697	0.586	36.00	5.77	11.82	0.853
Okinawa	Toyoda	1540	0.599	26.50	5.15	22.42	0.871
Malaysia	Goh	2381	0.359	4.00	6.11	26.73	0.727
Islamabad	Rasheed	205	0.819	33.43	8.07	21.34	0.522
Yangzhong	Zhu	5417	0.634	32.19	5.85	15.10	0.699
North Sulawesi	Miftahussurur	251	0.143	1.29	6.00	27.72	0.684
Arak	Afsharipour	525	0.742	34.10	8.09	13.65	0.751
Nahavand	Alizadeh	1518	0.710	34.11	7.55	10.83	0.735
Penang	Sasidharan	5370	0.142	5.24	6.75	27.00	0.723
Tehran	Nouraie	2326	0.690	35.40	8.25	17.00	0.703
Seoul	Kim	1485	0.649	37.33	5.77	11.82	0.853
Kota Bharu	Rahim	480	0.190	6.90	6.94	26.73	0.769
Hsinchu	Chen	3578	0.202	24.81	5.07	22.60	0.882
Xiangshui	Shi	1371	0.620	34.20	6.57	15.79	0.641
Korea	Lim	10,796	0.545	36.00	5.77	11.82	0.891
Beijing	Cheng	1232	0.468	40.15	7.52	11.80	0.812
Hangzhou	Xu	8820	0.438	30.30	5.42	15.79	0.723
Hokkaido	Ueda	1428	0.294	43.14	4.94	8.22	0.890
Aomori	Ueda	782	0.497	40.49	4.64	9.73	0.890
Yamagata	Ueda	3615	0.545	38.30	4.56	11.19	0.890

Table 1 The basic characteristics of included papers *(Continued)*

Region	Author	Number (n)	Positive rate	Latitude (°)	Temperature (°C)	Sunshine (h)	HDI
Gunma	Ueda	4914	0.323	36.40	5.42	13.91	0.890
Aichi	Ueda	2237	0.306	35.10	5.58	15.04	0.890
Kagawa	Ueda	442	0.378	34.30	5.80	15.35	0.890
America							
America	Everhart	7465	0.325	36.09	7.07	15.06	0.859
Nashville	Epplein	310	0.787	36.09	6.88	15.06	0.888
Seattle	Ioannou	6724	0.535	47.38	5.95	11.13	0.859
Ontario	Naja	1306	0.294	43.40	5.58	7.16	0.896
Aklavik	Cheung	194	0.660	68.13	3.54	−8.20	0.896
Nassau	Carter	204	0.578	24.15	7.91	24.85	0.778
São Paulo	Zaterka	993	0.657	23.33	5.49	19.20	0.720
Guadeloupe	Weill	854	0.552	16.15	7.60	26.30	0.848
São Paulo	Oba–Shinjo	942	0.484	23.33	4.75	19.26	0.688
Recife	Melo	405	0.314	8.30	6.75	25.46	0.683
Pelotas	Santos	359	0.644	31.46	6.14	17.50	0.709
Africa							
Belgium	Aguemon	446	0.740	6.21	6.44	27.22	0.413
Tunis	Mansour	250	0.632	36.48	7.69	20.00	0.689
Oceania							
Queensland	Pandeya	1316	0.230	27.30	7.50	21.40	0.904

HDI **Human Development Index**

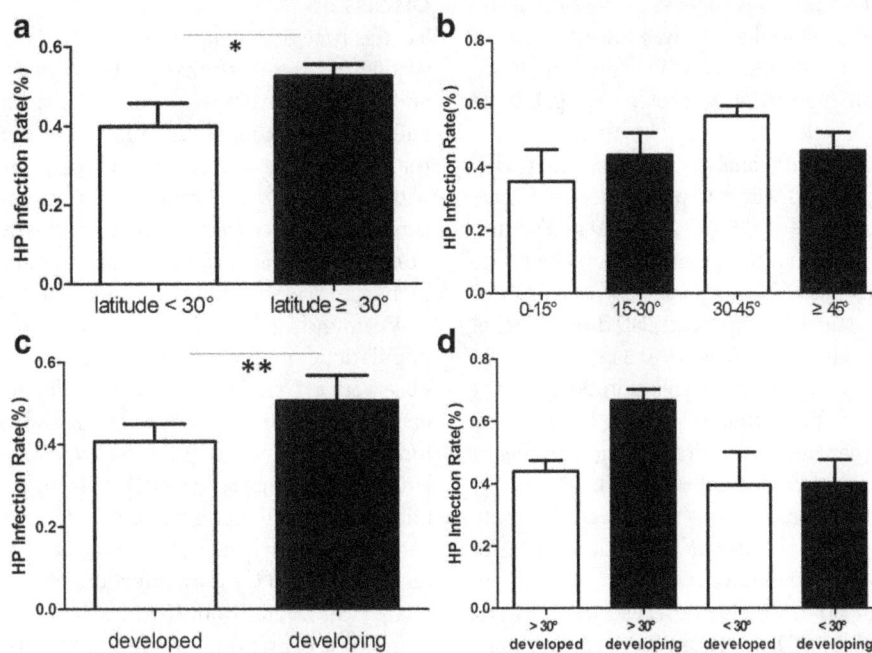

Fig. 2 a Comparison of the prevalence of *Helicobacter pylori* infection between low and mid-to-high latitude zones (39.92% ± 21.15% vs. 52.56% ± 19.88%, *P = 0.05); **b** Comparisons of the prevalence of *H. pylori* infection in each 15°-latitude zone; **c** Comparison of the prevalence of *H. pylori* infection between developed and developing regions (43.48% ± 17.73% vs. 57.42% ± 21.76%, **P = 0.009); **d** Comparisons of the prevalence of *H. pylori* infection in developed countries and mid-to-high latitude zones, developing countries and mid-to-high latitude zones, developed countries and low latitude, developing countries and low latitude zones (*P* < 0.001)

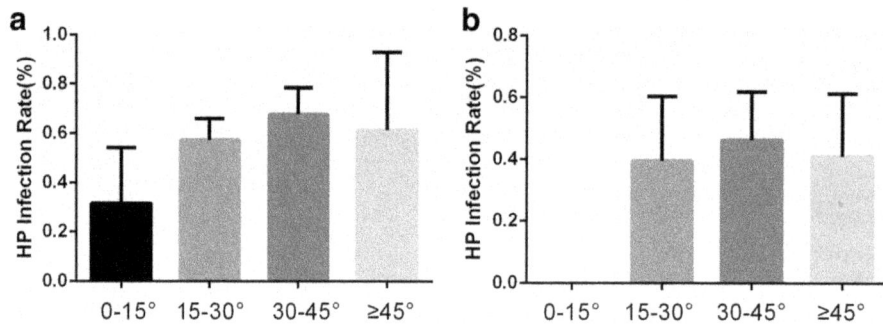

Fig. 3 a Comparisons of the prevalence of *Helicobacter pylori* infection for every 15°-latitude zone in developing regions; **b** Comparisons of the prevalence of *H. pylori* infection for every 15°-latitude zone in developed regions

45° (Fig. 3a and b). We also divided regions into developed and developing regions according to the HDI. Individuals living in developed regions showed a lower infection rate than those in the developing regions ($43.48\% \pm 17.73\%$ vs. $57.42 \pm 21.76\%$, $P = 0.009$) (Fig. 2c). To further confirm the relationship between HDI, latitude and *H. pylori* infection, we determined *H. pylori* infection rates in the following four groups of areas: I): $44.03\% \pm 17.60\%$ (developed countries & $> 30°$ latitude); II): $66.60\% \pm 15.08\%$ (developing countries & $> 30°$ latitude); III): $39.58\% \pm 20.88\%$ (developed countries & $< 30°$ latitude); and IV): $40.08\% \pm 22.53\%$ (developing countries & $< 30°$ latitude) (Fig. 2d); there were significant differences between each group ($P < 0.001$). The *H. pylori* infection rate was highest in developing regions at $> 30°$ latitude, while the rate was lowest in developed regions at $< 30°$ latitude. This indicated that low latitude regions with high HDI is protective against *H. pylori* infection.

Stepwise linear regression analysis revealed that HDI was significantly correlated with the prevalence of *H. pylori* infection (coefficient = $- 0.556$, $P < 0.001$). Furthermore, higher average annual temperature correlated with lower infection rates (coefficient = $- 0.577$, $P < 0.001$) and higher average daily sunshine time correlated with higher *H. pylori* infection rates (coefficient = 0.342, $P = 0.009$). However, there was no significant correlation between the prevalence of *H. pylori* infection and latitude. In European regions, we found that only HDI affected the prevalence of *H. pylori* infection (coefficient = $- 0.648$, $P = 0.003$), while the prevalence in Asian regions was affected by both HDI (coefficient = $- 0.584$, $P < 0.001$) and latitude (coefficient = 0.744, $P < 0.001$). Moreover, through adjustment and discretization of HDI, we also observed that latitude (coefficient = 0.774, $P < 0.001$) exerts an independent effect on the prevalence of *H. pylori* infection.

Based on existing data, we conducted meta-analysis to analyze the influences of age, sex, smoking and education on the *H. pylori* infection rate. *H. pylori*-infected individuals were found to be significantly older than

non-infected infected individuals (SMD = 0.26, 95% CI = 0.09–0.44, $I^2 = 94.2\%$, $P < 0.01$; Additional file 1) and males were 1.1 times more likely to be infected with *H. pylori* than females (OR = 1.1, 95% CI = 1.04–1.16, $I^2 = 72.1\%$, $P < 0.01$; Additional file 1). Furthermore, individuals with a high level of education were 0.58 times more likely to be infected with *H. pylori* than individuals with a low level of education (OR = 0.58, 95% CI = 0.41–0.84, $I^2 = 97.1\%$, $P < 0.01$; Additional file 1). In contrast, there were no significant differences in the *H. pylori infection rates* between smokers and non-smokers (OR = 0.99, 95% CI = 0.93–1.05, $I^2 = 43.3\%$, $P = 0.042$; Additional file 1).

Discussion

To the best of our knowledge, this is the first study investigating the relationships between *H. pylori* infection and latitude, average annual temperature and average daily sunshine time. Our multiple-factor analysis showed that higher average annual temperature was associated with lower *H. pylori* infection rates, while average daily sunshine time correlated positively with *H. pylori* infection. HDI was also found to be a significant factor, with higher HDI associated with lower infection rates.

We found higher *H. pylori* infection rates among the populations in high latitude regions. Furthermore, we observed a trend of increasing infection rates with increasing latitude. Vitamin D is known to be closely linked to ultraviolet radiation exposure [22] and lower latitudes are characterized by stronger ultraviolet radiation. Therefore, people living in low latitude zones may generate higher levels of vitamin D, which played a protective role in *H. pylori* infection, as shown by us previously [13]. In addition, Kwon et al. reported that vitamin D induced expression of vitamin D3-upregulated protein 1 (VDUP1), which reduced *H. pylori*-induced gastric carcinogenesis in mice [23]. The vitamin D nuclear receptor, which binds vitamin D, is detected in gastric mucosa [24]. Furthermore, the function of vitamin D in antimicrobial innate immune responses [25] indicates the possibility of a role in reducing *H. pylori* infection. In general, it can be speculated that different latitudes affect the synthesis of vitamin D, with a consequential influence on *H. pylori* infection rates. Our study also showed a suggestive correlation between latitude and infection rate, although no significant correlation was identified in our multiple-factor analysis. Interestingly, however, we observed that latitude independently affected *H. pylori* infection in Asian countries, indicating that latitude is an extremely important factor in *H. pylori* infection in these regions. Therefore, further studies are required to support the hypothesis that latitude influences *H. pylori* infection rates in different geographical regions.

In this study, we also found that average annual temperature was significantly related to *H. pylori* infection, a link that has not been reported previously. We propose that suitably warm temperatures provide more opportunities for people to engage in outside activities, with increased vitamin D synthesis resulting from the increased exposure to sunlight. However, this hypothesis requires verification in large-scale epidemiological studies and basic research.

Our results showed that more average daily sunshine time is associated with higher *H. pylori* infection rate, which was contrary to our expectation based on the positive correlation of daily sunshine time with vitamin D synthesis. Daily sunshine time is determined by several factors such as altitude, active area, environment. Our findings may provide evidence that ultraviolet light intensity based on latitude has a much more important influence on *H. pylori* infection than ultraviolet light exposure time. Furthermore, the *H. pylori* infection rate may also be influenced by other factors, such as sex, age, and education.

HDI, which represents the gold standard for measurement of human development, was found to be inversely related to *H. pylori* infection, which is consistent with a previous epidemiological study [26]. In our study, we found lower *H. pylori* infection rates in regions with latitude > 45°, which was not consistent with the trend of increasing *H. pylori* infection rates with latitude. Globally, regions higher than 45° latitude contain mainly the developed countries of North America and Northern Europe; thus, indicating that HDI plays a predominant role in the lower *H. pylori* infection rates found in these regions. ANCOVA showed a linear relationship between HDI and latitude and that HDI had a distinct influence on the effect of latitude on *H. pylori* infection rates. Furthermore, we observed the lowest infection rate among individuals living in developed regions with low latitude, which further illustrated that the importance of latitude and HDI on the rate of *H. pylori* infection.

Due to the lack of related reports, the results of our analysis of the influence of smoking were inconsistent with those of previous studies [27]; further investigations are required for clarification of the influence of this factor on the rate of *H. pylori* infection.

To our knowledge, this is the first study of the association of *H. pylori* infection with geographical latitude, average daily sunshine time, and average annual temperature.

Despite the strength of the numbers of participants, some limitations of our study should be noted. First, the studies included in our analysis predominantly used two diagnostic methods: the ^{13}C UBT and the serologic test; however, different diagnostic methods have different positive diagnostic rates [28]. The specificity and sensitivity of serologic tests were 100% and 82% respectively, while the corresponding values for the ^{13}C UBT were 100% and 92%, respectively [29]. Therefore, the differences in diagnostic approach may lead directly to selection bias in the included participants and consequently, to a greatly increased false positive rate. The ^{13}C UBT is the most effective noninvasive diagnostic method for detection of *H. pylori* infection with high specificity and sensitivity that is currently available. Second, our definition of latitude, average daily sunshine time and average annual temperature were based on the areas in which the research originated, while it was not certain that the participants really represented the area selected. Selected participants originating from different areas introduce a selection bias. In addition, although all the participants were healthy and without any digestive diseases during the study, it was not clear whether previous disease or other systemic diseases may have influenced *H. pylori* infection. Finally, several original studies failed to adjust for potentially confounding factors such as race, environmental factor, and gene polymorphisms. Any of these factors can lead to bias in the results.

Conclusions

In conclusion, we have demonstrated that *H. pylori* infection is significantly related to average annual temperature, average daily sunshine time and HDI. Higher average annual temperature and HDI correlated with lower *H. pylori* infection rates. Average daily sunshine time correlated positively with *H. pylori* infection rates; however, no correlation between the prevalence of *H. pylori* infection and latitude was observed in the multivariate analysis. Nevertheless, individuals living in high latitude regions showed a high infection rate. In consideration of the influence of HDI, a suggestive increasing trend of *H. pylori* infection rate with rising latitude also existed. Moreover, the combined statistically significant differences in infection rates at different latitudes and HDI scores suggest that latitude is also an influencing factor. Therefore, populations living in regions with low average annual temperature, low HDI and high latitude need to be alerted to the risk of *H. pylori* infection. We also believe that the global prevalence of *H. pylori* infection should be evaluated from a human development perspective. Our findings require further verification in large-scale epidemiological investigations.

Additional file

Additional file 1: Meta-analysis of analyzing the influences of age, sex, smoking and education on the *H. pylori* infection rate. *H. pylori*-infected individuals were older than non-infected infected individuals (SMD = 0.26, 95% CI = 0.09–0.44, I2 = 94.2%, $P < 0.01$) and males were 1.1 times more likely to be infected with *H. pylori* than females (OR = 1.1, 95% CI = 1.04–1.16, I2 = 72.1%, $P < 0.01$). High-educated individuals were 0.58 times more likely to be infected with *H. pylori* than low-educated individuals (OR = 0.58, 95% CI = 0.41–0.84, I2 = 97.1%, $P < 0.01$). There were no significant differences in the *H. pylori* infection rates between smokers and non-smokers (OR = 0.99, 95% CI = 0.93–1.05, I2 = 43.3%, $P = 0.042$).

Abbreviations

H. pylori: Helicobacter pylori; HDI: Human development index; RUT: Rapid urease test; UBT: Urea breath test; VDR: Vitamin D receptor; VDUP1: Vitamin D3-upregulated protein 1

Acknowledgments
We thank Hong Zhang (Statistics expert, Institute of Biostatistics, Fudan School of Life Sciences) for his outstanding statistical methods assistance.

Funding
This study was funded by the National Natural Science Foundation of China (81400606) and the Science and Technology Plan Projects of Zhejiang Province, China (2015C33102).

Availability of data and materials
The datasets generated during and/or analyzed during the current study are available in the PubMed (https://www.ncbi.nlm.nih.gov/pubmed/), ClinicalTrials.gov (https://clinicaltrials.gov/), EMBASE (https://www.sciencedirect.com/) and Web of Science (https://login.webofknowledge.com/) databases, or available from the corresponding author on reasonable request. In addition, data of annual average sunshine time and average annual temperature are available from the Hong Kong Observatory (http://gb.weather.gov.hk/contentc.htm). The HDI data (1990–2012) are available from the United Nations Development Programme website (http://hdr.undp.org/en/reports/).

Authors' contributions
LC, XP and YCH designed the study; LC and YY performed the research; LL collected and analyzed the data; LC gave statistical support; LC wrote the paper. All authors have read and approved the final manuscript.

Competing interests
The authors declare that they have no competing interests.

Author details
[1]Department of Gastroenterology, the First Affiliated Hospital, College of Medicine, Zhejiang University, No. 79 Qingchun Road, Hangzhou 310003, China. [2]Department of Rheumatology, the First Affiliated Hospital, College of Medicine, Zhejiang University, Hangzhou 310003, China.

References
1. Peek RM Jr, Blaser MJ. Pathophysiology of Helicobacter pylori-induced gastritis and peptic ulcer disease. Am J Med. 1997;102(2):200–7.
2. Eck M, Schmausser B, Haas R, Greiner A, Czub S, Muller-Hermelink HK. MALT-type lymphoma of the stomach is associated with Helicobacter pylori strains expressing the CagA protein. Gastroenterology. 1997;112(5):1482–6.
3. Huang JQ, Sridhar S, Chen Y, Hunt RH. Meta-analysis of the relationship between Helicobacter pylori seropositivity and gastric cancer. Gastroenterology. 1998;114(6):1169–79.
4. Konturek PC, Konturek SJ, Brzozowski T. Gastric cancer and Helicobacter pylori infection. J Physiol Pharmacol. 2006;57(Suppl 3):51–65.
5. Suerbaum S, Michetti P. Helicobacter pylori infection. N Engl J Med. 2002; 347(15):1175–86.
6. Cellini L. Helicobacter pylori: a chameleon-like approach to life. World J Gastroenterol. 2014;20(19):5575–82.
7. Yan TL, Hu QD, Zhang Q, Li YM, Liang TB. National rates of Helicobacter pylori recurrence are significantly and inversely correlated with human development index. Aliment Pharmacol Ther. 2013;37(10):963–8.
8. Chen TP, Hung HF, Chen MK, Lai HH, Hsu WF, Huang KC, et al. Helicobacter pylori infection is positively associated with metabolic syndrome in Taiwanese adults: a cross-sectional study. Helicobacter. 2015;20(3):184–91.
9. de Martel C, Parsonnet J. Helicobacter pylori infection and gender: a meta-analysis of population-based prevalence surveys. Dig Dis Sci. 2006;51(12): 2292–301.
10. Bures J, Kopacova M, Koupil I, Vorisek V, Rejchrt S, Beranek M, et al. Epidemiology of Helicobacter pylori infection in the Czech Republic. Helicobacter. 2006;11(1):56–65.
11. Calvet X, Ramirez Lazaro MJ, Lehours P, Megraud F. Diagnosis and epidemiology of Helicobacter pylori infection. Helicobacter. 2013;18(Suppl 1):5–11.
12. Fock KM, Ang TL. Epidemiology of Helicobacter pylori infection and gastric cancer in Asia. J Gastroenterol Hepatol. 2010;25(3):479–86.
13. Guo L, Chen W, Zhu H, Chen Y, Wan X, Yang N, et al. Helicobacter pylori induces increased expression of the vitamin d receptor in immune responses. Helicobacter. 2014;19(1):37–47.
14. Bouillon R, Carmeliet G, Verlinden L, van Etten E, Verstuyf A, Luderer HF, et al. Vitamin D and human health: lessons from vitamin D receptor null mice. Endocr Rev. 2008;29(6):726–76.
15. Gascon-Barre M, Demers C, Mirshahi A, Neron S, Zalzal S, Nanci A. The normal liver harbors the vitamin D nuclear receptor in nonparenchymal and biliary epithelial cells. Hepatology (Baltimore, Md). 2003;37(5):1034–42.
16. Holick MF. Environmental factors that influence the cutaneous production of vitamin D. Am J Clin Nutr. 1995;61(3 Suppl):638S–45S.
17. von Elm E, Altman DG, Egger M, Pocock SJ, Gotzsche PC, Vandenbroucke JP. The strengthening the reporting of observational studies in epidemiology (STROBE) statement: guidelines for reporting observational studies. J Clin Epidemiol. 2008;61(4):344–9.
18. Malfertheiner P, Megraud F, O'Morain CA, Atherton J, Axon AT, Bazzoli F, et al. Management of Helicobacter pylori infection-the Maastricht IV/Florence consensus report. Gut. 2012;61(5):646–64.
19. Szajewska H, Horvath A, Piwowarczyk A. Meta-analysis: the effects of Saccharomyces boulardii supplementation on Helicobacter pylori eradication rates and side effects during treatment. Aliment Pharmacol Ther. 2010;32(9):1069–79.
20. Klugman J. The real wealth of nations: pathways to human development, 20th anniversary edn. New York: United Nations Development Programme; 2010.
21. Benjamini Y, Yekutieli D. The control of the false discovery rate in multiple testing under dependency. Ann Stat. 2001;29:1165–88.
22. Holick MF. Sunlight, ultraviolet radiation, vitamin D and skin cancer: how much sunlight do we need? Adv Exp Med Biol. 2014;810:1–16.
23. Kwon HJ, Won YS, Nam KT, Yoon YD, Jee H, Yoon WK, et al. Vitamin D(3) upregulated protein 1 deficiency promotes N-methyl-N-nitrosourea and Helicobacter pylori-induced gastric carcinogenesis in mice. Gut. 2012;61(1):53–63.
24. Trowbridge R, Mittal SK, Sharma P, Hunter WJ, Agrawal DK. Vitamin D receptor expression in the mucosal tissue at the gastroesophageal junction. Exp Mol Pathol. 2012;93(2):246–9.
25. Wang TT, Nestel FP, Bourdeau V, Nagai Y, Wang Q, Liao J, et al. Cutting edge: 1,25-dihydroxyvitamin D3 is a direct inducer of antimicrobial peptide gene expression. J Immunol (Baltimore, Md : 1950). 2004;173(5):2909–12.

26. Malaty HM. Epidemiology of Helicobacter pylori infection. Best Pract Res Clin Gastroenterol. 2007;21(2):205–14.

27. Santibanez M, Aguirre E, Belda S, Aragones N, Saez J, Rodriguez JC, et al. Relationship between tobacco, cagA and vacA i1 virulence factors and bacterial load in patients infected by Helicobacter pylori. PLoS One. 2015; 10(3):e0120444.

28. Dunn BE, Cohen H, Blaser MJ. Helicobacter pylori. Clin Microbiol Rev. 1997; 10(4):720–41.

29. Logan RP, Polson RJ, Misiewicz JJ, Rao G, Karim NQ, Newell D, et al. Simplified single sample 13Carbon urea breath test for Helicobacter pylori: comparison with histology, culture, and ELISA serology. Gut. 1991;32(12): 1461–4.

Relationship between *Helicobacter pylori* infection and bone mineral density

Bo-Lin Pan[1], Chih-Fang Huang[1], Seng-Kee Chuah[2], Jui-Chin Chiang[1] and Song-Seng Loke[1*]

Abstract

Background: *Helicobacter pylori (H. pylori)* infection can induce individual inflammatory and immune reactions which associated with extra-digestive disorders. Our aim is to investigate the association between *H. pylori* infection and bone mineral density.

Methods: This retrospective cross-sectional study was performed by using the data from the health examination database in a medical center of southern Taiwan in 2013. We investigated the relationship between sex, age, body mass index (BMI), waist circumstance, lipid profile, *H. pylori* infection, the findings of upper gastrointestinal endoscopy and bone mineral density (BMD). Because of nonrandomized assignment and strong confounding effect of age on BMD, the 1:1 propensity score match was applied for age adjustment. The simple and multiple stepwise logistic regression analysis were performed to assess the risk factors of decreased BMD in these well-balanced pairs of participants.

Results: Of the 867 subjects in final analysis with the mean age of 55.9 ± 11.3 years, 381 (43.9%) subjects had *H. pylori* infection, and 556 (64.1%) subjects had decreased BMD. In decreased BMD group, the portion of woman was higher than a normal BMD group (37.2% versus 29.6%, $P = 0.023$), the age was significantly older (59.4 ± 9.8 versus 49.8 ± 11.3, $p < 0.001$) and BMI was significantly lower (24.7 ± 3.5 versus 25.4 ± 3.7, $p = 0.006$) than the normal BMD group. The prevalence of *H. pylori* infection was 39.9% and 46.2% in the normal BMD group and the decreased BMD group respectively ($P = 0.071$). The multivariate analysis which was used for these possible risk factors showed that only advanced age (OR 1.09, 95% CI 1.08–1.11, $P < 0.001$), and low BMI (OR 0.91, 95% CI 0.87–0.95, $P < 0.001$) were independently significantly associated with decreased BMD in this nonrandomized study. In the propensity score-matched participants, the multiple stepwise logistic regression analysis revealed *H. pylori* infection (OR 1.62, 95% CI 1.12–2.35, $P = 0.011$) and low BMI (OR 0.92, 95% CI 0.87–0.97, $P = 0.001$) were independently significantly associated with decreased BMD.

Conclusions: *H. pylori* infection and low BMI were independently significantly associated with decreased BMD in selected propensity score-matched populations after age adjustment.

Keywords: *Helicobacter pylori*, Bone mineral density, body mass index, Dual energy X-ray absorptiometry scan, Osteoporosis

* Correspondence: loke@adm.cgmh.org.tw
[1]Department of Family Medicine, Kaohsiung Chang Gung Memorial Hospital and Chang Gung University College of Medicine, 123, Dapi Road, Niaosong District, Kaohsiung 833, Taiwan

Background

Osteoporosis is a silent health problem characterized by decreased bone mineral density (BMD) with a risk of spine and hip fractures. Approximately half of the hip fractures globally result from osteoporosis. According to data from the National Health Insurance Research Database between 1996 and 2010 in Taiwan, the high annual incidence rate of hip fracture was 472.1 per 100,000 patients per year, higher than that in other Asian countries and even in the world. The in-hospital mortality rates were between 0.85 to 2.26% [1]. The spine and hip fractures resulted from osteoporosis could induce patients to become bedridden and needing care. Mortality and disability-associated osteoporosis have significant impact on prognosis and are a burden affecting patients, their families, society, and the health system. Early identification of the risk of decreased BMD and osteoporosis is very important. Previous study has revealed that the risk factors of osteoporosis include age, sex, low body mass index (BMI), steroid use and chronic alcohol consumption [2, 3]. Recently, several gastrointestinal diseases such as inflammatory bowel disease, peptic ulcer disease and atrophic gastritis have been suspected of being risk factors for osteoporosis [4–6].

Helicobacter pylori (*H. pylori*) infection is strongly associated with chronic gastritis, peptic ulcers, gastric cancer, and mucosa-associated lymphoid tissue lymphoma [7]. Several studies have reported *H. pylori* also plays a role in extra-digestive disorders including cardiovascular, neurological, skin disease and diabetes mellitus [8].

H. pylori infection can induce individual inflammatory and immune reactions, which can regulate bone turnover. Several research studies have reported that *H. pylori* infection is a risk factor of osteoporosis [9, 10], but this finding is controversial in other studies [11, 12]. To our knowledge, only one study has evaluated the relationship between *H. pylori* infection and osteoporosis in Taiwan, but the result was only found in elderly females [10]. Therefore, we aimed to investigate whether *H. pylori* infection was associated with decreased BMD in a general population undergoing routine health examination in Taiwan.

Methods

Subjects

This retrospective cross-sectional study was performed by using the data from the health examination database in a medical center of the southern Taiwan. We included subjects who were aged greater than 20 years, had undergone upper gastrointestinal endoscopy with the Campylobacter-like organism test (CLO test) and dual energy X-ray absorptiometry scan (DEXA) from January 2013 to December 2013. Subjects with missing data and gastric cancer were excluded. The study was approved by the Chang Gung Medical Foundation Institutional Review Board (IRB No.: 201701187B0).

Since this is a retrospective study, a written consent is waived by an IRB and is deemed unnecessary.

The medical records showed information on sex, age, waist circumstance, lipid profile, *H. pylori* testing, BMD, and the findings of upper gastrointestinal endoscopy. BMI was calculated as the weight in kilograms divided by the height in meters squared. Peptic ulcer or gastro-esophageal reflux disease (GERD) were diagnosed by upper gastrointestinal endoscopy.

Definition of *H. pylori* infection

The present of *H. pylori* infection was determined by CLO test via upper gastrointestinal endoscopy. CLO test is a rapid diagnostic test and is performed during upper gastrointestinal endoscopy. A biopsy of mucosa from the stomach is placed into the medium consisting of urea and an indicator. If *H. pylori* is present, the urease produced by *H. pylori* converts urea to ammonia, which increases the pH of the medium and then changes its color from yellow to red. In this health examination, all examinations were self-paid, CLO test was performed not only for peptic ulcer, but also performed under subjects request although no peptic ulcer was found by upper gastrointestinal endoscopy.

Determination of bone mineral density

BMD was measured by DEXA. The *T*-score is the number of standard deviations by which a given measurement differs from the mean for a normal young adult reference population. According to the World Health Organization definition [13], osteoporosis is defined as *T*-score ≤ – 2.5, and the osteopenia is defined as a T-score between – 1 and – 2.5. Decreased BMD in the present study included osteoporosis and osteopenia.

Statistical analysis

All data are described as the mean ± standard deviation for continuous variables and as numbers and percentages for categorical variables. SPSS software version 19.0 (IBM Corp., Armonk, NY, USA)) was used for the statistical analysis. The characteristics of subjects were compared by χ^2-test for the categorical variables and Student's t-test for the continuous variables. Univariate logistic regression analysis and multivariate logistic regression analysis were conducted to analyze the odds ratio (OR) of significant factors associated with decreased BMD. Besides, to minimize confounding effect of age due to nonrandomized assignment, propensity scores were calculated using a logistic regression model and the covariate, age. A 1:1 matched study group was created by the Greedy method with NCSS software (NCSS 10, NCSS Statistical software, Kaysville, Utah). After adjusting the age, univariate logistic regression analysis and multivariate logistic regression analysis were used to evaluate factors associated with decreased BMD. The strength of association was reported as OR with 95% confidential interval (CI) and P-values. All statistical assessments were two-sided and considered significant if $P < 0.05$.

Results

Prevalence of *H. pylori* infection and decreased BMD

We enroll 942 subjects who participated in the health examination and underwent biochemistry blood examination, upper gastrointestinal endoscopy with CLO test and the bone mineral density examinations. Seventy-five subjects were excluded due to missing data in some biochemical variables. Of the 867 subjects in final analysis with the mean age of 55.9 ± 11.3 years, 381(43.9%) subjects had *H. pylori* infection, and 556 (64.1%) subjects had decreased BMD. The numbers of female and male subjects were 299 (34.5%) and 568 (65.5%). Table 1 shows the baseline characteristics of all participants.

Differences between the subjects with normal and decreased BMD

Table 2 compares the characteristics between the normal BMD group and the decreased BMD group. In decreased BMD group, the portion of woman was higher than a normal BMD group (37.2% versus 29.6%, $P = 0.023$), the age was significantly older (59.4 ± 9.8 versus 49.8 ± 11.3, $p < 0.001$) and BMI was significantly lower (24.7 ± 3.5 versus 25.4 ± 3.7, $p = 0.006$) than the normal BMD group. Besides, lipid profiles except for triglyceride were significantly higher than in the normal BMD group. Comparing the gastrointestinal disorder between these

Table 1 Baseline characteristics

	Participants $N = 867$
Sex	
Female n, %	299(34.5%)
Male n, %	568(65.5%)
Age (years old)	55.9 ± 11.3
BMI(Kg/m^2)	24.9 ± 3.6
Waist circumference(cm)	85.1 ± 10.4
Total cholesterol(mg/dl)	195.7 ± 35.7
HDL cholesterol(mg/dl)	56.5 ± 15.6
Triglyceride(mg/dl)	131.9 ± 84.7
LDL cholesterol(mg/dl)	113.4 ± 32.4
Decreased BMD, n %	556(64.1%)
Peptic ulcer n, %	351(40.5%)
GERD n, %	187(21.6%)
H. pylori infection n, %	381(43.9%)

BMI body mass index, *LDL* low-density lipoprotein, *HDL* high-density lipoprotein, *BMD* bone mineral density, *GERD* gastro-esophageal reflux disease, H. pylori *Helicobacter pylori*

Table 2 Differences between normal BMD group and decreased BMD group

	Normal BMD $n = 311$	Decreased BMD $n = 556$	p value
Sex			0.023*
Male n, %	219(70.4%)	349(62.8%)	
Female n, %	92(29.6%)	207(37.2%)	
Age (years old)	49.8 ± 11.3	59.4 ± 9.8	< 0.001*
BMI(Kg/m^2)	25.4 ± 3.7	24.7 ± 3.5	0.006*
Waist circumference(cm)	85.9 ± 10.1	84.7 ± 10.5	0.08
Total cholesterol(mg/dl)	191.2 ± 34.5	198.2 ± 36.2	0.005*
HDL cholesterol(mg/dl)	54.4 ± 14.9	57.8 ± 15.8	0.002*
Triglyceride(mg/dl)	136.8 ± 83.8	129.2 ± 85.2	0.205
LDL cholesterol(mg/dl)	110.0 ± 31.5	115.3 ± 32.7	0.021*
Peptic ulcer n, %	111(35.7%)	240(43.2%)	0.032*
GERD n, %	69(22.2%)	118(21.2%)	0.741
H. pylori infection n, %	124(39.9%)	257(46.2%)	0.071

*Indicates a significant difference, p < 0.05
BMI body mass index, *LDL* low-density lipoprotein, *HDL* high-density lipoprotein, *BMD* bone mineral density, *GERD* gastro-esophageal reflux disease, H. pylori *Helicobacter pylori*

two groups, the prevalence of peptic ulcer was significantly higher in the decreased BMD group ($p = 0.032$), but the GERD was lower in the decreased BMD group ($p = 0.741$). The prevalence of *H. pylori* infection was 39.9% and 46.2% in the normal BMD group and decreased BMD group respectively ($P = 0.071$).

Simple and multiple stepwise logistic regression analyses of variables associated with decreased BMD

Simple logistic regression (Table 3) showed decreased BMD was significantly associated with the female gender (OR 0.71, 95% CI 0.53–0.94, $P = 0.023$), advanced age (OR 1.09, 95% CI 1.07–1.10, $P < 0.001$), low BMI (OR 0.95, 95% CI 0.91–0.99, $P = 0.006$), total cholesterol (OR 1.01, 95% CI 1.00–1.01, $P = 0.005$), low-density lipoprotein (LDL) cholesterol (OR 1.01, 95% CI 1.00–1.01, $P = 0.021$), high-density lipoprotein (HDL) cholesterol (OR 1.02, 95% CI 1.00–1.02, $P = 0.002$), and peptic ulcer disease (OR 1.37, 95% CI 1.03–1.82, $P = 0.032$). The multivariate analysis that was conducted with these risk factors revealed that only advanced age (OR 1.09, 95% CI 1.08–1.11, $P < 0.001$), and low BMI (OR 0.91, 95% CI 0.87–0.95, $P < 0.001$) were independently significantly associated with decreased BMD. The *H. pylori* infection was not independently significantly associated with decreased BMD (OR 1.30, 95% CI 0.98–1.71, $P = 0.071$).

Because the confounding effect of age was strong with nonrandomized assignment, propensity score-matching was used for age adjustment. The 234 well-balanced pairs of participants, with a 1:1 ratio after propensity score matching of age, were evaluated for risk factor of decreased

Table 3 Regression analysis for association of decreased BMD with different variables

Variables	Simple logistic regression OR (95% CI)	p value	multiple stepwise logistic regression OR (95% CI)	p value
Sex	0.71(0.53–0.94)	0.023*		
Age	1.09(1.07-1.10)	< 0.001*	1.09(1.08-1.11)	< 0.001*
BMI	0.95(0.91-0.99)	0.006*	0.91(0.87-0.95)	< 0.001*
Waist circumference	0.99(0.98–1.00)	0.08		
Total cholesterol	1.01(1.00–1.01)	0.005*		
HDL cholesterol	1.02(1.00–1.02)	0.002*		
TG	1.00(0.99-1.001)	0.207		
LDL cholesterol	1.01(1.00–1.01)	0.021*		
Peptic ulcer	1.37(1.03–1.82)	0.032*		
GERD	0.95(0.68-1.32)	0.74		
H. pylori infection	1.30(0.98–1.71)	0.071		

*Indicates a significant difference, p < 0.05
BMI body mass index, LDL, low-density lipoprotein, HDL high-density lipoprotein, BMD bone mineral density, GERD gastro-esophageal reflux disease, H. pylori Helicobacter pylori

BMD. In these propensity score-matched participants, the mean age was 53.3 ± 10.35 years in the normal BMD group and 53.4 ± 10.33 years in the decreased BMD group. There was no significant difference in age between the two groups ($p = 0.961$). The covariates of these well-balanced pairs of participants were conducted for simple and multiple stepwise logistic regression analysis. In simple logistic regression, the BMI (OR 0.92, 95% CI 0.87–0.97, $P = 0.001$), waist circumstance (OR 0.98, 95% CI 0.96–0.99, $P = 0.006$) and H. pylori infection (OR 1.60, 95% CI 1.11–2.30, $P = 0.012$) were significantly associated with decreased BMD. In multivariate analysis, H. pylori infection (OR 1.62, 95% CI 1.12–2.35, $P = 0.011$) and BMI (OR 0.92, 95% CI 0.87–0.97, $P = 0.001$) were independent significant risk factors of decreased BMD without confounding effect of age (Table 4).

Discussion

The main finding of this retrospective cross-sectional study revealed that advanced age and low BMI were significant risk factors of decreased BMD in the nonrandomized assignment. In addition, H. pylori infection was significantly associated with decreased BMD in selected propensity score-matched participants with respect to age. In other words, H. pylori infection was a risk factor of decreased BMD without the confounding effect of age, because the age corresponded to an increase in risk of osteoporosis [2].

This result was compatible with the past studies regarding the association between H. pylori infection and decreased BMD [10, 12, 14]. Several possible mechanisms might explain this finding. First, H. pylori infection may result in chronic gastritis and induce systemic

Table 4 Regression analysis for association between decreased BMD and different variables after propensity score matching

Variables	Simple logistic regression OR (95% CI)	p value	Multiple stepwise logistic regression OR (95% CI)	p value
Sex	0.80(0.54–1.19)	0.27		
BMI	0.92(0.87–0.97)	0.001*	0.92(0.87–0.97)	0.001*
Waist circumference	0.98(0.96–0.99)	0.006*		
Total cholesterol	1.00(0.99–1.01)	0.257		
HDL	1.01(1.00–1.02)	0.082		
TG	1.00(0.99–1.001)	0.672		
LDL	1.00(0.99–1.01)	0.425		
Peptic ulcer	1.10(0.75–1.60)	0.632		
GERD	0.88(0.56–1.38)	0.564		
H. pylori infection	1.60(1.11–2.30)	0.012*	1.62(1.12-2.35)	0.011*

*Indicates a significant difference, p < 0.05
BMI body mass index, LDL low-density lipoprotein, HDL high-density lipoprotein, BMD bone mineral density, GERD gastro-esophageal reflux disease, H. pylori Helicobacter pylori

inflammation with the release of cytokines, including tumor necrosis factor- , interleukin-1 and interleukin-6 [15]. These inflammatory cytokines are known to result in bone resorption, so *H. pylori* infection may affect bone turnover indirectly [16]. The second mechanism was that chronic *H. pylori* infection might cause the gastric mucosal atrophy which would decrease acid secretion. The hypochlorhydric stomach affects calcium absorption, calcium homeostasis and bone mass [17]. In addition, the low serum vitamin B12 level was found in the patients with *H. pylori* infection [18]. If the serum vitamin B12 levels are low, the folate becomes trapped as methyltetrahydrofolate and then interrupts for folate-related DNA synthesis. This reaction is an important factor of bone remodeling, so the low level of vitamin B12 may result in decreased BMD [19].

Besides, *H. pylori* infection was treated with the eradication therapy as triple or quadruple regimen, such as a proton pump inhibitor, clarithromycin, amoxicillin or tetracycline, and metronidazole, with or without bismuth. One study described cytokine gene expression as significantly decreasing after *H. pylori* was eradicated [20]. In a meta-analysis, mucosal atrophy of the stomach was improved after successful eradication therapy [21]. Because the cytokines result in bone resorption and gastric mucosal atrophy affects calcium metabolism, the improvement of gastric mucosa and decreased inflammatory cytokine by successful eradication therapy might be able to decrease the incidence of osteoporosis. Two studies support this hypothesis. Hong-Mo Shih et al. reported the incidence of osteoporosis relatively reduced in early eradication of *H. pylori* group, compared to the late eradication group by an analysis from the National Health Insurance Database in Taiwan [22]. In Japan, the success of *H. pylori* eradication may contribute to decrease the risk of osteoporosis. In our study, we found that *H. pylori* infection was independently significantly associated with decreased BMD after age adjustment, but eradication of *H. pylori* was not recorded in this health examination database. A further prospective cohort study is necessary to confirm that BMD would be improved after triple or quadruple *H. pylori* eradication therapy.

Advanced age and low BMI are well-known risk factors of osteoporosis and bone fracture [2]. From the National Health and Nutrition Examination Survey (NHANES) 2005–2006 in US, 49% of US women age 50 years and older had decreased BMD, and 30% of older men had decreased BMD [23]. The prevalence rates of BMD from Nutrition and Health Survey in Taiwan 2005–2008 was higher in advanced age. In females, the prevalence rate was 50.3% in the 60 years and older group, and increased to 63.7% in the 70 years and older group. In male, the prevalence rate was 18.6% in the 60 years and older group, and increased to 45.4% in those aged 70 years and older

[24]. One research showed that the weight loss appears to increase the rate of hip bone loss, even in obese men undergoing voluntary weight reduction [25]. This present study reported a similar result where the advanced age and low BMI had the strong association with the decreased BMD.

Several researches have reported that the GERD was associated with osteoporosis. However, the vertebral fractures or kyphosis were also found in these studies [26–28]. In the present study, the GERD was not significantly associated with decreased BMD. Because this study was derived from the health examinations, these subjects may be healthy relatively without any bone deformities. Besides, two studies revealed peptic ulcer disease was an independent risk factor for osteoporosis [6, 29]. The mechanism of this association was not clear. The malabsorption of calcium and macroelements due to the defective stomach and duodenal epithelium in which inflammation at these sites results may play a role in bone metabolism. Our result showed the peptic ulcer was not a risk factor of decreased BMD, but it tended to be associated with decreased BMD in univariate logistic regression analysis. The disorder of the small intestine may affect the absorption of these substances more than disorders of the stomach and duodenum.

There were several limitations in our study. First, our study was conducted in a single hospital, which might not be representative of other settings. Second, retrospective studies based on abstraction of medical records are constrained by the accuracy and completeness of such records. Third, some laboratory data, including serum calcium, serum phosphorus, serum specific alkaline phosphatase or serum vitamin D level were unavailable, because this study was retrospective from the health examination.

Conclusions

In conclusion, advanced age and low BMI were independent significant risk factors of decreased BMD in this retrospective study. Besides low BMI, *H. pylori* infection was independently significantly associated with decreased BMD in selected propensity score-matched participants with respect to age. Further prospective cohort studies including the potential important factors are required to confirm this association in the Taiwan population.

Abbreviations
BMD: Bone mineral density; BMI: Body mass index; CI: Confidential interval; CLO test: Campylobacter-like organism test; DEXA: Dual energy X-ray absorptiometry scan; GERD: Gastro-esophageal reflux disease; *H. pylori*: *Helicobacter pylori*; HDL: High-density lipoprotein; LDL: Low-density lipoprotein

Acknowledgments
We appreciated the Biostatistics Center, Kaohsiung Chang Gung Memorial Hospital for statistics work.

Funding
This study was not supported by any grant.

Authors' contributions

PBL analyzed the data and drafted the paper; HCF, CSK, CJC performed the research; LSS designed the research and revised the paper. All authors read and approved the final manuscript.

Competing interests

CSK is a member of the editorial board of this journal. All other authors declare that they have no competing interests.

Author details

[1]Department of Family Medicine, Kaohsiung Chang Gung Memorial Hospital and Chang Gung University College of Medicine, 123, Dapi Road, Niaosong District, Kaohsiung 833, Taiwan. [2]Division of Hepatogastroenterology, Department of Internal Medicine, Kaohsiung Chang Gung Memorial Hospital and Chang Gung University College of Medicine, 123, Dapi Road, Niaosong District, Kaohsiung 833, Taiwan.

References

1. Wu TY, Hu HY, Lin SY, Chie WC, Yang RS, Liaw CK. Trends in hip fracture rates in Taiwan: a nationwide study from 1996 to 2010. Osteoporos Int. 2017;28(2):653–65.
2. Nih Consensus Development Panel on Osteoporosis Prevention D, Therapy. Osteoporosis prevention, diagnosis, and therapy. JAMA. 2001;285(6):785–95.
3. Kouda K, Iki M, Fujita Y, Tamaki J, Yura A, Kadowaki E, Sato Y, Moon JS, Morikawa M, Tomioka K, et al. Alcohol intake and bone status in elderly Japanese men: baseline data from the Fujiwara-kyo osteoporosis risk in men (FORMEN) study. Bone. 2011;49(2):275–80.
4. Ali T, Lam D, Bronze MS, Humphrey MB. Osteoporosis in inflammatory bowel disease. Am J Med. 2009;122(7):599–604.
5. Kim HW, Kim YH, Han K, Nam GE, Kim GS, Han BD, Lee A, Ahn JY, Ko BJ. Atrophic gastritis: a related factor for osteoporosis in elderly women. PLoS One. 2014;9(7):e101852.
6. Sawicki A, Regula A, Godwod K, Debinski A. Peptic ulcer disease and calcium intake as risk factors of osteoporosis in women. Osteoporos Int. 2003;14(12):983–6.
7. Atherton JC. The pathogenesis of Helicobacter pylori-induced gastro-duodenal diseases. Annu Rev Pathol. 2006;1:63–96.
8. Goni E, Franceschi F. Helicobacter pylori and extragastric diseases. Helicobacter. 2016;21(Suppl 1):45–8.
9. Asaoka D, Nagahara A, Shimada Y, Matsumoto K, Ueyama H, Matsumoto K, Nakagawa Y, Takeda T, Tanaka I, Sasaki H, et al. Risk factors for osteoporosis in Japan: is it associated with Helicobacter pylori? Ther Clin Risk Manag. 2015;11:381–91.
10. Lin SC, Koo M, Tsai KW. Association between Helicobacter pylori infection and risk of osteoporosis in elderly Taiwanese women with upper gastrointestinal diseases: a retrospective patient record review. Gastroenterol Res Pract. 2014;2014:814756.
11. Kakehasi AM, Mendes CM, Coelho LG, Castro LP, Barbosa AJ. The presence of Helicobacter pylori in postmenopausal women is not a factor to the decrease of bone mineral density. Arq Gastroenterol. 2007;44(3):266–70.
12. Fotouk-Kiai M, Hoseini SR, Meftah N, Ghadimi R, Bijani A, Noreddini H, Nematollahi H, Shokri-Shirvani J. Relationship between Helicobacter pylori infection (HP) and bone mineral density (BMD) in elderly people. Caspian J Intern Med. 2015;6(2):62–6.
13. Kanis JA. Assessment of fracture risk and its application to screening for postmenopausal osteoporosis: synopsis of a WHO report. WHO Study Group Osteoporos Int. 1994;4(6):368–81.
14. Asaoka D, Nagahara A, Hojo M, Sasaki H, Shimada Y, Yoshizawa T, Osada T, Watanabe S. The relationship between H. Pylori infection and osteoporosis in Japan. Gastroenterol Res Pract. 2014;2014:340765.
15. Noach LA, Bosma NB, Jansen J, Hoek FJ, van Deventer SJ, Tytgat GN. Mucosal tumor necrosis factor-alpha, interleukin-1 beta, and interleukin-8 production in patients with Helicobacter pylori infection. Scand J Gastroenterol. 1994;29(5):425–9.
16. Pacifici R. Cytokines, estrogen, and postmenopausal osteoporosis–the second decade. Endocrinology. 1998;139(6):2659–61.
17. Kakehasi AM, Rodrigues CB, Carvalho AV, Barbosa AJ. Chronic gastritis and bone mineral density in women. Dig Dis Sci. 2009;54(4):819–24.
18. Kalkan C, Karakaya F, Tuzun A, Gencturk ZB, Soykan I. Factors related to low serum vitamin B12 levels in elderly patients with non-atrophic gastritis in contrast to patients with normal vitamin B12 levels. Geriatr Gerontol Int. 2016;16(6):686–92.
19. Tucker KL, Hannan MT, Qiao N, Jacques PF, Selhub J, Cupples LA, Kiel DP. Low plasma vitamin B12 is associated with lower BMD: the Framingham osteoporosis study. J Bone Miner Res. 2005;20(1):152–8.
20. Moss S, Legon S, Davies J, Calam J. Cytokine gene expression in Helicobacter pylori associated antral gastritis. Gut. 1994;35(11):1567–70.
21. Rokkas T, Pistiolas D, Sechopoulos P, Robotis I, Margantinis G. The long-term impact of Helicobacter pylori eradication on gastric histology: a systematic review and meta-analysis. Helicobacter. 2007;12(Suppl 2):32–8.
22. Shih H-M, Hsu T-Y, Chen C-Y, Lin C-L, Kao C-H, Chen C-H, Yang T-Y, Chen W-K. Analysis of patients with Helicobacter pylori infection and the subsequent risk of developing osteoporosis after eradication therapy: a Nationwide population-based cohort study. PLoS One. 2016;11(9):e0162645.
23. Looker AC, Melton LJ 3rd, Harris TB, Borrud LG, Shepherd JA. Prevalence and trends in low femur bone density among older US adults: NHANES 2005-2006 compared with NHANES III. J Bone Miner Res. 2010;25(1):64–71.
24. Lin YC, Pan WH. Bone mineral density in adults in Taiwan: results of the nutrition and health survey in Taiwan 2005-2008 (NAHSIT 2005-2008). Asia Pac J Clin Nutr. 2011;20(2):283–91.
25. Ensrud KE, Fullman RL, Barrett-Connor E, Cauley JA, Stefanick ML, Fink HA, Lewis CE, Orwoll E. Osteoporotic fractures in men study research G: voluntary weight reduction in older men increases hip bone loss: the osteoporotic fractures in men study. J Clin Endocrinol Metab. 2005;90(4):1998–2004.
26. Miyakoshi N, Kasukawa Y, Sasaki H, Kamo K, Shimada Y. Impact of spinal kyphosis on gastroesophageal reflux disease symptoms in patients with osteoporosis. Osteoporos Int. 2009;20(7):1193–8.
27. Sugimoto M, Hasegawa T, Nishino M, Sahara S, Uotani T, Ichikawa H, Kagami T, Sugimoto K, Yamato Y, Togawa D, et al. Improvement of gastroesophageal reflux disease in Japanese patients with spinal kyphotic deformity who underwent surgical spinal correction. Dig Endosc. 2016;28(1):50–8.
28. Yamane Y, Yamaguchi T, Tsumori M, Yamauchi M, Yano S, Yamamoto M, Honda C, Kinoshita Y, Sugimoto T. Elcatonin is effective for lower back pain and the symptoms of gastroesophageal reflux disease in elderly osteoporotic patients with kyphosis. Geriatr Gerontol Int. 2011;11(2):215–20.
29. Wu CH, Tung YC, Chai CY, Lu YY, Su YF, Tsai TH, Kuo KL, Lin CL. Increased risk of osteoporosis in patients with peptic ulcer disease: a Nationwide population-based study. Medicine (Baltimore). 2016;95(16):e3309.

15

Prevalence of clarithromycin resistance in *Helicobacter pylori* in Santiago, Chile, estimated by real-time PCR directly from gastric mucosa

Patricio Gonzalez-Hormazabal[1][*] (iD), Maher Musleh[2,3], Susana Escandar[2], Hector Valladares[2,3], Enrique Lanzarini[2,3], V. Gonzalo Castro[1], Lilian Jara[1] and Zoltan Berger[2]

Abstract

Background: Current available treatments for *Helicobacter pylori* eradication are chosen according to local clarithromycin and metronidazole resistance prevalence. The aim of this study was to estimate, by means of molecular methods, both clarithromycin and metronidazole resistance in gastric mucosa from patients infected with *H.pylori*.

Methods: A total of 191 DNA samples were analyzed. DNA was purified from gastric mucosa obtained from patients who underwent an upper gastrointestinal endoscopy at an university hospital from Santiago, Chile, between 2011 and 2014. *H.pylori* was detected by real-time PCR. A 5'exonuclease assay was developed to detect A2142G and A2143G mutations among *H.pylori*-positive samples. *rdxA* gene was sequenced in samples harboring A2142G and A2143G mutations in order to detect mutations that potentially confer dual clarithromycin and metronidazole resistance.

Results: Ninety-three (93) out of 191 DNA samples obtained from gastric mucosa were H.pylori-positive (48.7%). Clarithromycin-resistance was detected in 29 samples (31.2% [95%CI 22.0–41.6%]). The sequencing of *rdxA* gene revealed that two samples harbored truncating mutations in *rdxA*, one sample had an in-frame deletion, and 11 had amino acid changes that likely cause metronidazole resistance.

Conclusions: We estimated a prevalence of clarithomycin-resistance of 31.8% in Santiago, Chile. Three of them harbor inactivating mutations in *rdxA* and 11 had missense mutations likely conferring metronidazole resistance. Our results require further confirmation. Nevertheless, they are significant as an initial approximation in re-evaluating the guidelines for *H.pylori* eradication currently used in Chile.

Keywords: Helicobacter pylori, Clarithromycin, Metronidazole, 23S rRNA, rdxA, Mutation

Background

Helicobacter pylori is a gram-negative bacillus that colonizes the gastric mucosa. The infection is associated with both gastric and extragastric diseases such as peptic ulcer disease, gastric atrophy, gastric adenocarcinoma, gastric MALT (mucosa-associated lymphoid tissue) lymphoma, and iron deficiency anemia. The evidence strongly suggests that *H.pylori* eradication is beneficial in treatment or prevention of those diseases [1]. One treatment for *H.pylori* eradication is the triple-therapy that comprises clarithromycin, amoxicillin, and proton pump inhibitor (PPI), nevertheless, triple-therapy is not recommended in regions with high clarithomycin resistance rate [1]. Global claritrhomycin-resistance rates in adults are contrasted among various countries, from 1% in The Netherlands to 37.6% in Italy [2]. In light of this observation, the last Maastricht V/Florence consensus

---
* Correspondence: patriciogonzalez@uchile.cl
[1]Human Genetics Program, Institute of Biomedical Sciences, School of Medicine, University of Chile, Av. Independencia 1027, 8380453 Santiago, CL, Chile

on management of *H.pylori* [1] recommends that in high-clarithromycin resistance regions (> 15% resistance prevalence), quadruple therapy is necessary. If dual clarithromycin and metronidazole resistance is > 15%, bismuth-containing quadruple therapy is the recommended first-line treatment.

Clarithromycin belongs to the class of macrolide antibiotics. The mechanism of action is the inhibition of protein synthesis of bacteria by binding to the 23S ribosomal subunit (23S rRNA). Mutations in the peptidyltransferase region encoded in domain V of 23S rRNA are responsible for macrolide resistance [3]. Three mutations in the 23S rRNA gene account for nearly all clarithromycin-resistant (ClaR) strains: A2143G, A2142G and A2142C to a small extent [3]. Standard method (antibiogram), after culture or molecular tests, can be used to detect *H.pylori* and clarithromycin resistance directly from the gastric biopsy [1]. Epidemiological studies evaluating regional clarithromycin resistance have been conducted based on detection of A2142G and A2143G in DNA isolated from gastric biopsies [4, 5]. Commercial tests detecting both mutations are available [3], performing at a sensitivity rate of > 94% and a specificity rate of > 98.5% compared to the culture susceptibility test. Recently, Tamayo et al. [6] found a high concordance between Etest for clarithromycin and 23S rRNA mutations. To date, only Garrido and Toledo [7] have evaluated primary resistance of *H.pylori* to clarithromycin in clinical isolates from Santiago, Chile. They found primary resistance in 10 out of 50 isolates by agar dilution. Resistant isolates harbor A2142G or A2143G mutations.

Metronidazole is a nitroimidazole synthesized as an inactive antibiotic prodrug. The bactericidal effect of the drug is mainly explained by the cytotoxic effect of molecules resulting from a reduction of metronidazole intracellularly in facultative anaerobic bacteria. Reduction of metronidazole in *H.pylori* is mediated mainly by a nonessential oxygen-insensitive NADPH nitroreductase encoded by the *rdxA* gene. NADPH-flavin-oxidoreductase (FrxA) is also involved in the reduction of metronidazole [3]. Various authors found that metronidazole resistance arises from inactivating mutations in *rdxA* found only in resistant isolates, and missense mutations have also been involved in metronidazole resistance [8]. On the other hand, the role of inactivating mutations in the *frxA* gene is controversial since truncating mutations have been found in sensitive isolates, and some studies report that *frxA* mutations alone may not be enough to confer resistance [8]. Vallejos et al. [9] studied resistance to clarithromycin and metronidazole in 50 isolates obtained from patients in Santiago, Chile. Forty-five and twenty percent respectively were resistant, resulting in 13.2% of the prevalence of dual clarithromycin and metronidazole resistance.

The aim of the present study was to estimate clarithromycin resistance in 93 clinical isolates from Santiago,

Chile. To do so, we developed a test to detect A2142G and A2143G mutations in 23S gene by 5'nuclease assay. We also aimed to detect mutations in the *rdxA* gene among ClaR isolates.

Methods

Subjects

Subjects invited to participate were patients who underwent a physician-requested upper gastrointestinal endoscopy, at the Department of Gastroenterology at the University of Chile Clinical Hospital between July 2011 and July 2014. Participants were asked to donate a sample of gastric mucosa obtained from antrum and corpus. This study was approved by the Ethical Committee of the following institutions: University of Chile School of Medicine (#023/2011), and University of Chile Clinical Hospital (#029/2011). The study was performed in accordance with the Declaration of Helsinki. DNA was isolated from gastric mucosa using FavorPrep Tissue DNA Extraction Mini Kit (Favorgen Biotech Corp, Taiwan, China). Samples were identified as *H.pylori*-positive or *H.pylori*-negative by detection of the 16S rRNA gene by real-time PCR as described by Kobayashi et al. [10].

Analysis of 23S rRNA mutations

A segment of the 23S rRNA gene from position 1911 to 2200 was amplified by PCR using primers described by Agudo et al. [11], and sequenced by Sanger sequencing (Service provided by Macrogen Inc., Korea). A 5'exonuclease assay was developed to detect A2142G and A2143G mutations. We designed primers and probes for each allele in highly conserved regions from position 1911 to 2200, comparing sequences obtained from 44 randomly selected *H.pylori*-positive subjects recruited for this study. Both mutations were tested in separate assays. Primers were: F: 5'-GAGCTGTCTCAACCAGAG-3' and R: 5'-GCGCATGATATTCCCATTA-3'. Probes detecting 2142G (5'-CAAGACGGGAAGACCCC-3') and 2143G (5'-CAAGACGGAGAGACCCC-3') alleles were dual-labeled with 5'FAM-3'BHQ1, and the probe complementary to the 2142A - 2143A allele (5'-CAAGACGGAAAGACCCCG-3') was dual-labeled with 5'HEX-3'BHQ1. Primers and probes were synthesized at Macrogen Inc. (Korea). The 5'exonuclease was carried out in a StepOne Real Time PCR system (Applied Biosystems, USA) using 5X HOT FIREPol Probe qPCR Mix Plus (ROX) (Solis BioDyne, Estonia) according to manufacturer's directions.

Detection of mutations in *rdxA* gene

The sequence of *rdxA* was obtained from samples harboring 23S 2142G or 2143G. Primers for PCR amplification of *rdxA* (F: 5'-CRTTAGGGATTTTTATTGTATGC-3' R: 5'-CTCTTRCCCAAWGCGATC-3') were designed with AliView 1.18 for Linux in conserved regions after comparing 83 sequences of *H.pylori* obtained from GenBank. PCR was performed using Q5 Hot Start High Fidelity DNA Polymerase (New England Biolabs, USA) according to manufacturer's directions, using an annealing temperature of 56 °C. Electrophoretograms were obtained by Sanger sequencing (Service provided by Macrogen Inc., Korea).

Results

A total of 191 subjects were included in this study, 124 were female (64.9%) and 67 male (35.1%). The median age was 46 years (range 19 years to 82 years). None of them was treated for *H.pylori* eradication.

Ninety-three (93) out of 191 DNA samples obtained from gastric mucosa were *H.pylori*-positive (48.7%). Clarithomycin resistance was detected using a 5'exonuclease assay in 29 samples (31.2% [95%CI 22.0–41.6%]). Of them, 9 harbored 2142G (31.0%) and 20 (69.0%) harbored 2143G. All ClaR samples were confirmed by Sanger sequencing. Both Sanger sequencing and 5'exonuclease allowed us to detect heteroresistance, i.e., the coexistence of resistant and susceptible bacterial strains in the same patient [12]. Sixteen (16) out of 93 *H.pylori* subjects were homoresistant to clarithromycin (17.2%). In addition, we detected heteroresistance in 13 out of 93 patients (14.0%).

Table 1 Missense changes and truncating mutations in the *rdxA* gene among 28 clarithromycin-resistant samples

Sample	Amino acid position[a]																					
	6	16	31	49	53	62	67	73	75	88	90	97	98	118	123	151	162	166	172	175	183
26695[b]	Q	R	T	T	H	L	A	N	E	S	R	H	G	A	V	V	G	P	V	E	A
EN02	H	.	E	.	.	.	.	.	.	.	K	T	.	.	.	.	.	.	I	Q[d]	.
EN05	.	.	E	.	.	.	.	.	.	.	.	.	.	.	.	.	.	A	I	.	.
EN07	H	.	E	.	.	.	V[d]	.	.	.	K	.	.	T	.	.	.	.	.	.	.
EN11	.	.	.	.	.	.	.	.	.	.	K	.	.	.	.	.	.	.	I	.	.
EN15	H	.	.	.	R	V	.	.	.	P	.	.	S	.	.	.	L	.	I	.	.
EN16	H	.	.	.	R	V	.	.	.	P	.	T	.	.	.	.	.	.	.	.	.
EN20	.	H	.	.	.	.	.	.	.	.	.	.	.	.	T	.	.	.	I	.	.
EN30	.	.	.	.	.	.	.	.	.	.	.	Y	.	.	.	.	.	S	.	.	V
EN33	H	.	.	.	.	.	.	Q	.	.	.	.	.	.	.	.	.	.	.	.	.
EN36	H	.	.	X[d]	.	.	.	.	.	.	.	.	.	.	.	.	.	.	.	.	.
EN42	.	.	.	.	.	.	.	.	.	.	.	.	S	.	.	.	.	.	I	Q	.
EN61	.	.	E	.	.	.	.	.	.	.	K	.	.	.	.	.	.	.	I	Q	.
EN70	H	.	E	.	.	.	.	.	.	.	K	.	.	.	.	.	.	.	I	Q	V
EN82[c]	.	.	.	.	.	.	.	.	.	.	.	.	.	.	.	.	.	.	.	.	.
EN89	.	.	E	.	.	.	.	.	.	.	.	Y	.	T	.	.	.	.	.	.	.
EN97	H	.	.	.	.	.	.	.	.	.	K	.	S	.	.	T	.	.	I	Q	.
EN115	H	.	.	.	.	V[d]	.	.	.	.	.	.	.	.	.	.	.	.	.	.	.
EN117	.	.	E	.	.	.	.	.	.	.	.	.	.	.	.	.	.	.	I	Q	.
EN125	.	.	.	.	.	.	.	.	.	.	.	.	.	.	.	T	.	.	I	Q	.
EN131	.	.	.	.	.	.	.	.	.	.	.	.	.	.	.	.	.	.	.	.	.
EN137	.	.	E	.	.	.	.	.	.	.	.	Y	.	.	.	T	.	.	.	.	.
EN148	.	.	E	.	.	.	.	.	.	.	.	.	.	.	.	.	.	.	I	Q	V
EN155	H	.	.	.	.	.	X[d]	.	.	.	.	.	.	.	.	.	.	.	.	.	.
EN161	H	.	.	.	R	V	.	.	.	P	.	.	S	.	.	.	L	.	I	.	.
EN167	H	.	E	.	.	.	.	.	.	.	.	Y	.	.	T	.	R[d]	.	.	.	.
EN179	H	.	E	.	.	.	.	.	.	.	.	.	.	T	.	.	.	.	I	Q	V
EN187	.	.	.	M	.	.	.	.	.	.	.	.	.	.	.	.	.	.	.	.	.
EN190	H	H	E	.	.	.	.	.	.	.	K	.	.	T	.	.	.	.	.	.	.

[a](.): same amino acid as for reference strain
[b]Corresponds to amino acid sequence of RdxA from strain 26,695
[c]In-frame deletion of 39 nucleotides which causes the deletion of amino acids 80 to 92
[d]Coexistence of both nucleotide substitutions in the same sample. X: Stop codon

Prevalence of clarithromycin resistance in Helicobacter pylori in Santiago, Chile, estimated by real-time...

115

The *rdxA* gene was sequenced in 28 ClaR samples. One ClaR sample was not available at the time of analysis. A nonsense substitution (H53stop) was found in one sample; and an insertion of A at nucleotide 186, leading to a frameshift resulting in N73stop, was found in a different sample. Therefore, two samples harbored truncating mutations in *rdxA*. One sample had an in-frame deletion of 39 nucleotides which causes the deletion of amino acids 80 to 92 (ASALMVVCSLKPS). Table 1 shows the amino acid variations in *rdxA* found in ClaR samples.

Discussion

A total of 29 out of the 93 *H.pylori* positive samples resulted resistant to clarithomycin (31.2%). This estimation is higher than the 20% of ClaR reported by Garrido and Toledo in Chile [7]. Taken together, ClaR resistance reported for Chile is above the suggested 15% threshold to abandon triple-therapy, according to the recommendation of Maastricht V/Florence consensus [1].

Among 28 ClaR samples, two of them harbored truncating mutations and one an in-frame deletion in *rdxA*, and therefore are likely resistant to metronidazole. A total of 22 amino acid substitutions was found. Thirteen of them (Q6H, T31E, H53R, L62 V, R90K, H97T, H97Y, G98S, A118T, V123 T, V172I, E175Q, A183V) have been previously observed in metronidazole-resistant (MtzR) as well as in metronidazole-sensitive strains [13–17]. Therefore, those substitutions probably do not confer resistance to metronidazole. Four substitutions (R16H, A67V, S88P and G162R) were found in 8 samples. R16H and S88P have been observed only in MtzR strains [13–15]. In fact, Arg 16 is one of the residues of RdxA that interacts with the cofactor flavin mononucleotide (FMN) [18]. A67V corresponds to the replacement of a small alanine by a bulky valine in the protein core, and is associated with resistance [8, 19]. Analysis from the crystallographic data of RdxA reveals that G162 is involved in FMN binding [18]. Hence, missense mutations R16H, A67V, S88P and G162R likely cause MtzR. Nevertheless, phenotypic testing is needed to confirm that those mutations actually cause MtzR.

Five amino acid changes in RdxA (T49 M, E75Q, V151 L, P166A and P166S) have not been described previously in the literature. None of them have been observed as an important amino acid for the RdxA function. We predicted the effect of those substitutions using the crystallographic data of RdxA protein (Protein Data Bank accession number 3QDL) in the I-Mutant Suite server [20], which estimates protein stability changes (expressed as delta delta G values) upon single-point mutations from the protein structure. Delta-delta G values and the prediction were as follows: T49 M = − 0.41 (neutral stability),

E75Q = − 0.78 (large decrease of stability), V151 L = − 0.44 (neutral stability), P166A = − 1.28 (large decrease in stability), P166S = − 1.50 (large decrease in stability). Thus, we propose that E75Q (1 sample), P166A (1 sample), and P166S (1 sample) could confer MtzR. However, a phenotypic testing shloud be carry out to confirm it.

Conclusions

We estimated a prevalence of ClaR of 31.2% in Santiago, Chile, which is above the suggested 15% threshold to abandon triple-therapy, according to the recommendation of Maastricht V/Florence consensus. Three out of 28 ClaR samples harboring inactivating mutations in *rdxA* may be clearly MtzR, and 11 of them had missense mutations in *rdxA* likely confering MtzR. Further phenotypic testing is needed to obtain a clinically significant conclusion from *rdxA* sequencing results. Nevertheless, the estimated prevalence of ClaR is significant as an approximation in re-evaluating the triple-therapy for *H.pylori* eradication currently used in Chile.

Abbreviations
ClaR: Clarithromycin-resistant; PPI: Proton pump inhibitor

Acknowledgements
We would like to acknowledge Paul Zuckerman for his help in proofreading the manuscript.

Funding
This work was supported by Fondo Nacional de Desarrollo Científico y Tecnológico -Chile- (FONDECYT) [1151015]. The authors declare that the funding body had no participation in the design of the study and collection, analysis, and interpretation of data and in writing the manuscript.

Authors' contributions
PGH conceived, designed the study and drafted the manuscript. PGH, MM and ZB were responsible for analysis and interpretation of data. VGC and LJ performed molecular analysis. MM, SE, HV and EL were involved in acquisition of samples and data. All authors read and approved the final manuscript.

Competing interests
The authors declare that they have no competing interests.

Author details
[1]Human Genetics Program, Institute of Biomedical Sciences, School of Medicine, University of Chile, Av. Independencia 1027, 8380453 Santiago, CL, Chile. [2]Department of Gastroenterology, University of Chile Clinical Hospital, Santiago, Chile. [3]Department of Surgery, University of Chile Clinical Hospital, Santiago, Chile.

References

1. Malfertheiner P, Megraud F, O'Morain CA, Gisbert JP, Kuipers EJ, Axon AT, et al. Management of Helicobacter pylori infection-the Maastricht V/ Florence consensus report. Gut. 2017;66:6–30.

2. De Francesco V, Giorgio F, Hassan C, Manes G, Vannella L, Panella C, et al. Worldwide H. pylori antibiotic resistance: a systematic review. J Gastrointestin Liver Dis. 2010;19:409–14.

3. Nishizawa T, Suzuki H. Mechanisms of helicobacter pylori antibiotic resistance and molecular testing. Front Mol Biosci. 2014;1:19.

4. Navarro-Jarabo JM, Fernández-Sánchez F, Fernández-Moreno N, Hervas-Molina AJ, Casado-Caballero F, Puente-Gutierrez JJ, et al. Prevalence of primary resistance of helicobacter pylori to clarithromycin and levofloxacin in southern Spain. Digestion. 2015;92:78–82.

5. Park JY, Dunbar KB, Mitui M, Arnold CA, Lam-Himlin DM, Valasek MA, et al. Helicobacter pylori clarithromycin resistance and treatment failure are common in the USA. Dig Dis Sci. 2016;61:2373–80.

6. Tamayo E, Montes M, Fernández-Reyes M, Lizasoain J, Ibarra B, Mendarte U, et al. Clarithromycin resistance in Helicobacter pylori and its molecular determinants in Northern Spain, 2013–2015. J Glob Antimicrob Resist. 2017;9:43–6.

7. Garrido L, Toledo H. Novel genotypes in helicobacter pylori involving domain V of the 23S rRNA gene. Helicobacter. 2007;12:505–9.

8. Jones KR, Cha J-H, Merrell DS. Who's winning the war? Molecular mechanisms of antibiotic resistance in helicobacter pylori. Curr Drug Ther. 2008;3:190–203.

9. Vallejos C, Garrido L, Cáceres D, Madrid AM, Defilippi C, Defilippi C, et al. Prevalencia de la resistencia a metrodinazol, claritromicina y tetraciclina en *Helicobacter pylori* aislado de pacientes de la Región Metropolitana. Rev Med Chil. 2007;135:287–93.

10. Kobayashi D, Eishi Y, Ohkusa T, null l, Suzuki T, Minami J, et al. Gastric mucosal density of helicobacter pylori estimated by real-time PCR compared with results of urea breath test and histological grading. J Med Microbiol. 2002;51:305–11.

11. Agudo S, Pérez-Pérez G, Alarcón T, López-Brea M. Rapid detection of clarithromycin resistant helicobacter pylori strains in Spanish patients by polymerase chain reaction-restriction fragment length polymorphism. Rev. Espanola Quimioter. Publicacion of. Soc. Espanola Quimioter. 2011;24:32–6.

12. De Francesco V, Giorgio F, Ierardi E, D'Ercole C, Hassan C, Zullo A. Helicobacter pylori clarithromycin resistance assessment: are gastric antral biopsies sufficient? Gastroenterol Insights. 2012;4:2.

13. Solcà NM, Bernasconi MV, Piffaretti JC. Mechanism of metronidazole resistance in helicobacter pylori: comparison of the rdxA gene sequences in 30 strains. Antimicrob Agents Chemother. 2000;44:2207–10.

14. Bereswill S, Krainick C, Stähler F, Herrmann L, Kist M. Analysis of the rdxA gene in high-level metronidazole-resistant clinical isolates confirms a limited use of rdxA mutations as a marker for prediction of metronidazole resistance in helicobacter pylori. FEMS Immunol Med Microbiol. 2003;36:193–8.

15. Matteo MJ, Pérez CV, Domingo MR, Olmos M, Sanchez C, Catalano M. DNA sequence analysis of rdxA and frxA from paired metronidazole-sensitive and -resistant helicobacter pylori isolates obtained from patients with heteroresistance. Int J Antimicrob Agents. 2006;27:152–8.

16. Albert JM, Al-Mekhaizeem K, Neil L, Dhar R, Dhar PM, Al-Ali M, et al. High prevalence and level of resistance to metronidazole, but lack of resistance to other antimicrobials in helicobacter pylori, isolated from a multiracial population in Kuwait. Aliment Pharmacol Ther. 2006;24:1359–66.

17. Kim SY, Joo YM, Lee HS, Chung I-S, Yoo Y-J, Merrell DS, et al. Genetic analysis of helicobacter pylori clinical isolates suggests resistance to metronidazole can occur without the loss of functional rdxA. J Antibiot (Tokyo). 2009;62:43–50.

18. Martínez-Júlvez M, Rojas AL, Olekhnovich I, Espinosa Angarica V, Hoffman PS, Sancho J. Structure of RdxA--an oxygen-insensitive nitroreductase essential for metronidazole activation in helicobacter pylori. FEBS J. 2012;279:4306–17.

19. Secka O, Berg DE, Antonio M, Corrah T, Tapgun M, Walton R, et al. Antimicrobial susceptibility and resistance patterns among helicobacter pylori strains from the Gambia, West Africa. Antimicrob Agents Chemother. 2013;57:1231–7.

20. Capriotti E, Calabrese R, Casadio R. Predicting the insurgence of human genetic diseases associated to single point protein mutations with support vector machines and evolutionary information. Bioinformatics. 2006;22:2729–34.

16

Absence of *Helicobacter pylori* high tetracycline resistant 16S rDNA AGA926-928TTC genotype in gastric biopsy specimens from dyspeptic patients of a city in the interior of São Paulo, Brazil

Rodrigo Buzinaro Suzuki[1,3†], Cristiane Maria Almeida[2†] and Márcia Aparecida Sperança[2,3*]

Abstract

Background: Treatment effectiveness of *Helicobacter pylori* varies regionally and is decreasing worldwide, principally as a result of antibiotic resistant bacterium. Tetracycline is generally included in second line *H. pylori* eradication regimens. In Brazil, a high level of tetracycline resistance (TetR) is mainly associated with AGA926-928TTC 16 S rDNA nucleotide substitutions. As *H. pylori* culture is fastidious, we investigated the primary occurrence of *H. pylori* 16 S rDNA high level TetR genotype using a molecular approach directly on gastric biopsies of dyspeptic patients attending consecutively at Hospital das Clinicas of Marilia, São Paulo, Brazil.

Methods: Gastric biopsy specimens of 68 peptic ulcer disease (PUD) and 327 chronic gastritis (CG) patients with a positive histological diagnosis of *H. pylori* were investigated for TetR 16 S rDNA genotype through a molecular assay based on amplification of a 16 S rDNA 545 bp fragment by polymerase chain reaction and H*infl* restriction fragment length polymorphism (PCR/RFLP). Through this assay, AGA926-928TTC 16 S rDNA TetR genotype resulted in a three DNA fragment restriction pattern (281, 227 and 37 bp) and its absence originated two DNA fragments (264 and 281 bp) due to a 16 S rDNA conserved H*inf I* restriction site.

Results: The 545 bp 16 S rDNA PCR fragment was amplified from 90% of gastric biopsies from histological *H. pylori* positive patients. H*infl* RFLP revealed absence of the AGA926–928TTC *H. pylori* genotype and PCR products of two patients showed absence of the conserved 16 S rDNA H*infl* restriction site. BLASTN sequence analysis of four amplicons (two conserved and two with an unpredicted H*infl* restriction pattern) revealed a 99% homology to *H. pylori* 16 S rDNA from African, North and South American bacterial isolates. A nucleotide substitution abolished the conserved H*infl* restriction site in the two PCR fragments with unpredicted H*infl* RFLP, resulting in an *EcoRI* restriction site.

Conclusions: *H. pylori* AGA926-928TTC 16 S rDNA gene substitutions were not found in our population. More research is required to investigate if *H. pylori* TetR has a different genetic background in our region and if the nucleotide substitutions of the uncultured *H. pylori* 16 S rRNA partial sequences have biological significance.

Keywords: *Helicobacter pylori*, Tetracycline resistance, *Helicobacter pylori* 16 S rDNA, Nucleic acid based diagnosis, *Helicobacter pylori* 16 S rDNA polymorphism

* Correspondence: marcia.speranca@ufabc.edu.br
†Equal contributors
[2]Department of Molecular Biology, Marilia Medical School, Marilia, SP, Brazil
[3]Center of Natural and Human Sciences, Universidade Federal do ABC, Rua Santa Adélia, 166 Bloco A, Torre 3, 6° andar, Sala 625, CEP 09210-170 Bairro Bangu, Santo André, SP, Brazil

Background

It is widely accepted that *Helicobacter pylori*, a Gram negative microaerophilic bacterium, is associated with several digestive tract diseases such as chronic gastritis, peptic and duodenal ulcers, gastric cancer and lymphoproliferative disorders [1]. There is no standardized treatment regimen for *H.pylori* infection [2] and once the bacterium is detected in altered gastric mucosa, the indicated treatment consists of a triple antibiotic regimen including metronidazole, clarithromycin, amoxicillin, tinidazole, tetracycline and fluoroquinolones associated with a proton pump inhibitor such as omeprazole, lansoprazole or pantoprazole [3-5], according to antibiotic prescription policies for local medical care.

H. pylori eradication rates with a number of combined agents and regimens are close to 80% [6,7], varying from country to country and regionally within countries [8]. Several factors contribute to this low rate of *H. pylori* healing including the inefficiency of the antibiotic penetration in the gastric mucosa, inactivation of the antibiotic by the acid secretion of the stomach [9], lack of patient compliance [10] and principally, emergency cases and increase in *H. pylori* antibiotic resistant strains [11]. Thus, regional *H. pylori* resistance surveillance is of great importance for test and treatment strategies.

In Brazil, a country of continental dimensions, the majority of practicing clinicians include tetracycline in a second line treatment regimen after failure of the classical triple regimen composed of claritromycin, amoxicillin and a proton pump inhibitor for seven days to overcome *H. pylori* infection [12].

H. pylori resistance to tetracycline (TetR) is low in most countries [13-15], conversely, in Latin America, according to a small number of studies, it has been shown to be high in Chile [16] and in Brazil [17]. Moreover, for some years the incidence of TetR has been increasing [15,18-21]. Accordingly, considering the clinical importance of primary *H. pylori* resistance to antibiotics, it should be considered regionally before being included in eradication regimens.

The gold standard method for determination of *H. pylori in vitro* susceptibility to antibiotics corresponds to the isolation of the microorganism by culture. However, because of the slow growth and the particular requirements of *H. pylori* culture, this approach is not reliable for use in most routine clinical laboratories, principally in developing countries. Hence, molecular tests targeting resistance associated gene mutations directly from biopsy specimens have the potential for use in large scale studies [22-25].

The molecular mechanism of TetR consists of its binding to a specific 16 S rRNA region, interacting stoically with the aminoacyl-tRNA transferase to the A site of the ribosome. This binding site has been defined by atomic resolution in ribosomes of *Thermus thermophilus* being formed by two domains of the 16 S rRNA fraction consisting of helix 34 and the loop next to helix 31 [26,27]. In *H. pylori* isolates, the high degree of TetR is mainly due to three base mutations, from AGA926-928 to TTC, in the 16 S rRNA genes rrnA/B [28,29]. Mutations in one or two of these positions result in a low level of TetR [30,31].

In Brazil, studies performed on patients from Bragança Paulista, São Paulo, showed that triple AGA926-928 to TTC mutations are found in all TetR *H. pylori* isolates [32]. Thus, using a molecular approach based on a polymerase chain reaction associated with restriction fragment length polymorphism (PCR-RFLP) assay, we investigated the primary incidence of *H. pylori* high level TetR directly in gastric biopsy specimens obtained from dyspeptic patients submitted to gastroscopy at Hospital das Clínicas of Marília, São Paulo, Brazil, from January 2003 to July 2006.

Results and discussion

Gastric disease outcome of 1102 patients attending the gastroenterology outpatient clinic of Hospital das Clínicas of Marília was investigated by endoscopy and histopathology. Endoscopic finding of peptic or duodenal ulcer disease (PUD) were present in 119 patients. Different degrees of chronic gastritis (CG) were observed by histopathology in 693 patients and other alterations corresponding mostly to gastroesophageal reflux disease (GERD) and normal gastric mucosa, were found in 290 patients. Some patients presented more than one alteration, with the most severe pathology being considered in the analysis.

Detection of *H. pylori* was performed directly from biopsy specimens by histology, the gold standard *H. pylori* diagnostic test employed in our clinical routine which together with histopathological analysis is used to decide for *H. pylori* eradication therapy. Of 119 PUD, 693 CG and 290 GERD samples, 76, 359 and 2, respectively, were positive for *H. pylori* by histology.

Once detected in gastric mucosa, a classical *H. pylori* eradication triple regimen is prescribed in our gastroenterology health care clinics. When first choice regimen therapy fails to eradicate *H. pylori*, a second line regimen containing tetracycline is the most indicated. *H. pylori* antibiotic TetR varies regionally, being very low in Europe and North America [2,33,34]. However, in Asia [15,19,35] and Latin America, including Brazil [16,32], a high rate of *H. pylori* TetR has been found. Thus, in order to improve the choice of *H. pylori* associated disease therapy, principally in case of first eradication failure, we investigated the regional high level of *H. pylori* TetR using a molecular approach based on PCR and RFLP directly from the same gastric biopsy used for rapid urease test. Only biopsy samples from the patients with positive *H.*

pylori diagnosis by histology were included. A 545 bp *H. pylori* 16SrDNA PCR fragment was obtained from 89.5% (68/76) and 91.1% (327/359) of gastric biopsies from PUD and CG patients, respectively. As both tests were performed on a single and different gastric biopsy and *H. pylori* infection presents a focal characteristic of infection [36], to improve sensitivity of this method, multiple biopsy sampling is recommended.

Sequentially, in order to detect the major related point mutations, AGA to TTC at the positions 926, 927 and 928 of the *H. pylori* 16 S rDNA associated with a high level of TetR, and a unique genotype characterized in Brazilian TetR *H. pylori* isolates [32], the 545 bp 16 S rDNA PCR fragment was restricted with H*inf*I. In this *H. pylori* 16 S rDNA amplicon there is a conserved H*inf*I restriction site, which provides an internal control of enzyme digestion, resulting in a two DNA fragment restriction pattern, when the triple AGA926-928TTC nucleotide substitution is absent. Of 395 PCR samples, 393 presented the two DNA fragment restriction pattern and two PCR products obtained from a PUD (Hp16S563Mar) patient and a CG (Hp16S587bp) patient were not digested by H*inf*I. The high tetracycline resistant AGA926-928TTC genotype dependent on *H. pylori* 16 S rDNA was not present in our population. These results can be indicative of *H. pylori* high level TetR absence or that in our region other 16 S rDNA nucleotide substitutions or different genetic factors are involved in tetracycline resistance, as found by other studies [21]. More research has to be carried out to confirm or exclude these hypotheses.

In order to confirm the specificity of the 545 bp *H. pylori* 16 S rDNA PCR products amplified from gastric biopsies, the 545 bp PCR fragments obtained from two *H. pylori* positive PUD patients used as controls in PCR reactions (Hp16S248Mar and Hp16S644Mar), and the 545 bp PCR fragments with unpredicted H*inf*I restriction pattern named Hp16S563Mar and Hp16S587bp, were sequenced and analyzed by basic BLASTN search [37]. All four sequences presented 99% homology to the 16 S rDNA from West and South African, South and North American *H.pylori* isolates. The point mutations found in each analyzed PCR sequence compared to the *H. pylori* 16 S rDNA reference sequences presenting higher homology to the obtained amplicons are summarized in Table 1. Abolishment of the H*inf*I restriction site of Hp16S563 and 587Mar resulted from a nucleotide substitution at position 958, originating in an *Eco*RI restriction site. Thus, the nucleotide substitutions in these 16 S 545 bp PCR fragments were confirmed by *Eco*RI restriction analysis (data not shown). The biological significance of nucleotide substitutions found in our 16 S uncultured *H. pylori* PCR fragments needs to be investigated.

Conclusions

The high level TetR *H. pylori* genotype dependent on AGA926-929TTC 16 S rDNA gene substitutions was not found in our population. More research is required to investigate if *H. pylori* high rate TetR is absent or if it is associated with a different bacterial genetic background in our region. Also, the biological significance of the unpredicted nucleotide substitutions of the Marilia uncultured *H. pylori* 16 S rDNA partial sequence needs further investigation.

Methods
Patients
1102 adult patients resident in Marilia city, São Paulo State, Brazil, aged 19 to 91 years, who had consecutively undergone esophagogastroduodenoscopy (EGD) for upper abdominal pain or dyspeptic symptoms from January 2003 through July 2006 at the gastroenterology outpatient clinic of the Hospital das Clínicas of Marília Medical School, were enrolled in this study.

Endoscopy, biopsies
The EGD was accomplished by fibroendoscope (GIF-XP20, GIF-XQ20) or video-endoscope (GIF-100) both from Olympus. Gastric or duodenal ulcer diagnosis was defined by endoscopy and two fragments of the antrum were collected to perform the rapid urease and histopathological tests. The biopsy used for the rapid urease test was further submitted to DNA extraction. The protocol used is in agreement with the Helsinki Declaration and was approved by the Ethical Committee in Human Research from Marilia Medical School, under reference number 388/01.

Histology
One antral specimen was fixed in formol solution at 10% and embedded in paraffin. Sections were Giemsa stained for *H. pylori* evaluation and were stained with hematoxilin and eosin for assessment of histopathologic alterations [38].

DNA extraction and Polymerase chain reaction
Polymerase chain reaction and restriction analysis were set up with the same biopsy used for the rapid urease test. This was submitted to DNA extraction with the employment of the GFx DNA extraction kit purchased from Amersham/Pharmacia Biotech, following the manufacturer's instructions. DNA was quantified in agarose gel electrophoresis using the Invitrogem low mass ladder and 50-100ηg were used in the PCR reactions with the primer set Hp16Sr1 (sense),): 5' AAC ATT ACT GAC GCT GAT TG 3'; Hp16S r2 (antisense): 5' TGG CTC CAC TTC GCA GTA TT 3', which amplify a conserved fragment of 545 bp corresponding to the *H.*

Table 1 Comparison of *Helicobacter pylori* 545 bp 16 S rDNA nucleotide polymorphisms among references and uncultured bacterium strains

H. pylori strain+	16 S rDNA nucleotide positions#							
	926-928	947	954-959	981	988	1092	1093	1097
SouthAfrica07	AGA	A	GAATCC	A	T	T	C	G
2017WestAfrica	AGA	A	GAATCC	A	T	T	C	G
EU544200USA	AGA	A	GAATCC	A	T	T	T	G
Puno/Peru	AGA	A	GAATCC	G	C	T	C	G
Hp16S248Mar	AGA	G	GAATCC	A	T	T	C	A
Hp16S644Mar	AGA	A	GAATCC	A	T	G	C	G
Hp16S563Mar	AGA	A	GAATTC	A	T	T	T	G
Hp16S587Mar	AGA	A	GAATTC	G	C	T	C	G

based on *H. pylori* reference strain 26995; + accession numbers of the *H. pylori* sequence strains for SouthAfrica07, 2017WestAfrica, EU544200USA, Puno/Peru, Hp16S248Mar, Hp16S644mar, Hp16S563Mar and Hp16S567Mar are, respectively: [Genbank:CP002336.1, Genbank:CP002571.1, Genbank:EU544200.1, Genbank: CP002982.1, Genbank:JQ315410, Genbank:JQ315411, Genbank:JQ315412 and Genbank:JQ315413].

pylori 16 S rRNA gene between nucleotide positions 700 and 1245 (numbered according to the rrnA gene of *H. pylori* strain 26695), modified from [32]. In all PCR reactions a negative and a positive control were used corresponding to, respectively, sterile water and two different urease *H. pylori* positive gastric biopsies from PUD patients. PCR condition was 94°C 5′ followed by 40 cycles of 94°C 1′/55°C 1′/72°C 1′ and one cycle at 72°C 7′, with a total volume of 25 µl containing 1x PCR buffer, 200 µM dNTPs, 2.0 mM MgCl$_2$, 1µM oligoHp16Sr1, 1µM oligo Hp16Sr2, 1.25 U Taq DNA Polymerase Platinum Brazil (Invitrogen), 2.5% DMSO, 50ηg DNA. The PCR products were resolved in 1.5% agarose gels stained with ethidium bromide and photographed under UV light.

Restriction and sequencing analysis

The 16 S rDNA 545 bp amplicons obtained by PCR from biopsy specimens were digested with H*inf* I (biolab – New England) according to the manufacturer's instructions. The predictable restriction pattern for tetracycline susceptible *H. pylori* strains corresponds to two fragments of 264 and 281 bp and for *H. pylori* strains with high tetracycline resistance corresponds to three fragments of 281, 227 and 37 bp. The products of restriction analysis were resolved in 8% acrylamide gels, stained with ethidium bromide and photographed under UV light. 16 S rRNA 545 bp PCR amplicons from the two *H. pylori* positive control gastric biopsies (Hp16S248Mar and 644Mar) and the two amplicons presenting unexpected H*inf* I restriction patterns (Hp16S563Mar and Hp16S587bp) were submitted to sequencing with DyeTM Terminator v3.0 cycle Sequencing Ready Reaction kit and an ABI-3100 machine purchased from Applied Biosystem, according to the manufacturer's instructions. Nucleotide sequence determination was performed in duplicate and comparative

analysis was carried out by basic nucleotide BLAST alignment [37].

Abbreviations

PUD: Peptic ulcer disease; CG: Chronic gastritis; GERD: Gastroesophageal reflux disease; PCR: Polymerase chain reaction; RFLP: Restriction fragment length polymorphism; TetR: Tetracycline resistance.

Competing interests

We do not have any to declare.

Author's contributions

RBS and CMA carried out the molecular studies and contributed to the acquisition and interpretation of data; MAS designed the experiments, contributed to data analysis and drafted the manuscript. All authors read and approved the final manuscript.

Acknowledgments

We are grateful to Dr. Adriana Augusta Pimenta de Barros for her care to all of the patients included in the study and to Dr. David Howe for his contribution in the edition of the manuscript language. This work was supported by the Fundação de Amparo a Pesquisa do Estado de São Paulo (FAPESP), Research Grant 2006/01223-0; Fellowship CMA 2005/04087-7.

Author details

[1]Department of Genotyping, Hemocenter, Marilia Medical School, Marilia, SP, Brazil. [2]Department of Molecular Biology, Marilia Medical School, Marilia, SP, Brazil. [3]Center of Natural and Human Sciences, Universidade Federal do ABC, Rua Santa Adélia, 166 Bloco A, Torre 3, 6° andar, Sala 625, CEP 09210-170 Bairro Bangu, Santo André, SP, Brazil.

References

1. Megraud F: **Helicobacter pylori infection: review and practice.** *Presse Med* 2010, **39**(7–8):815–822.
2. Rimbara E, Fischbach LA, Graham DY: **Optimal therapy for Helicobacter pylori infections.** *Nat Rev Gastroenterol Hepatol* 2011, **8**(2):79–88.
3. Chisholm SA, Teare EL, Davies K, Owen RJ: **Surveillance of primary antibiotic resistance of Helicobacter pylori at centres in England and Wales over a six-year period (2000–2005). Euro surveillance: bulletin europeen sur les maladies transmissibles.** *European communicable disease bulletin* 2007, **12**(7):E3–4.
4. Coelho LG, Zaterka S: **Second brazilian consensus conference on helicobacter pylori infection.** *Arq Gastroenterol* 2005, **42**(2):128–132.
5. McNamara D, O'Morain C: **Consensus guidelines: agreement and debate surrounding the optimal management of Helicobacter pylori infection.**

Canadian journal of gastroenterology. *Journal canadien de gastroenterologie* 2000, 14(6):511–517.

6. Malfertheiner P, Megraud F, O'Morain C, Bazzoli F, El-Omar E, Graham D, Hunt R, Rokkas T, Vakil N, Kuipers EJ: **Current concepts in the management of Helicobacter pylori infection: the Maastricht III Consensus Report.** *Gut* 2007, 56(6):772–781.

7. Chey WD, Wong BC: **American College of Gastroenterology guideline on the management of Helicobacter pylori infection.** *Am J Gastroenterol* 2007, 102(8):1808–1825.

8. Graham DY, Fischbach L: **Helicobacter pylori infection.** *N Eng J Med* 2010, 363(6):595–596. author reply 596.

9. Qasim A, O'Morain CA: **Review article: treatment of Helicobacter pylori infection and factors influencing eradication.** *Aliment Pharmacol Ther* 2002, 16(Suppl 1):24–30.

10. Wermeille J, Cunningham M, Dederding JP, Girard L, Baumann R, Zelger G, Buri P, Metry JM, Sitavanc R, Gallaz L, *et al*: **Failure of Helicobacter pylori eradication: is poor compliance the main cause?** *Gastroenterol Clin Biol* 2002, 26(3):216–219.

11. Egan BJ, Marzio L, O'Connor H, O'Morain C: **Treatment of Helicobacter pylori infection.** *Helicobacter* 2008, 13(Suppl 1):35–40.

12. Frota LC, da Cunha Mdo P, Luz CR, de Araujo-Filho AH, Frota LA, Braga LL: **Helicobacter pylori eradication using tetracycline and furazolidone versus amoxicillin and azithromycin in lansoprazole based triple therapy: an open randomized clinical trial.** *Arq Gastroenterol* 2005, 42(2):111–115.

13. Cuchi Burgos E, Forne Bardera M, Quintana Riera S, Lite Lite J, Garau Alemany J: **[Evolution of the sensitivity of 235 strains of Helicobacter pylori from 1995 to 1998 and impact of antibiotic treatment].** *Enferm Infecc Microbiol Clin* 2002, 20(4):157–160.

14. Parsons HK, Carter MJ, Sanders DS, Winstanley T, Lobo AJ: **Helicobacter pylori antimicrobial resistance in the United Kingdom: the effect of age, sex and socio-economic status.** *Aliment Pharmacol Ther* 2001, 15(9):1473–1478.

15. Kim JJ, Reddy R, Lee M, Kim JG, El-Zaatari FA, Osato MS, Graham DY, Kwon DH: **Analysis of metronidazole, clarithromycin and tetracycline resistance of Helicobacter pylori isolates from Korea.** *J Antimicrob Chemother* 2001, 47(4):459–461.

16. Vallejos C, Garrido L, Caceres D, Madrid AM, Defilippi C, Toledo H: **Prevalence of metronidazole, clarithromycin and tetracycline resistance in Helicobacter pylori isolated from Chilean patients.** *Rev Med Chil* 2007, 135(3):287–293.

17. Mendonca S, Ecclissato C, Sartori MS, Godoy AP, Guerzoni RA, Degger M, Pedrazzoli J Jr: **Prevalence of Helicobacter pylori resistance to metronidazole, clarithromycin, amoxicillin, tetracycline, and furazolidone in Brazil.** *Helicobacter* 2000, 5(2):79–83.

18. Boyanova L, Mitov I: **Geographic map and evolution of primary Helicobacter pylori resistance to antibacterial agents.** *Expert Rev Anti Infect Ther* 2010, 8(1):59–70.

19. Kwon DH, Kim JJ, Lee M, Yamaoka Y, Kato M, Osato MS, El-Zaatari FA, Graham DY: **Isolation and characterization of tetracycline-resistant clinical isolates of Helicobacter pylori.** *Antimicrob Agents Chemother* 2000, 44(11):3203–3205.

20. Realdi G, Dore MP, Piana A, Atzei A, Carta M, Cugia L, Manca A, Are BM, Massarelli G, Mura I, *et al*: **Pretreatment antibiotic resistance in Helicobacter pylori infection: results of three randomized controlled studies.** *Helicobacter* 1999, 4(2):106–112.

21. Wu JY, Kim JJ, Reddy R, Wang WM, Graham DY, Kwon DH: **Tetracycline-resistant clinical Helicobacter pylori isolates with and without mutations in 16 S rRNA-encoding genes.** *Antimicrob Agents Chemother* 2005, 49(2):578–583.

22. Woo HY, Park DI, Park H, Kim MK, Kim DH, Kim IS, Kim YJ: **Dual-priming oligonucleotide-based multiplex PCR for the detection of Helicobacter pylori and determination of clarithromycin resistance with gastric biopsy specimens.** *Helicobacter* 2009, 14(1):22–28.

23. Chisholm SA, Owen RJ, Teare EL, Saverymuttu S: **PCR-based diagnosis of Helicobacter pylori infection and real-time determination of clarithromycin resistance directly from human gastric biopsy samples.** *J Clin Microbiol* 2001, 39(4):1217–1220.

24. Tajbakhsh S, Samarbaf-Zadeh AR, Moosavian M: **Comparison of fluorescent in situ hybridization and histological method for the diagnosis of Helicobacter pylori in gastric biopsy samples.** *Medical science monitor: international medical journal of experimental and clinical research* 2008, 14(9):BR183–BR187.

25. Burucoa C, Garnier M, Silvain C, Fauchere JL: **Quadruplex real-time PCR assay using allele-specific scorpion primers for detection of mutations conferring clarithromycin resistance to Helicobacter pylori.** *J Clin Microbiol* 2008, 46(7):2320–2326.

26. Brodersen DE, Clemons WM Jr, Carter AP, Morgan-Warren RJ, Wimberly BT, Ramakrishnan V: **The structural basis for the action of the antibiotics tetracycline, pactamycin, and hygromycin B on the 30S ribosomal subunit.** *Cell* 2000, 103(7):1143–1154.

27. Pioletti M, Schlunzen F, Harms J, Zarivach R, Gluhmann M, Avila H, Bashan A, Bartels H, Auerbach T, Jacobi C, *et al*: **Crystal structures of complexes of the small ribosomal subunit with tetracycline, edeine and IF3.** *EMBO J* 2001, 20(8):1829–1839.

28. Gerrits MM, de Zoete MR, Arents NL, Kuipers EJ, Kusters JG: **16 S rRNA mutation-mediated tetracycline resistance in Helicobacter pylori.** *Antimicrob Agents Chemother* 2002, 46(9):2996–3000.

29. Trieber CA, Taylor DE: **Mutations in the 16 S rRNA genes of Helicobacter pylori mediate resistance to tetracycline.** *J Bacteriol* 2002, 184(8):2131–2140.

30. Gerrits MM, Berning M, Van Vliet AH, Kuipers EJ, Kusters JG: **Effects of 16 S rRNA gene mutations on tetracycline resistance in Helicobacter pylori.** *Antimicrob Agents Chemother* 2003, 47(9):2984–2986.

31. Dailidiene D, Bertoli MT, Miciuleviciene J, Mukhopadhyay AK, Dailide G, Pascasio MA, Kupcinskas L, Berg DE: **Emergence of tetracycline resistance in Helicobacter pylori: multiple mutational changes in 16 S ribosomal DNA and other genetic loci.** *Antimicrob Agents Chemother* 2002, 46(12):3940–3946.

32. Ribeiro ML, Gerrits MM, Benvengo YH, Berning M, Godoy AP, Kuipers EJ, Mendonca S, van Vliet AH, Pedrazzoli J Jr, Kusters JG: **Detection of high-level tetracycline resistance in clinical isolates of Helicobacter pylori using PCR-RFLP.** *FEMS Immunol Med Microbiol* 2004, 40(1):57–61.

33. Boyanova L, Stancheva I, Spassova Z, Katzarov N, Mitov I, Koumanova R: **Primary and combined resistance to four antimicrobial agents in Helicobacter pylori in Sofia, Bulgaria.** *J Med Microbiol* 2000, 49(5):415–418.

34. Megraud F: **Resistance of Helicobacter pylori to antibiotics.** *Aliment Pharmacol Ther* 1997, 11(Suppl 1):43–53.

35. Wu H, Shi XD, Wang HT, Liu JX: **Resistance of helicobacter pylori to metronidazole, tetracycline and amoxycillin.** *J Antimicrob Chemother* 2000, 46(1):121–123.

36. Morris A, Ali MR, Brown P, Lane M, Patton K: **Campylobacter pylori infection in biopsy specimens of gastric antrum: laboratory diagnosis and estimation of sampling error.** *J Clin Pathol* 1989, 42(7):727–732.

37. Altschul SF, Madden TL, Schaffer AA, Zhang J, Zhang Z, Miller W, Lipman DJ: **Gapped BLAST and PSI-BLAST: a new generation of protein database search programs.** *Nucleic Acids Res* 1997, 25(17):3389–3402.

38. Rotimi O, Cairns A, Gray S, Moayyedi P, Dixon MF: **Histological identification of Helicobacter pylori: comparison of staining methods.** *J Clin Pathol* 2000, 53(10):756–759.

17

Association of polymorphism of *PTPN* 11 encoding SHP-2 with gastric atrophy but not gastric cancer in *Helicobacter pylori* seropositive Chinese population

Jing Jiang[1], Zhi-Fang Jia[1], Fei Kong[1], Mei-Shan Jin[2], Yin-Ping Wang[2], Suyan Tian[1], Jian Suo[3] and Xueyuan Cao[3*]

Abstract

Background: The interaction between Src homology 2 domain-containing protein tyrosine phosphatase (SHP-2) of gastric epithelial cells and cagA from *H. pylori* plays a crucial role in developments of gastric atrophy and gastric cancer. This study aimed to investigate the association of haplotype tagging SNPs (htSNPs) in the *PTPN11* gene encoding SHP-2 with gastric atrophy and gastric cancer in Chinese population.

Methods: The subjects comprised 414 patients with gastric cancer, 109 individuals with gastric atrophy and 923 healthy controls. Blood was collected from October 2008 to October 2010. Five htSNPs rs2301756, rs12423190, rs12229892, rs7958372 and rs4767860 from the *PTPN11* gene were selected and genotyped by Taqman assay. Serum Ig G antibodies to *H. pylori* were detected by ELISA. Gastric atrophy was screened by the levels of serum pepsinogenIandII, and confirmed by endoscopy and histopatholgical examinations. Odds ratio (ORs) and 95% confidence intervals (CIs) were calculated by a multivariate logistic regression.

Results: Among *H. pylori* seropositive subjects, age and gender-adjusted OR of gastric atrophy was 2.47 (95%CI 1.13-4.55, $P = 0.02$) for CC genotype compared with CT/TT genotypes, suggesting a recessive model of genetic risk for rs12423190. The prevalence of *H. pylori* seropositivity were significantly higher in groups of gastric cancer and gastric atrophy compared to the control group (70.3% vs. 75.2% vs. 49.7%, $P < 0.001$). However, the distributions of genotypes and haplotypes in patients with gastric cancer were not significantly different from healthy controls.

Conclusions: Our study provides the first evidence that rs12423190 polymorphism of the *PTPN11* gene is significantly associated with an increased risk of gastric atrophy in *H. pylori* infected Chinese Han population, suggesting that rs12423190 polymorphism could be used as a useful marker of genetic susceptibility to gastric atrophy among *H. pylori* infected subjects. The biological roles of this polymorphism require a further investigation.

Background

Gastric cancer is the most common malignancy of gastrointestinal tract in East Asian populations and the third most common cause of cancer-related deaths in China [1,2]. *Helicobacter pylori* (*H. pylori*) infection has been established as a major risk factor for gastric cancer, through the induction of gastric atrophy and progression of precancerous lesions by numerous studies [3,4]. Although *H. pylori* is estimated to inhabit at least half of the world's human population, just few subjects develop to gastric precancerous lesions and adenocarcinoma. The extent of gastric damages induced by *H. pylori* infection seems to vary from one subject to another, suggesting that the combination of host genetic traits and bacterial virulence plays important roles in long-term outcomes of *H. pylori* infection [5-7].

Several studies have provided evidences that infection with cagA-positive *H. pylori* associates with higher grades of gastric inflammation and is more virulent than the cagA-negative strains [8]. The CagA protein is delivered into gastric epithelial cells via the bacterial type IV secretion system, where it undergoes tyrosine phosphorylation

* Correspondence: ccmzc32jdyycao@yahoo.com.cn
[3]Department of Gastric and Colorectal Surgery, Jilin University First Hospital, Changchun, China

by Src and Abl kinases. Tyrosine-phosphorylated CagA then acquires capability to interact with and deregulate SHP-2 phosphatase, a bona-fide oncoprotein [9]. The formation of cagA/SHP-2 complex induces abnormal proliferation and migration of gastric epithelial cells, consequently resulting in gastric atrophy and gastric carcinoma [10-12]. In addition, gain-of-function mutations of the SHP-2 have recently been found in human malignancies [13-15]. Kim et al also revealed that gastric cancers displayed higher levels of SHP-2 protein compared to normal cells, suggesting that neo-expression of this signalling protein in cells might play a role in the gastric carcinogenesis [16]. Since the protein-tyrosine phosphatase nonreceptor-type 11 (*PTPN11*) gene encodes protein containing two tandem Src homology-2 domains, which function as phospho-tyrosine binding domains. SHP-2 closely interacts with the CagA protein, therefore, it is speculated that functional polymorphisms in the *PTPN11* may mediate the interaction of this protein with its substrates and affect its regulatory role in various cell signalling events, such as mitogenic activation, metabolic control, transcription regulation, cell migration, and malignant transformation in *H. pylori* infected subjects.

The *PTPN11* gene is on chromosome 12, containing 16 exons. Several single–nucleotide polymorphisms (SNPs) rs11066322, rs11066320 and rs2301756 have been identified in Caucasian females to be associated with apoB levels and LDL-C levels [17]. Another study demonstrated that the rs11066322 was associated with increased plasma HDL-C levels [18]. These results suggested that genetic variants influencing SHP-2 activities may modulate biological functions of the protein. In gastric cancer, Japanese group has found that a prevalent SNP in intron3 (rs2301756) was associated with an increased risk of gastric atrophy in Japanese population with *H. pylori* infection [19-22]. The aim of the present study is to determine whether polymorphisms of *PTPN11* gene are associated with clinical outcomes of *H. pylori* infection in Chinese population.

Methods

Study populations

Four hundred and fourteen Gastric cancer cases were selected from the department of gastric and colorectal surgery, the First Hospital, Jilin University, from 2008 to 2010. All patients underwent tumor resection with histologically confirmed diagnosis of gastric adenocarcinoma. The gastric atrophy individuals and health controls were recruited from the healthy check-up centre of the same hospital from 2009 to 2010. A total 1080 persons (630 males and 450 females, aged 35 to 80 years old) participated in the study without history of cancer. The examinees were Han inhabitants in Changchun city. The informed consent was obtained from all subjects and the study protocol was approved by the ethics committee of

the first affiliated hospital, Jilin University. The examinees received serum anti-*H. pylori* IgG titre and pepsinogen examinations for screening *H. pylori* infection and gastric atrophy.

Tests for *H. pylori* infection and diagnosis of gastric Atrophy

Serum immunoglobulin (Ig) G antibodies to *H. pylori* were detected by enzyme-linked immunosorbent assay (ELISA) using *H. pylori* -IgG ELISA kit (Biohit, Helsink, Finland). The antibody titres were defined by optical density (OD) values according to the manufacturer's protocol and titres higher than the cut off value of 30EIU, were considered as positive for *H. pylori* infection. PepsinogenIand II (PGIand PGII) in serum were measured using ELISA kits (Biohit, Helsink, Finland). For screening gastric atrophy, we decided to use cut-off points of <82.3 ng/ml for PGIand <6.05 for PGI/PGIIratio due to no universally accepted cut-off points for dichotomising PGI or the PGI/PGII ratio, which have been validated against histological confirmatory studies for gastric atrophy [23]. The kit quality control samples showed Coefficient of variations (CVs) of 4.5, 4.3 and 4.7% for *H. pylori*, PGI and PGII, respectively. All suspected cases with gastric atrophy by serum screening were re-determined by endoscopic, biopsy and histological examinations for a definite diagnosis.

Selection of tagging SNPs

The principal hypothesis underlying this experiment is that one or more common SNPs in *PTPN11* gene are associated with an altered risk of gastric atrophy and/or gastric cancer. Thus, the aim of the SNP tagging is to identify a set of SNPs that efficiently tags all known SNPs. We postulate that such SNPs are also likely to tag any hitherto unidentified SNPs in *PTPN11* gene. Haplotype tagging SNPs (htSNPs) were selected from the Han Chinese data in the HapMap Project (06-02-2009 HapMap) using the SNPbrowser™ Software v4.0 to capture SNPs with a minimum minor allele frequency (MAF) of 0.05 with a pair-wise r square of 0.8 or greater [24]. There are 9 SNPs at minor allele frequencies >0.05 in the *PTPN11* gene in Chinese on HapMap, all of which are located in noncoding regions of the *PTPN11* gene (Figure 1). Finally, five htSNPs rs2301756, rs12423190, rs12229892, rs7958372 and rs4767860 were selected and four of them are shown to be in a complete linkage disequilibrium (LD) with Tag SNP (D' = 1 and r^2 >0.8).

Genotyping

Genomic DNA from whole blood was extracted with an AxyPrep blood Genomic DNA extraction Kit (AP-MN-BL-GDNA-250, Axygen Biosciences, Union City, USA). Polymerase chain reactions (PCR) were carried out on

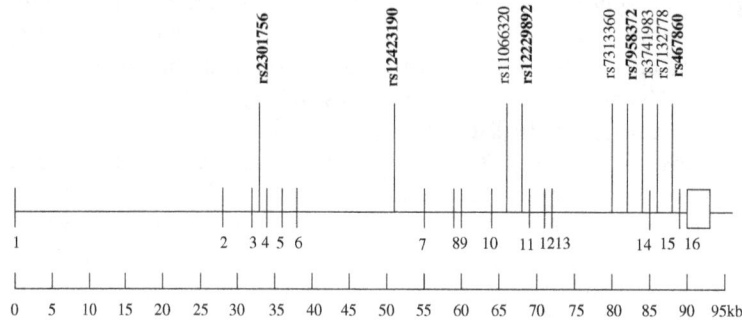

Figure 1 Genomic map of *PTPN11* gene. Validated SNPs are illustrated and htSNPs genotyped in the present study are indicated in bold. Vertical Lines and a box represent exons.

genomic DNA (10 ng) using a TaqMan universal PCR master mix (Applied Biosystems). Forward and reverse primers and FAM and VIC labelled probes were designed by Applied Bio systems (ABI Assay-by-Designs) in a 5ul reaction. Sequences of primers and probes are available on request. Amplification conditions on BIO-RAD S1000™ thermal cyclers (Bio-Rad Laboratories, Hercules, California) were as follows: 1 cycle of 95°C for 10 min, followed by 40 cycles of 95°C for 15 s and 60°C for 1 min. The completed PCR products were read on an ABI PRISM 7900 Sequence Detector in end-point mode using the Allelic Discrimination Sequence Detector Software V2.3 (Applied Biosystems). For the software to recognize genotypes, two non-template controls were included in each 384-well plate. All patients' and normal control samples were arrayed together in four 384-well plates and the fifth plate contained eight duplicate samples from each of four plates to ensure the quality of genotyping (the concordance was >99% for all SNPs).

Statistics analysis

For each polymorphism, the deviation of genotype frequencies in controls from those expected under Hardy-Weinberg equilibrium was assessed by a goodness-of-fit x^2-test. Linkage disequilibrium (LD) between pairs of biallelic loci was determined using two measures, D' and r^2. Either Chi-square test or Fisher's exact test was performed by comparing distributions of genotype frequencies between patients and controls. Risks associated with rare genotypes were estimated as odds ratios (ORs). Corresponding 95% confidence intervals (CIs) by an unconditional logistic regression were adjusted by age (scale variable) and sex (nominal variable). For haplotypes with frequencies >1%, risks were compared to the reference haplotype(major haplotype in control group) using an unconditional logistic regression model with the HAPSTAT 3.0 software, according to Lin et al [Copyright (c) 2006–2008 Tammy Bailey, Danyu Lin and the University of North Carolina, NC, USA.] [25,26]. HAPSTAT allows the user to estimate or test haplotype

effects and haplotype-environment interactions by maximum likelihood estimation and the EM algorithm. All statistical tests were two-tailed and *P*-values were considered to be statistically significant when ≦0.05. All analyses were performed using a statistical analysis software for windows, version 9.2 (SAS Institute, Cary, NC, USA). The statistical power calculations were performed using the QUANTO software program (Version 1.2.3).

Results

Characteristics of subject allele frequencies of the htSNPs

A total of 414 patients gastric cancer (300 males and 114 females) aged 35 to 80 years old were included in this study. Of 1080 examinees, 148 individuals were screened for gastric atrophy using serum PG examination; 109 patients were confirmed with gastric atrophy by biopsy and histopathological examinations; 17 people were diagnosed as pseudopositive for gastric atrophy and excluded from the study; 22 people who rejected endoscopic examination were excluded from the study. Nine hundred and thirty-two individuals were included in the control group. Nine persons were excluded, due to the failure to detected anti-*H. pylori* Ig G and/or genotyps in blood samples. Finally, 923 subjects were included and analysed as control. The characteristics of subjects are summarized in Table 1. The mean age was older in gastric cancer patients than that in controls (61.5 vs. 50.7 years; *P* <0.001). There were more females in the control group (*P* <0.001). Prevalence of *H. pylori* seropositivity were significantly higher in groups of gastric cancer and gastric atrophy than that in the healthy control (70.3% vs. 49.7%, *P* <0.001; 75.2% vs. 49.7%, *P* = 0.01).

The linkage disequilibrium structure of the 5 polymorphic loci is shown in Figure 2. All D' values are above 0.93, and the pair-wise comparison among rs12423190 and rs12229892 revealed a complete LDs (|D'| = 1 and r^2 = 0.285). The genotype distribution for five htSNPs in the control group were in Hardy-Weinberg equilibrium (*P* value were 0.54, 0.94, 0.78, 0.68 and 0.87 respectively). In the present study, the distribution

Table 1 Characteristics of the subjects and the *PTPN11* polymorphisms

	Gastric cancer (%)	Gastric atrophy (%)	Control (%)	P value
N	414	109	923	
Sex				
Male	300(72.5)	64(58.7)	539(58.4)	<0.001
Female	114(27.5)	45(41.3)	384(41.6)	
Age				
≤45	32(7.7)	19(17.4)	276(29.9)	<0.001
46-65	224(54.1)	80(73.4)	579(62.7)	
>65	158(38.2)	10(9.2)	68(7.4)	
Anti-*H.pylori* IgG				
Negative	123(29.7)	27(24.8)	464(50.3)	<0.001
Postive	291(70.3)	82(75.2)	459(49.7)	
SNPs				
rs2301756				
GG	305(73.7)	86(78.9)	687(74.4)	0.462
GA	95(22.9)	22(20.2)	216(23.4)	
AA	14(3.4)	1(0.9)	20(2.2)	
rs12423190				
TT	214(51.7)	55(50.5)	476(51.6)	0.047
TC	166(40.1)	36(33.0)	373(40.4)	
CC	34(8.2)	18(16.5)	74(8.0)	
rs12229892				
GG	137(33.1)	40(36.7)	308(33.4)	0.963
GA	205(49.5)	50(45.9)	454(49.2)	
AA	72(17.4)	19(17.4)	161(17.4)	
rs7958372				
TT	305(73.7)	87(79.8)	685(74.2)	0.747
TC	102(24.6)	21(19.3)	222(24.1)	
CC	7(1.7)	1(0.9)	16(1.7)	
rs4767860				
AA	137(33.1)	39(35.8)	306(33.2)	0.386
AG	206(49.8)	44(40.4)	453(49.1)	
GG	71(17.1)	26(23.9)	164(17.8)	

		|D'|				
r^2		rs2301756A>G	rs12423190T>C	rs12229892G>A	rs7958372T>C	rs4767860A>G
	rs2301756A>G	-	0.956	0.950	0.931	0.953
	rs12423190T>C	0.036	-	1.000	0.933	0.969
	rs12229892G>A	0.105	0.285	-	0.983	0.978
	rs7958372T>C	0.859	0.055	0.112	-	0.971
	rs4767860A>G	0.199	0.205	0.509	0.503	-

Figure 2 Linkage disequilibrium coefficients (|D'| and r2) between *PTPN11 htSNPs*.

of rs12423190 genotype was found to be statistically different between groups (P = 0.047), however, distributions of rest four SNPs were not significantly different between groups.

Association between htSNPs and *H. pylori* seropositivity, gastric atrophy and gastric cancer

The age and sex-adjusted ORs of gastric atrophy among *H. pylori* seropositive subjects were 0.93 (95%CI 0.55-1.57, P = 0.78) for CT and 2.20 (95%CI 1.06-4.55, P = 0.03) for CC genotype compared with rs12423190

TT genotype. In a recessive model, the age- and sex-adjusted OR was 2.47 (95%CI 1.13-4.55, P = 0.02) for CC genotype versus rs12423190 CT/TT genotypes (Table 2). However, the age and sex-adjusted ORs of gastric cancer among *H. pylori* seropositive subjects was 1.18 (95%CI 0.64-2.18, P = 0.60) for CT and 1.30 (95%CI 0.93-1.83, P = 0.13) for CC genotype compared with rs12423190 TT genotype. The haplotypes with frequencies ≥1% are shown in Table 2. The most frequent haplotypes were GTATA (rs2301756G, rs12423190T, rs12229892A, rs7958372T, rs4767860A) and four major haplotypes were accounted for over 95% of distribution. There was no significant association between haplotypes and gastric atrophy. The OR of GCGTG haplotype was 1.36 (95%CI 0.92-2.02, P = 0.12) versus the GTATA haplotype (Table 2). The association between the SNPs of *PTPN11* and the *H. pylori* infection was examined in health controls (Table 3), but no significant association between five htSNPs of *PTPN11* and *H. pylori* seropositivity was found. Distributions of *PTPN11* haplotypes were not correlated with *H. pylori* seropositivity. No association between htSNPs and gastric atrophy in *H. pylori* seronegative subjects was found either (data not shown). In a subgroup analysis, we did not find any association of htSNPs with Lauren's classification, tissue differentiation and TNM staging (data not shown).

Discussions

CagA-secreting *H. pylori* infection plays an important role in gastric carcinogenesis via a sequential CagA signal transduction pathway. CagA initially binds to seven protein components to activate aberrant cellular responses that promote the development of gastric cancer. Since the function of CagA protein is regulated by its binding partners, therefore genes that encode CagA interacting molecules may modify the risk of gastric cancer. In the present study, 5 htSNPs of the *PTPN11* gene were investigated for their associations with *H. pylori* infection, gastric atrophy and gastric cancer in Chinese Hans population. We found that subjects bearing

Table 2 *PTPN11* polymorphisms among *H. pylori* (+) subjects

Genotype	Control (%) n = 459	Gastric atrophy (%) n = 82	OR(95%CI)*	P value	Gastric cancer (%) n = 291	OR(95%CI)*	P value
rs2301756							
GG	74.3	76.8	Reference		73.9	Reference	
GA	23.5	22.0	0.90(0.51-1.59)	0.72	37.9	0.92(0.62-1.35)	0.66
A/A	2.2	1.2	0.51(0.06-4.09)	0.53	3.4	1.26(0.47-3.37)	0.65
rs12423190							
TT	52.5	50.0	Reference		50.9	Reference	
TC	40.1	34.1	0.93(0.55-1.57)	0.78	41.2	1.18(0.64-2.18)	0.60
CC	7.4	15.9	2.20(1.06-4.55)	0.03	7.9	1.30(0.93-1.83)	0.13
TT/TC	92.6	84.1	Reference		92.1	Reference	
CC	7.4	15.9	2.47(1.13-4.55)	0.02	7.9	1.21(0.89-1.76)	0.15
rs12229892							
GG	32.2	36.6	Reference		30.6	Reference	
GA	51.2	47.6	0.82(0.49-1.39)	0.46	52.2	1.04(0.72-1.51)	0.82
AA	16.6	15.9	0.86(0.42-1.75)	0.67	17.2	1.02(0.63-1.67)	0.93
rs7958372							
TT	74.1	78.0	Reference		74.2	Reference	
TC	24.4	20.7	0.80(0.45-1.43)	0.46	24.1	0.94(0.64-1.37)	0.74
CC	1.5	1.2	0.83(0.10-7.01)	0.86	1.7	1.16(0.30-4047)	0.83
rs4767860							
AA	33.8	34.1	Reference		31.9	Reference	
AG	49.5	40.2	1.54(0.82-2.91)	0.18	51.9	1.04(0.70-1.88)	0.59
GG	16.8	25.6	0.80(0.46-1.38)	0.43	16.2	1.32(0.92-1.90)	0.14
Haplotpe							
GTATA	41.3	39.6	Reference		41.2	Reference	
GCGTG	26.0	32.3	1.36(0.92-2.02)	0.12	27.6	1.12(0.80-1.57)	0.51
GTGTA	16.0	14.0	0.96(0.58-1.61)	0.89	14.4	1.14(0.88-1.47)	0.32
ATGCG	12.4	11.6	1.03(0.59-1.78)	0.92	13.1	0.96(0.71-1.32)	0.82
Others	4.3	2.5			3.7		

*OR for each genotype and hapolotype were calculated by age and sex adjusted logistic regression model.

rs12423190 CC genotype at intron 6 had a significantly higher risk in *H. pylori*-seropositive gastric atrophy. The OR for gastric cancer was increased in those carrying the GCGTG haplotype versus the GTATA (OR = 1.30, 95%CI: 0.93-1.83), however, the *P* value was 0.09, not statistically significant. In this study, the allele frequencies of rs12423190 were 71.8% for the T allele and 28.2% for the C allele among control subjects. The frequency of the C allele was similar to that reported in the HapMap Project (31.4%). Compared to the NCBI SNP database, we found that the frequency of the C allele is obviously higher in Chinese population than other populations (23.3% in Japanese; 11.5% in Utah residents with Northern and Western European ancestry). As incidences of gastric cancer are high in Chinese, Japanese and Koreans, high frequencies of this polymorphism in Asian populations

may be part of explanation. Our findings indicated that the C allele contributes to genetic predisposition to *H. pylori*-induced gastric atrophy in Chinese population. A further study is required to confirm associations of the *PTPN11* rs12423190 polymorphism with gastric atrophy in diverse ethnic populations.

Recent studies revealed significant associations between the rs2301756 AA genotype in intron3 and reduced risk of gastric atrophy among *H. pylori*-seropositive Japanese subjects [7,19,22]. Our study found a similar trend of decreased risk of OR for rs2301756, however, the OR of atrophy was not significantly lower compared with the GA genotype (OR = 0.90, 95%CI: 0.51-1.59) and AA genotype (OR = 0.51, 95%CI: 0.06-4.09). In controversy, the association study for rs2301756 and gastric atrophy showed a completely opposite result

Table 3 PTPN11 polymorphisms for H. pylori seropositivity in control

Genotype	Hp + (%) (n = 459)	Hp-(%) (n = 464)	OR(95%CI)*	P value
rs2301756				
GG	74.7	75.2	Reference	
GA	23.3	22.8	1.18(0.51-2.72)	0.71
AA	2.0	2.0	1.52(0.49-4.66)	0.47
rs12423190				
T/T	52.1	50.7	Reference	
T/C	39.2	40.1	0.98(0.55-1.76)	0.95
C/C	8.7	9.2	0.92(0.29-2.93)	0.89
rs12229892				
G/G	32.9	34.6	Reference	
G/A	50.6	46.8	1.25(0.93-1.70)	0.15
A/A	16.5	18.5	1.01(0.65-1.57)	0.97
rs7958372				
T/T	74.7	74.9	Reference	
T/C	23.8	23.2	0.84(0.40-1.77)	0.65
C/C	1.5	1.8	0.61(0.13-2.79)	0.53
rs4767860				
A/A	33.8	33.0	Reference	
A/G	48.1	48.3	1.11(0.36-3.45)	0.86
G/G	18.1	18.7	1.00(0.55-1.84)	0.99
Haplotpe				
GTATA	41.0	41.6	Reference	
GCGTG	26.9	28.4	0.97(0.79-1.20)	0.77
GTGTA	15.7	14.8	1.08(0.83-1.40)	0.56
ATGCG	12.3	13.0	0.94(0.71-1.24)	0.66
Others	4.1	2.2		

*OR for each genotype and hapolotype were calculated by age and sex adjusted logistic regression model.

in Uzbekistan population [20]. Zhu F and colleagues also demonstrated that the rs2301756 A allele was associated with low risk of intestinal metastasis (IM) indicating that H. pylori infection induces gastric precancerous lesions, such as gastric atrophy (OR = 0.46, 95%CI: 0.21-0.99) in H. pylori seropositive individuals. Meantime, an inverse association was shown in H. pylori-seronegative subjects in the same study (OR =2.51, 95%CI: 1.21-4.43) [27]. There were no statistically differences in the frequency of rs2301756 in our study and others [21,28]. Inconsistent results from different studies may be due to different environmental backgrounds and ethnic groups. In our study, gastric atrophy was only identified in 82 cases of H. pylori- seropositive subjects, the minor allele of rs2301756 was relatively rare (MAF = 0.139). The statistical power maybe not sufficient (power = 0.10)

to examine the association. A further investigation of association between rs2301756 and gastric atrophy is needed in a large population and other ethnic groups.

The functions of PTPN11 polymorphisms are still unknown. SHP-2 contains two tandem SH2 domains, a PTP domain, and other functional motifs. Genetic mutations in PTPN11 exon 3(encoding the N-SH2 domain), exon 4(encoding the C-SH2 domain), Exons 7, 8 and 12 (encoding the PTP domain) have been identified in Noonan syndrome, juvenile myelomonocytic leukemia, LEOPARD syndrome, lung cancer, liver cancer and colon cancer [29]. The interaction of tyrosine phosphorylated Cag-A with the SH2 domain of the protein is supposed to induce a conformational change in SHP-2 that weakens the inhibitory interaction between PTP and N-SH2 domain, and results in activation of SHP-2's catalytic activity [10,30]. The rs12423190 polymorphism is located in the intron 6, 1408 bp upstream exon 7, encoding part of PTP domain. Using a free bioinformatic tool (http://fastsnp. ibms.sinica.edu.tw/pages/inputCandidateGeneSearch.jsp) the rs12423190 is predicted to locate in the side of an intronic enhancer which could affect the gene transcriptional regulation. SHP-2 has several biological functions. The gain-of-function of SHP-2 may accelerate the downregulation of T-cell and B-cell activation through CTLA-4/PD-1 as well as IL-6/STAT3 signalings, eventually leading to a decrease in inflammation. Meantime, it might act as a signal promoter in inflammation. SHP-2 promotes growth factor induced activation of phosphatidylinositol 3-kinase (PI3-K)/Akt, the extracellular signal-related kinases (ERKs) and nuclear factor-kappa B (NF-κB). SHP-2 can either negatively or positively regulate the activation of Janus kinase 2 (Jak2)/signal transducer and activator of transcription (STAT) and the c-Jun-amino terminal kinases (JNKs) depending on different circumstances. rs12423190 may promote the over-expression of SHP-2, further involvement in the up-regulation of inflammatory cytokines through MAPKs and NF-κB signaling pathways, eventually leading to increase in inflammation related to atrophy [31]. However, the rs2301756 does not appear to reside in transcription factor binding sites or splicing sites, but is in the LD with associated haplotypes. The rs12423190 polymorphism is also in a linkage disequilibrium, which may contain other unidentified causative SNPs. Further studies of PTPN11 sequence variants and their biologic functions may shed light in understanding the association of PTPN11 polymorphisms and the risk of GA.

In addition, we demonstrated that gastric cancer patients had high prevalence of both H. pylori seropositivity and gastric atrophy; the prevalence of H. pylori seropositivity was significantly higher in subjects with gastric atrophy compared to controls without gastric atrophy, implying the important links with of *H. pylori* infection, gastric atrophy, and gastric cancer. Genetic factors, such as *PTPN11* polymorphisms may contribute to gastric atrophy, through affecting the connection of Cag A and SHP-2 protein.

The first limitation in our study is the *H. pylori* infection status being determined by serology, not by the serum CagA antibody test. In East Asia countries, almost all *H. pylori* strains reported from infected patients were East Asian CagA positive strains [32-34], therefore *H. pylori* strains in infected patients most likely possess CagA in our study. The second limitation is the PG criteria for GA screening, the criterion for GA is PGI <82.3 ng/ml and PGI/II ratio <6.05. These parameters for atrophy are used in China and have been validated in only one histological confirmatory study [23], it is may be insufficient to draw a reliable diagnosis, thus more confirmatory studies are needed. Finally, a small sample size of gastric atrophy, especially for the cohort of *H. pylori* (+) gastric atrophy individuals is due to a low incidence of gastric atrophy in China. A large-scale study for recruiting more patients with gastric atrophy is required to confirm our findings in the future.

Conclusions

In conclusion, our study provides the first evidence that rs12423190 polymorphism of the *PTPN11* gene is significantly associated with an increased risk of gastric atrophy in *H. pylori* infected Chinese population, suggesting that rs12423190 polymorphism could be used as a biomarker of genetic susceptibility to gastric atrophy.

Competing interests
No competing interests to be disclosed.

Authors' contributions
JJ and CX designed and carried out most of study; JZF, KF, JMS, WYP and TSY participated data acquisition and analysis; JJ and JZF wrote the first draft of manuscript. All authors contributed to and approved the final manuscript by providing constructive suggestions.

Acknowledgements
This study has been supported by National Natural Science Foundation of China (30940060 and 81072369). The authors would like to thank everybody participating in this study, particularly to Mr Chang-Song Guo and Ms Ying Song for their technical support.

Author details
[1]Division of Clinical Epidemiology, Jilin University First Hospital, Changchun, China. [2]Division of Pathology, Jilin University First Hospital, Changchun, China. [3]Department of Gastric and Colorectal Surgery, Jilin University First Hospital, Changchun, China.

References

1. Hamiliton SR, Aaltonen L (Eds): *WHO classification of tumors.* Lyon: IARC Press; 2000.

2. Dai M, Ren JS, Li N, Li Q, Yang L, Chen YH: Estimation and prediction on cancer related incidence and mortality in China, 2008. *Zhonghua Liu Xing Bing Xue Za Zhi* 2012, **33**(1):57–61.

3. Lochhead P, El-Omar EM: Helicobacter pylori infection and gastric cancer. *Best Pract Res Clin Gastroenterol* 2007, **21**(2):281–297.

4. Kabir S: Effect of Helicobacter pylori eradication on incidence of gastric cancer in human and animal models: underlying biochemical and molecular events. *Helicobacter* 2009, **14**(3):159–171.

5. Amieva MR, El-Omar EM: Host-bacterial interactions in Helicobacter pylori infection. *Gastroenterology* 2008, **134**(1):306–323.

6. Snaith A, El-Omar EM: Helicobacter pylori: host genetics and disease outcomes. *Expert Rev Gastroenterol Hepatol* 2008, **2**(4):577–585.

7. Hishida A, Matsuo K, Goto Y, Hamajima N: Genetic predisposition to Helicobacter pylori-induced gastric precancerous conditions. *World J Gastrointest Oncol* 2010, **2**(10):369–379.

8. Kuipers EJ, Perez-Perez GI, Meuwissen SG, Blaser MJ: Helicobacter pylori and atrophic gastritis: importance of the cagA status. *J Natl Cancer Inst* 1995, **87**(23):1777–1780.

9. Yamazaki S, Yamakawa A, Ito Y, Ohtani M, Higashi H, Hatakeyama M, Azuma T: The CagA protein of Helicobacter pylori is translocated into epithelial cells and binds to SHP-2 in human gastric mucosa. *J Infect Dis* 2003, **187**(2):334–337.

10. Hatakeyama M: The role of Helicobacter pylori CagA in gastric carcinogenesis. *Int J Hematol* 2006, **84**(4):301–308.

11. Hatakeyama M: Helicobacter pylori and gastric carcinogenesis. *J Gastroenterol* 2009, **44**(4):239–248.

12. Hatakeyama M: Relationship between Helicobacter pylori CagA-SHP-2 interaction and gastric cancer. *Nihon Rinsho* 2005, **63**(Suppl 11):48–52.

13. Chan G, Kalaitzidis D, Neel BG: The tyrosine phosphatase Shp2 (PTPN11) in cancer. *Cancer Metastasis Rev* 2008, **27**(2):179–192.

14. Grossmann KS, Rosario M, Birchmeier C, Birchmeier W: The tyrosine phosphatase Shp2 in development and cancer. *Adv Cancer Res* 2010, **106**:53–89.

15. Jongmans MC, van der Burgt I, Hoogerbrugge PM, Noordam K, Yntema HG, Nillesen WM, Kuiper RP, Ligtenberg MJ, van Kessel AG, van Krieken JH, *et al*: Cancer risk in patients with Noonan syndrome carrying a PTPN11 mutation. *Eur J Hum Genet* 2011, **19**(8):870–874.

16. Kim JS, Shin OR, Kim HK, Cho YS, An CH, Lim KW, Kim SS: Overexpression of protein phosphatase non-receptor type 11 (PTPN11) in gastric carcinomas. *Dig Dis Sci* 2010, **55**(6):1565–1569.

17. Jamshidi Y, Gooljar SB, Snieder H, Wang X, Ge D, Swaminathan R, Spector TD, O'Dell SD: SHP-2 and PI3-kinase genes PTPN11 and PIK3R1 may influence serum apoB and LDL cholesterol levels in normal women. *Atherosclerosis* 2007, **194**(2):e26–e33.

18. Lu Y, Dolle ME, Imholz S, van 't Slot R, Verschuren WM, Wijmenga C, Feskens EJ, Boer JM: Multiple genetic variants along candidate pathways influence plasma high-density lipoprotein cholesterol concentrations. *J Lipid Res* 2008, **49**(12):2582–2589.

19. Goto Y, Ando T, Yamamoto K, Tamakoshi A, El-Omar E, Goto H, Hamajima N: Association between serum pepsinogens and polymorphismof PTPN11 encoding SHP-2 among Helicobacter pylori seropositive Japanese. *Int J Cancer* 2006, **118**(1):203–208.

20. Hamajima N, Rahimov B, Malikov Y, Abdiev S, Ahn KS, Bahramov S, Kawai S, Nishio K, Naito M, Goto Y: Associations between a PTPN11 polymorphism and gastric atrophy–opposite in Uzbekistan to that in Japan. *Asian Pac J Cancer Prev* 2008, **9**(2):217–220.

21. Hishida A, Matsuo K, Goto Y, Naito M, Wakai K, Tajima K, Hamajima N: Associations of a PTPN11 G/A polymorphism at intron 3 with Helicobactor pylori seropositivity, gastric atrophy and gastric cancer in Japanese. *BMC Gastroenterol* 2009, **9**:51.

22. Kawai S, Goto Y, Ito LS, Oba-Shinjo SM, Uno M, Shinjo SK, Marie SK, Ishida Y, Nishio K, Naito M, *et al*: Significant association between PTPN11 polymorphism and gastric atrophy among Japanese Brazilians. *Gastric Cancer* 2006, **9**(4):277–283.

23. Cao Q, Ran ZH, Xiao SD: Screening of atrophic gastritis and gastric cancer by serum pepsinogen, gastrin-17 and Helicobacter pylori immunoglobulin G antibodies. *J Dig Dis* 2007, **8**(1):15–22.

24. De La Vega FM: Selecting single-nucleotide polymorphisms for association studies with SNPbrowser software. *Methods Mol Biol* 2007, **376**:177–193.

25. Lin DY, Zeng D, Millikan R: **Maximum likelihood estimation of haplotype effects and haplotype-environment interactions in association studies.** *Genet Epidemiol* 2005, **29**(4):299–312.
26. Zeng D, Lin DY, Avery CL, North KE, Bray MS: **Efficient semiparametric estimation of haplotype-disease associations in case-cohort and nested case–control studies.** *Biostatistics* 2006, **7**(3):486–502.
27. Zhu F, Loh M, Hill J, Lee S, Koh KX, Lai KW, Salto-Tellez M, Iacopetta B, Yeoh KG, Soong R: **Genetic factors associated with intestinal metaplasia in a high risk Singapore-Chinese population: a cohort study.** *BMC Gastroenterol* 2009, **9**:76.
28. Zhang LWP, Liang H, Wen J, Jiang J, Zhang Z, Wei S, Liu C: **Correlation of PTPN11 polymorphism at intron 3 with gastric cancer.** *Med J chin PLA* 2011, **36**(5):474–477.
29. Zheng H, Alter S, Qu CK: **SHP-2 tyrosine phosphatase in human diseases.** *Int J Clin Exp Med* 2009, **2**(1):17–25.
30. Higashi H, Tsutsumi R, Muto S, Sugiyama T, Azuma T, Asaka M, Hatakeyama M: **SHP-2 tyrosine phosphatase as an intracellular target of Helicobacter pylori CagA protein.** *Science* 2002, **295**(5555):683–686.
31. Chong ZZ, Maiese K: **The Src homology 2 domain tyrosine phosphatases SHP-1 and SHP-2: diversified control of cell growth, inflammation, and injury.** *Histol Histopathol* 2007, **22**(11):1251–1267.
32. Ito Y, Azuma T, Ito S, Miyaji H, Hirai M, Yamazaki Y, Sato F, Kato T, Kohli Y, Kuriyama M: **Analysis and typing of the vacA gene from cagA-positive strains of Helicobacter pylori isolated in Japan.** *J Clin Microbiol* 1997, **35**(7):1710–1714.
33. Miehlke S, Kibler K, Kim JG, Figura N, Small SM, Graham DY, Go MF: **Allelic variation in the cagA gene of Helicobacter pylori obtained from Korea compared to the United States.** *Am J Gastroenterol* 1996, **91**(7):1322–1325.
34. Pan ZJ, van der Hulst RW, Feller M, Xiao SD, Tytgat GN, Dankert J, van der Ende A: **Equally high prevalences of infection with cagA-positive Helicobacter pylori in Chinese patients with peptic ulcer disease and those with chronic gastritis-associated dyspepsia.** *J Clin Microbiol* 1997, **35**(6):1344–1347.

18

Assessment of *Helicobacter pylori* eradication in patients on NSAID treatment

Harald E Vonkeman[1*], HTJI deLeest[2†], MAFJ van deLaar[1], J vanBaarlen[3], KSS Steen[2], WF Lems[2], JWJ Bijlsma[4], EJ Kuipers[5], HHML Houben[6], M Janssen[7] and BAC Dijkmans[2]

Abstract

Background: In this post-hoc analysis of a randomized, double blind, placebo controlled trial, we measured the sensitivity and specificity of *Helicobacter pylori* IgG-antibody titer changes, hematoxylin and eosin (H&E) stains, immunohistochemical (IHC) stains and culture results in NSAID using patients, following *H. pylori* eradication therapy or placebo.

Methods: 347 NSAID using patients who were *H. pylori* positive on serological testing for *H. pylori* IgG-antibodies were randomized for *H. pylori* eradication therapy or placebo. Three months after randomization, gastric mucosal biopsies were taken for *H. pylori* culture and histological examination. At 3 and 12 months, blood samples were taken for repeated serological testing. The gold standard for *H. pylori* infection was based on a positive culture or both a positive histological examination and a positive serological test. Sensitivity, specificity and receiver operating curves (ROC) were calculated.

Results: *H. pylori* eradication therapy was successful in 91% of patients. Culture provided an overall sensitivity of 82%, and 73% after eradication, with a specificity of 100%. Histological examination with either H&E or IHC stains provided sensitivities and specificities between 93% and 100%. Adding IHC to H&E stains did not improve these results. The ROC curve for percent change in *H. pylori* IgG-antibody titers had good diagnostic power in identifying *H. pylori* negative patients, with an area under the ROC curve of 0.70 (95 % CI 0.59 to 0.79, $P = 0.085$) at 3 months and 0.83 (95% CI 0.76 to 0.89, $P < 0.0001$) at 12 months. A cut-off point of at least 21% decrease in *H. pylori* IgG-antibody titers at 3 months and 58% at 12 months provided a sensitivity of 64% and 87% and a specificity of 81% and 74% respectively, for successful eradication of *H. pylori*.

Conclusions: In NSAID using patients, following *H. pylori* eradication therapy or placebo, histological examination of gastric mucosal tissue biopsies provided good sensitivity and specificity ratios for evaluating success of *H. pylori* eradication therapy. A percentual *H. pylori* IgG-antibody titer change has better sensitivity and specificity than an absolute titer change or a predefined *H. pylori* IgG-antibody titer cut-off point for evaluating success of *H. pylori* eradication therapy.

Background

Helicobacter pylori (*H. pylori*) infection has been shown to be related to the development of peptic ulcer disease, chronic gastritis, MALT lymphoma and gastric cancer [1-4]. Accurate diagnosis of *H. pylori* infection has clinical consequences as *H. pylori* eradication improves outcome and recurrence of peptic ulcer disease. *H. pylori* infection can be detected using non-invasive tests such as serological tests, 13C-urea breath test and stool tests, and invasive tests requiring endoscopically obtained gastric mucosal tissue biopsies, such as tissue culture, examination of histological stains and the rapid urease test. Serological tests based on the detection of antibodies to *H. pylori* have been shown to have high sensitivity and are therefore useful in screening for *H. pylori* infection [5-7]. However, because serological tests merely detect an immune response, they do not discriminate between current or previous infection. *H. pylori*

* Correspondence: h.vonkeman@mst.nl

†Equal contributors

[1]Arthritis Center Twente, Department of Rheumatology and Clinical Immunology, Medisch Spectrum Twente Hospital and University of Twente, P.O. Box 50.000, 7500 KA Enschede, The Netherlands

infection of the gastric mucosa causes a chronic local inflammatory cell infiltration, which in turn gives rise to a serological response, in which *H. pylori* specific antibodies are almost always detectable [8,9]. After successful *H. pylori* eradication therapy, the level of *H. pylori* specific antibodies decreases progressively over a period of several months, possibly parallel to the slowly healing inflammation of the gastric mucosa [10]. As a result, evaluating success of *H. pylori* eradication therapy using repeated serological tests has only been shown to be useful if a period of several months is maintained between tests [11-13].

Culture of *H. pylori* in biopsy specimens has very high specificity and allows testing for antibiotic susceptibility but has relatively low sensitivity and is labour-intensive [14]. Histological identification of *H. pylori* in biopsy specimens has long been considered to be the clinical standard for the diagnosis of *H. pylori* infection. A high density of *H. pylori* is readily apparent on routine hematoxylin and eosin (H&E) stains but detection of a lower density of bacteria may require additional staining techniques [15]. *H. pylori* is more easily visualised with immunohistochemical *H. pylori* antibody stains than with the standard H&E staining. However, the use of immunohistochemical (IHC) stains adds time and expense to the diagnostic evaluation for *H. pylori* and is therefore not routinely performed.

The interaction between *H. pylori* infection and the use of non-steroidal anti-inflammatory drugs (NSAIDs) in the development of gastroduodenal ulcers remains unclear. In a meta-analysis of 16 endoscopic studies in NSAID users from various countries, uncomplicated gastric ulcer disease was twice as common in *H. pylori* positive patients as in *H. pylori* negative patients [16]. However, the rate of *H. pylori* infection in patients with NSAID associated gastric ulcers is significantly lower than in those with non-NSAID associated gastric ulcers [17]. Furthermore, while eradication of *H. pylori* infection in NSAID-naïve patients prior to NSAID therapy reduces the risk of ulcer development, it does not do so in current NSAID users [18-20]. This was also confirmed in a recent randomized, double blind, placebo controlled clinical trial, in which we found that eradication of *H. pylori* infection did not reduce the incidence of endoscopic gastroduodenal ulcers in *H. pylori* seropositive patients currently taking NSAIDs for rheumatic diseases [21].

H. pylori infection has been shown to induce cyclooxygenase (COX)-2 expression in the gastric mucosa, which persists during active *H. pylori* infection [22-25]. It has been suggested that COX-2 plays an immunosuppressive role in *H. pylori* gastritis [26]. Conversely, in *H. pylori* infected mice, NSAID treatment has been shown to significantly decrease the degree of gastric inflammation

[27]. It is therefore possible that in patients with *H. pylori* infection, concurrent NSAID treatment may affect levels of gastric inflammation and may consequently affect the serological response. While several studies have investigated the time course of *H. pylori* antibody titers after *H. pylori* eradication therapy, none have been conducted in NSAID users [9,11-13,28].

This study presents a post-hoc investigation into *H. pylori* IgG-antibody titer changes following *H. pylori* eradication therapy in NSAID users. In patients participating in the before mentioned *H. pylori* eradication in NSAID users trial, we measured *H. pylori* IgG-antibody titers and titer changes in order to diagnose successful *H. pylori* eradication [29]. We further compared *H. pylori* IgG-antibody titers, H&E stains, IHC stains and *H. pylori* culture results in follow-up biopsies from *H. pylori*-positive NSAID-users randomized to eradication treatment or placebo, to determine the sensitivity and specificity of these different methods in NSAID users. Furthermore, we determined whether adding IHC stains to H&E stains improves the histological identification of *H. pylori* in these patients.

Methods
Study design
The methods of the primary randomized, double blind, placebo controlled clinical trial have been previously described in more detail[21]. Between May 2000 and June 2002, patients between the ages of 40 and 80 years with a rheumatic disease requiring NSAID treatment, were recruited and included in the study if tested positive for *H. pylori* on serological testing. During the study, no change in NSAID-therapy was permitted, but there was no restraint on other medication. Exclusion criteria were previous *H. pylori* eradication therapy and severe concomitant disease.

After stratification by concurrent use of gastroprotective agents (proton pump inhibitors, H2 receptor antagonists or misoprostol, but not prokinetics, or antacids), patients were randomly assigned to receive either *H. pylori* eradication therapy with omeprazole 20 mg, amoxycillin 1000 mg, and clarithromycin 500 mg (OAC) twice daily for 7 days or placebo. Patients with an allergy for amoxycillin were randomized in a separate stratum to receive omeprazole 20 mg, metronidazol 500 mg and clarithromycin 250 mg (OMC) or placebo therapy twice daily for one week. Randomization to consecutive patient numbers was done in proportions of 1:1, in blocks of four from a computer-generated list. The study centers were provided with individually sealed packages containing the treatment for each patient. Each centre received entire blocks to be used sequentially. Rheumatologists were not practicing in more than one center. The study medication was given in a double blind, double dummy manner. Active and placebo preparations were identical in appearance. The employees of the VU University Medical Center pharmacy who packaged the medication only knew the assignment. It was disclosed to the treating physician only in case of emergency. All study personnel and participants were blinded to treatment assignment for the duration of the study.

After 3 months patients underwent gastroduodenal endoscopy, during which 4 antrum biopsies and 4 corpus biopsies were taken for culture and histological examination. After 3 and 12 months, blood samples were taken for repeated serological testing. Immunohistochemical staining was only available for a subset of patients recruited at the Medisch Spectrum Twente hospital in Enschede, the Netherlands. The study protocol was approved by the Institutional Ethical Review Board of all participating hospitals and all patients gave written informed consent.

Serology

Serological testing for *H. pylori* IgG-antibodies was performed using a commercially available enzyme-linked immunosorbent assay (ELISA) kit (Pyloriset® new EIA-G, Orion Diagnostica, Espoo, Finland). Results were considered positive if the antibody titers were ≥250 International Units per mL (IU/mL), according to the manufacturer's guidelines. This assay has been assessed, in a population similar to the population in the presented trial, and has proven a sensitivity and specificity in the Netherlands of 98-100% and 79-85%, even in patients on acid suppressive therapy [11,30,31].

Culture

Biopsy specimens of corpus and antrum taken during endoscopy were inoculated onto Columbia agar (Becton Dickinson, Cockeysville, MD, USA) with 10% lysed horse blood (Bio Trading, Mijdrecht, The Netherlands), and onto Columbia agar with *H. pylori* selective supplement (Oxoid, Basingstoke, UK). Media were then incubated for 72 hours at 37°C under microaerophilic conditions (5% O_2, 10% CO_2 and 85% N_2). The isolated colonies of *H. pylori* were identified by Gram stain showing spiral-shaped Gram-negative rods, producing urease rapidly, with positive catalase and oxidase tests.

Histology

Biopsy specimens were stained for Hematoxylin and Eosin (H&E) according to the standard procedure. For immunohistochemical (IHC) staining, the slides were heated in an autoclave (Kavoklave, Prestige Medical Ltd, UK) in a citric-acid solution (pH = 6 to 121–126°C during 30 minutes for antigen retrieval. The slides were then incubated in a Shandon Sequenza Immunostaining Center (Thermo Electron Corporation, the Netherlands)

with a polyclonal rabbit IgG anti-Helicobacter pylori antibody (DakoCytomation, Denmark, dilution 1:300), followed by biotinylated goat anti-polyvalent antibody (LabVision Corporation, USA), strepavidin peroxidase (LabVision Corporation, USA) and Liquid DAB + substrate chromogen system (DakoCytomation, Denmark), and counterstained with hematoxylin.

All stained biopsy specimens of corpus and antrum taken during endoscopy were examined by a single expert pathologist who was blinded for clinical data, treatment allocation and other test results.

Gold standard definition

As the gold standard for *H. pylori* infection in this study, at 3 months a patient was defined as being *H. pylori* positive on the basis of a positive culture for *H. pylori* or, in the case of a negative culture, a positive examination of either H&E or IHC stains in combination with *H. pylori* IgG-antibody titers persistently ≥ 250 IU/mL. At 12 months, a patient was defined as being *H. pylori* positive on the basis of a positive culture for *H. pylori* or, in the case of a negative culture, a positive examination of either H&E or IHC stains in biopsy samples at 3 months in combination with *H. pylori* IgG-antibody titers persistently ≥ 250 IU/mL at 12 months.

Statistical analysis

Continuous variables with a normal distribution were expressed as mean with standard deviation (SD), and continuous variables with a non-normal distribution as median with interquartile range (IQR). Differences between groups were analysed using Students t-test, Mann–Whitney U test, Pearson's Chi-square test or Fisher's Exact test in case of low expected values. For all analyses $P < 0.05$, two sided, was considered significant. All analyses were performed with SPSS for Windows, version 19.0 (SPSS, Chicago, IL, USA). Receiver Operating Characteristic (ROC) curves and likelihood ratios were analysed with MedCalc for windows, version 12.1.3.0. Differences in the proportions of patients were analyzed with 95% confidence interval using the Confidence Interval Analysis software for Windows (version 2.2.0).

Results

A total of 347 patients were included in the present study. The treatment groups (172 patients in the eradication group and 175 patients receiving placebo) were similar in terms of demographics, rheumatic disease, NSAIDs and other drug use. Our eligibility criteria resulted in a study group with mainly inflammatory rheumatic diseases (rheumatoid arthritis 61%, spondyloarthropathy 8%, psoriatic arthritis 7%, osteoarthritis 9%, other 15%). The most commonly used NSAIDs were diclofenac (29%), naproxen (18%), and ibuprofen (13%). The mean age was 60 years (SD 10), 61% was female. Twenty-two patients had a known allergy for amoxicillin and received metronidazole instead (10 patients) or placebo (12 patients). Forty-eight percent used a gastroprotective drug (7% H2 receptor antagonists (H2RA), 37% proton pump inhibitors (PPI), 7% misoprostol, 3% used a combination of these).

At baseline, Anti-*H. pylori* IgG antibodies were present in all 347 patients (median titre 1689 (IQR 700–3732). At three months, data on both culture and histology were available in 305 patients; 152 in the eradication group and 153 in the placebo group. In two cases only culture data were available and in 1 case only histology was available. All three cases met the criteria for *H. pylori*-positivity and were found in the placebo group. A total of 32 patients (with no significant differences between eradication and placebo groups) refused the 3-month endoscopy, withdrew informed consent, or could not undergo endoscopy because of adverse events. Seven patients used anticoagulant therapy, ruling out biopsy sampling in accordance with the study protocol, and in one patient no biopsy specimens could be obtained because of discomfort requiring early completion of the procedure.

The results of *H. pylori* detection by each of the different tests are shown in Table 1. Out of the 152 patients who had been treated with *H. pylori* eradication therapy, 141 (93%) had a negative culture, and of the 153 patients who had been receiving placebo, 54 (35%) had a negative culture (*P* < 0.001). Out of the 152 patients who had been treated with *H. pylori* eradication therapy, 133 (88%) had a negative H&E stain, compared to 41 (27%) of the 153 patients who had been receiving placebo (*P* < 0.001). In the subgroup (with statistically similar

baseline characteristics as the whole population, data not shown) of 68 patients in which IHC stains were performed, 29 (85%) of the 34 patients who had been treated with *H. pylori* eradication therapy had a negative IHC stain, compared to 7 (21%) of the 34 patients in the placebo group (*P* < 0.001). There were no differences between patients using gastroprotection compared to patients who did not take gastroprotective drugs for the presence of *H. pylori* by culture or histology (p = 0.454).

According to the gold standard criteria, a patient could be either *H. pylori* positive or *H. pylori* negative. The sensitivity, specificity, positive predictive values (PPV) and negative predictive values (NPV) of each test were calculated for the whole group and also differentiated for preceding *H. pylori* eradication therapy or placebo, as is shown in Table 2. For the combined analysis of H&E and IHC stains, results were positive if either test was positive or results were negative if both tests were negative. According to the gold standard criteria for *H. pylori* infection, *H. pylori* eradication was successful in 133 (89.9%) of the 148 patients who had been treated with *H. pylori* eradication therapy, while 120 (78.9%) of the 152 patients who had been receiving placebo remained *H. pylori* positive. Gold standard criteria could not be calculated in 4 patients in the eradication group en 1 in the placebo group because of missing or negative

Table 1 Results of *H. pylori* detection by each test

Test		Positives (%)	Negatives (%)
T=3months			
Culture (N=305)	Eradication	11 (7)	141 (93)
	Placebo	99 (65)	54 (35)
H&E stains (N=305)	Eradication	19 (12)	133 (88)
	Placebo	112 (73)	41 (27)
IHC stains (N=68)	Eradication	29 (85)	5 (15)
	Placebo	7 (20)	27 (79)
Serology (N=203)	Eradication	92 (91)	9 (9)
	Placebo	94 (92)	8 (8)
T=12months			
Serology (N=304)	Eradication	96 (64)	55 (36)
	Placebo	138 (90)	15 (10)

H&E: hematoxylin and eosin, IHC: immunohistochemistry. Positive serology was defined as *H. pylori* IgG-antibody titers ≥ 250 IU/mL.

Table 2 Results of the sensitivity, specificity, positive predictive value (PPV) and negative predictive value (NPV) of each test; for the total study group and differentiated for preceding *H. pylori* eradication therapy or placebo

Test	Sensitivity (%)	Specificity (%)	PPV (%)	NPV (%)
Culture				
Total	82	100	100	87
Eradication	73	100	100	97
Placebo	83	100	100	62
H&E stains				
Total	93	99	99	94
Eradication	93	99	93	99
Placebo	92	100	100	78
Subgroup of 68 patients				
IHC stains				
Total	100	95	94	100
Eradication	100	94	60	100
Placebo	100	100	100	100
H&E+IHC				
Total	100	92	91	100
Eradication	100	90	50	100
Placebo	100	100	100	100

H&E: hematoxylin and eosin, IHC: immunohistochemistry.

culture results, or missing serology data in combination with available histology results.

Serology

At baseline, *H. pylori* IgG-antibody titers varied from 250 IU/mL to 19029 IU/mL with a median of 1689 IU/mL (interquartile range (IQR) 700 to 3732 IU/mL) with no significant differences in titers between the groups assigned to *H. pylori* eradication therapy or to placebo (P = 0.39). At endoscopy at 3 months, *H. pylori* IgG-antibody titers varied from 126 IU/mL to 12800 IU/mL, with a median of 1190 IU/mL (IQR 500 to 2820 IU/mL). Patients who had been treated with *H. pylori* eradication therapy had lower *H. pylori* IgG-antibody titers than those treated with placebo; eradication group (n = 101) median 730 IU/mL (IQR 415 to 1461 IU/mL) and placebo group (n = 102) median 2026 IU/mL (IQR 700 to 3571 IU/mL) (median difference −907, 95% CI −1356 to −460, P < 0.001 Figure 1). At serological testing at 12 months, patients who had been treated with *H. pylori* eradication therapy had lower *H. pylori* IgG-antibody titers than those treated with placebo; eradication group (n = 151) median 370 IU/mL (IQR 200 to 672 IU/mL) and placebo group (n = 153) median 1340 IU/mL (IQR 490 to 3272 IU/mL) (median difference −778, 95% CI −1128 to −466, P < 0.001 Figure 1).

At 3 months, *H. pylori* IgG-antibody titers had dropped below the 250 IU/mL threshold for positivity in 17/203 (8.4%) patients; 9/101 (9%) in the eradication group and 8/102 (8%) in the placebo group (P = 0.78). At 12 months, *H. pylori* IgG-antibody titers had dropped

below the 250 IU/mL threshold for positivity in 70/304 (23%) patients; 55/151 (36%) in the eradication group and 15/153 (10%) in the placebo group (P < 0.05), Table 1.

The absolute change in *H. pylori* IgG-antibody titers from baseline to 3 months (titer at baseline minus titer at 3 months) did differ significantly between the groups; eradication group median change 980 IU/mL (IQR 190 to 2720 IU/mL) and placebo group median change −26 IU/mL (IQR −605 (elevation of titer) to 870 IU/mL) (median difference 1006, 95% CI 654 to 1471, P < 0.001). The change in *H. pylori* IgG-antibody titers from baseline to 12 months also differed significantly between the groups; eradication group median change 1010 IU/mL (IQR 363 to 2917 IU/mL) and placebo group median change 167 IU/mL (IQR −337 (elevation of titer) to 1625 IU/mL) (median difference 913, 95% CI 547 to 1362, P < 0.001).

Compared to baseline, at 3 months *H. pylori* IgG-antibody titers were median 55% lower (IQR 24% to 72%) in the eradication group and median 0.9% lower (IQR −32% to 40%) in the placebo group (median difference 46%, 95% CI 34% to 60%, P < 0.001). Compared to baseline, at 12 months *H. pylori* IgG-antibody titers were median 77 % lower (IQR 48% to 88%) in the eradication group and median 22 % lower (IQR −34% to 56%) in the placebo group (median difference 46%, 95% CI 36 to 58, P < 0.001).

Using the predefined *H. pylori* IgG-antibody titer cut-off point of ≥250 IU/mL, serological testing for *H. pylori* IgG-antibodies at endoscopy at 3 months was found to be highly sensitive (99%) but with very poor specificity (15%), especially following *H. pylori* eradication therapy (10%). Arguably, the absolute or percent change in *H. pylori* IgG-antibody titers from baseline represent better methods for evaluating success of *H. pylori* eradication. Figure 2 presents the Receiver Operating Characteristic (ROC) curves for absolute and percent change in *H. pylori* IgG-antibody titers after 3 and 12 months, associated with a negative result for the gold standard criteria for *H. pylori* infection. Percent change scores had better diagnostic power in identifying *H. pylori* negative patients at both 3 and 12 months, with area under the ROC curves (AUCs) of 0.62 (95% CI 0.52 to 0.72, P = 0.343) for absolute change and 0.70 (95% CI 0.59 to 0.79, P = 0.085) for percent change at 3 months and 0.73 (95% CI 0.65 to 0.80, P = 0.0016) for absolute change and 0.83 (95% CI 0.76 to 0.89, P < 0.0001) for percent change at 12 months. The optimal cut-off point at 3 months for percent change in *H. pylori* IgG-antibody titers was 21 %, corresponding to a sensitivity of 64% (95% CI 31% to 89%) and specificity of 81% (95% CI 71% to 89%), negative Likelihood ratio 0.45 (95% CI 0.2 to 1.1), positive Likelihood ratio 3.3 (95% CI 2.1 to 5.2).

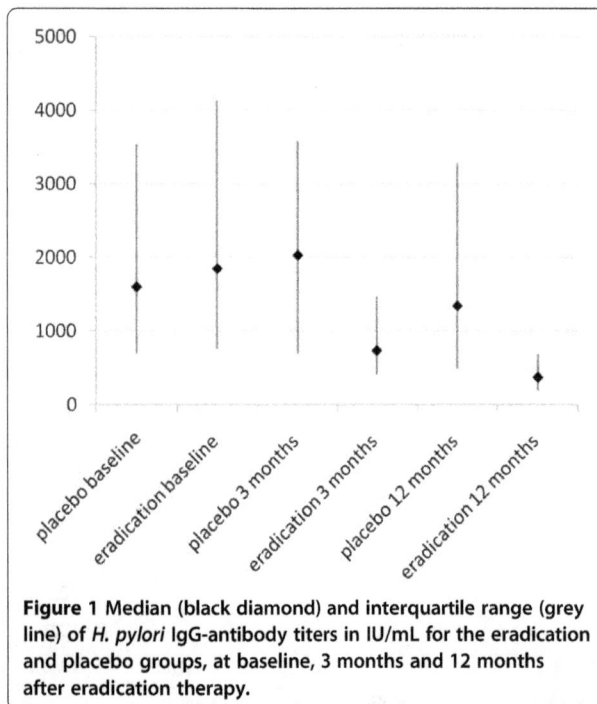

Figure 1 Median (black diamond) and interquartile range (grey line) of *H. pylori* IgG-antibody titers in IU/mL for the eradication and placebo groups, at baseline, 3 months and 12 months after eradication therapy.

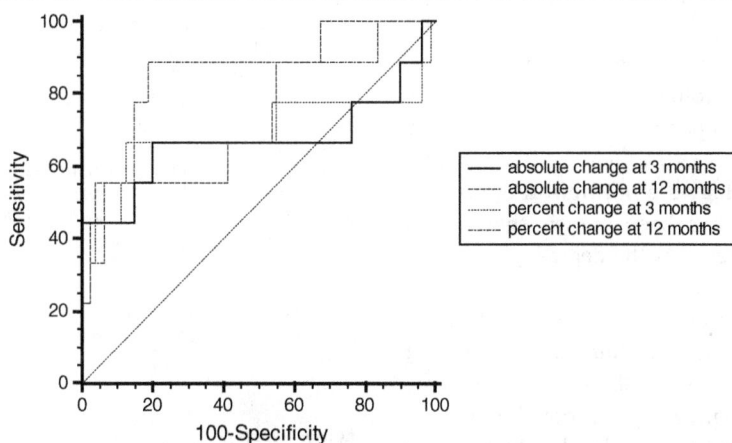

Figure 2 Comparison of ROC curves for absolute and percent change of *H. pylori*-IgG antibody titers at 3 and 12 months after eradication therapy.

The optimal cut-off point at 12 months for percent change in *H. pylori* IgG-antibody titers was 58%, corresponding to a sensitivity of 87% (95% CI 60% to 98%) and specificity of 74% (95% CI 65% to 81%), negative Likelihood ratio 0.18 (95% CI 0.05 to 0.7), positive Likelihood ratio 3.3 (95% CI 2.6 to 4.1).

Discussion

Following *H. pylori* eradication therapy or placebo, histological examination of gastric mucosal tissue biopsies provided good sensitivity and specificity ratios for evaluating success of *H. pylori* eradication therapy. In the subgroup with both IHC and H&E staining, IHC was slightly superior to H&E. Following eradication therapy both staining methods provided 100% sensitivity and also very high specificity. A combined analysis of H&E and IHC stains, in which results were positive if either test was positive or results were negative if both tests were negative, did not improve sensitivity while the number of false positive test results increased. Culture of *H. pylori* in gastric biopsy specimens has very high specificity but relatively low sensitivity [5,32]. In the present study, culture provided 100% specificity and 82% sensitivity. However, after *H. pylori* eradication therapy sensitivity dropped to 73% due to an increasing percentage of false negative cultures. Culture of *H. pylori* therefore does not appear to be very useful for evaluating success of *H. pylori* eradication therapy. In clinical practice, invasive tests for confirmation of eradication should only be used in cases where repeat endoscopy is indicated, for example in patients with gastric ulcer. In all other cases non-invasive test should be employed for follow-up after *H. pylori* eradication treatment [33].

The choice of a gold standard affects test results of all other tests. According to the guidelines for clinical trials in *H. pylori* infection, a reliable gold standard should consist of at least 2 methods based on different principles for detecting *H. pylori* infection [5,34]. In the present study, a patient was also considered *H. pylori* positive if culture alone was positive, in view of its absolute specificity. The gold standard in the present study corresponds to acceptable criteria.

Other accurate and relatively inexpensive non-invasive tests that may also be considered for the evaluation of success of *H. pylori* eradication therapy are serology, 13C-urea breath tests and stool antigen tests [33]. While the 13C-urea breath test may have better accuracy (>90%), the serology test used in this study was less expensive and readily available in all study centres [35]. At the time of the study, stool antigen tests were not yet widely available in the Netherlands. PPI usage (in this study 48 % of the population) may result in false negative test results in both invasive and non-invasive tests, such as culture, histology and 13C-urea breath testing, and should therefore be stopped two weeks before testing [36]. This does not apply for serological testing. Besides, stopping PPI in a population of chronic NSAID users would be non-ethical in a trial setting.

This study shows that in NSAID users, percent change in *H. pylori* IgG-antibody titers has better diagnostic power in identifying *H. pylori* negative patients at both 3 and 12 months than absolute change in *H. pylori* IgG-antibody titers. Repeated serological testing using a cut-off point of 21% decrease in *H. pylori* IgG-antibody titers after 3 months and 58% after 12 months has sufficiently high sensitivity and specificity to be useful for evaluating the success of *H. pylori* eradication therapy. Other groups have found high sensitivity and specificity ratios for percent decrease in *H. pylori* IgG-antibody titers using cut-off points of 25% at 6 months and 40% at 3 to 6 months [10,11,37]. Using a predefined *H. pylori* IgG-antibody titer cut-off point of 250 IU/mL, repeated serological testing for *H. pylori* IgG-antibodies was found to have little diagnostic value.

Overall, NSAID use did not seem to influence *H. pylori* eradication rates or serological testing for *H. pylori* IgG-antibodies, when compared to other studies with patients who do not take NSAIDs [5,32]. Although studies on *H. pylori* IgG serology are not new, there is some data available in which has been shown that NSAID treatment significantly decreases the degree of gastric inflammation [22-25]. However in some studies aspirin and NSAID possibly suppresses the growth of *H. pylori* and may influence diagnostic testing and increase its susceptibility to the antibiotics [38-40]. It is therefore possible that in patients with *H. pylori* infection, concurrent NSAID treatment may affect levels of gastric inflammation and may consequently affect the serological response. While several studies have investigated the time course of *H. pylori* antibody titers after *H. pylori* eradication therapy, none have been conducted in NSAID users yet. Theoretically, if NSAID treatment decreases the degree of gastric inflammation and subsequently affects the serological response, one would not expect to find many false positive test results. However, such an effect still cannot be ruled out because in the present study, a relatively strong decline in *H. pylori* IgG-antibodies was noted 3 months after *H. pylori* eradication (median 55% decline at 3 months and median 77% decline at 12 months), compared to other studies. A previous longitudinal analysis of *H. pylori* IgG-antibody titers following successful *H. pylori* eradication demonstrated a mean decline of 26% at 3 months, 43% at 6 months, and 55% at nine months follow-up, after which titers appeared to plateau at approximately 50% compared to baseline [28].

Conclusions

In the present study in NSAID taking patients, following *H. pylori* eradication therapy or placebo, histological examination of gastric mucosal tissue biopsies provided good sensitivity and specificity ratios. The H&E and IHC staining methods provided comparable high sensitivity and specificity but combining IHC and H&E did not improve results. A percentual *H. pylori* IgG-antibody titer change has better sensitivity and specificity than an absolute titer change or a predefined *H. pylori* IgG-antibody titer cut-off point for evaluating success of *H. pylori* eradication therapy.

Competing interests
The author(s) declare that they have no competing interests.

Authors' contributions
HEV carried out analyses and drafted the manuscript. HDL participated in the design of the study and coordination, carried out the analyses and drafted the manuscript. MVL conceived of the study, and participated in its design and coordination and helped to draft the manuscript. JVB carried out pathological assessments. KSS participated in the design of the study and helped to draft the manuscript. WFL conceived of the study, and participated in its design and coordination and helped to draft the manuscript. JWB conceived of the study, and participated in its design and coordination and helped to draft the manuscript. EJK conceived of the study, and participated in its design and coordination and helped to draft the manuscript. HMH participated in the design of the study and helped to draft the manuscript. MJ participated in the design of the study and helped to draft the manuscript. BAD conceived of the study, and participated in its design and coordination and helped to draft the manuscript. All authors read and approved the final manuscript.

Acknowledgements
Funded by: Health Care Insurance Board, the Netherlands; Grant Number: OG-98-22.

Author details
[1]Arthritis Center Twente, Department of Rheumatology and Clinical Immunology, Medisch Spectrum Twente Hospital and University of Twente, P.O. Box 50.000, 7500 KA Enschede, The Netherlands. [2]Department of Rheumatology, VU University Medical Center and Jan van Breemen Institute, Amsterdam, The Netherlands. [3]Laboratorium Pathologie Oost-Nederland, Enschede, The Netherlands. [4]Department of Rheumatology and Clinical Immunology, University Medical Center Utrecht, Utrecht, The Netherlands. [5]Department of Gastroenterology and Hepatology, Erasmus MC University Medical Center, Rotterdam, The Netherlands. [6]Department of Rheumatology, Atrium Medical Center, Heerlen, The Netherlands. [7]Department of Rheumatology, Rijnstate Hospital, Arnhem, The Netherlands.

References
1. Marshall BJ, Warren JR: **Unidentified curved bacilli in the stomach of patients with gastritis and peptic ulceration.** *Lancet* 1984, **1:**1311–1315.
2. Rauws EA, Tytgat GN: **Cure of duodenal ulcer associated with eradication of Helicobacter pylori.** *Lancet* 1990, **335:**1233–1235.
3. Montalban C, Manzanal A, Boixeda D, Redondo C, Bellas C: **Treatment of low-grade gastric MALT lymphoma with Helicobacter pylori eradication.** *Lancet* 1995, **345:**798–799.
4. Parsonnet J, Friedman GD, Vandersteen DP, Chang Y, Vogelman JH, Orentreich N, Sibley RK: **Helicobacter pylori infection and the risk of gastric carcinoma.** *N Engl J Med* 1991, **325:**1127–1131.
5. Kullavanijaya P, Thong-Ngam D, Hanvivatvong O, Nunthapisud P, Tangkijvanich P, Suwanagool P: **Analysis of eight different methods for the detection of Helicobacter pylori infection in patients with dyspepsia.** *J Gastroenterol Hepatol* 2004, **19:**1392–1396.
6. Talley NJ, Newell DG, Ormand JE, Carpenter HA, Wilson WR, Zinsmeister AR, Perez-Perez GI, Blaser MJ: **Serodiagnosis of Helicobacter pylori: comparison of enzyme-linked immunosorbent assays.** *J Clin Microbiol* 1991, **29:**1635–1639.
7. Oksanen A, Veijola L, Sipponen P, Schauman KO, Rautelin H: **Evaluation of Pyloriset Screen, a rapid whole-blood diagnostic test for Helicobacter pylori infection.** *J Clin Microbiol* 1998, **36:**955–957.
8. Perez-Perez GI, Dworkin BM, Chodos JE, Blaser MJ: **Campylobacter pylori antibodies in humans.** *Ann Intern Med* 1988, **109:**11–17.
9. Lahner E, Bordi C, Di GE, Caruana P, D'Ambra G, Milione M, Grossi C, Delle FG, Annibale B: **Role of Helicobacter pylori serology in atrophic body gastritis after eradication treatment.** *Aliment Pharmacol Ther* 2002, **16:**507–514.
10. Bergey B, Marchildon P, Peacock J, Megraud F: **What is the role of serology in assessing Helicobacter pylori eradication?** *Aliment Pharmacol Ther* 2003, **18:**635–639.
11. Lerang F, Moum B, Mowinckel P, Haug JB, Ragnhildstveit E, Berge T, Bjorneklett A: **Accuracy of seven different tests for the diagnosis of Helicobacter pylori infection and the impact of H2-receptor antagonists on test results.** *Scand J Gastroenterol* 1998, **33:**364–369.
12. Bermejo F, Boixeda D, Gisbert JP, Sanz JM, Canton R, Defarges V, Martin-de-Argila C: **Concordance between noninvasive tests in detecting Helicobacter pylori and potential use of serology for monitoring eradication in gastric ulcer.** *J Clin Gastroenterol* 2000, **31:**137–141.

13. Kawai T, Kawakami K, Kudo T, Ogiahara S, Handa Y, Moriyasu F: A new serum antibody test kit (E plate) for evaluation of Helicobacter pylori eradication. *Intern Med* 2002, **41**:780–783.

14. Fabre R, Sobhani I, Laurent-Puig P, Hedef N, Yazigi N, Vissuzaine C, Rodde I, Potet F, Mignon M, Etienne JP, *et al*: Polymerase chain reaction assay for the detection of Helicobacter pylori in gastric biopsy specimens: comparison with culture, rapid urease test, and histopathological tests. *Gut* 1994, **35**:905–908.

15. Marzio L, Angelucci D, Grossi L, Diodoro MG, Di CE, Cellini L: Anti-Helicobacter pylori specific antibody immunohistochemistry improves the diagnostic accuracy of Helicobacter pylori in biopsy specimen from patients treated with triple therapy. *Am J Gastroenterol* 1998, **93**:223–226.

16. Huang JQ, Sridhar S, Hunt RH: Role of Helicobacter pylori infection and non-steroidal anti-inflammatory drugs in peptic-ulcer disease: a meta-analysis. *Lancet* 2002, **359**:14–22.

17. Kamada T, Hata J, Kusunoki H, Sugiu K, Tanimoto T, Mihara M, Hamada H, Kido S, Dongmei Q, Haruma K: Endoscopic characteristics and Helicobacter pylori infection in NSAID-associated gastric ulcer. *J Gastroenterol Hepatol* 2006, **21**:98–102.

18. Chan FK, Sung JJ, Chung SC, To KF, Yung MY, Leung VK, Lee YT, Chan CS, Li EK, Woo J: Randomised trial of eradication of Helicobacter pylori before non-steroidal anti-inflammatory drug therapy to prevent peptic ulcers. *Lancet* 1997, **350**:975–979.

19. Chan FK, To KF, Wu JC, Yung MY, Leung WK, Kwok T, Hui Y, Chan HL, Chan CS, Hui E, *et al*: Eradication of Helicobacter pylori and risk of peptic ulcers in patients starting long-term treatment with non-steroidal anti-inflammatory drugs: a randomised trial. *Lancet* 2002, **359**:9–13.

20. Hawkey CJ, Tulassay Z, Szczepanski L, van Rensburg CJ, Filipowicz-Sosnowska A, Lanas A, Wason CM, Peacock RA, Gillon KR: Randomised controlled trial of Helicobacter pylori eradication in patients on non-steroidal anti-inflammatory drugs: HELP NSAIDs study. *Helicobacter Eradication for Lesion Prevention. Lancet* 1998, **352**:1016–1021.

21. de Leest HT, Steen KS, Lems WF, Bijlsma JW, Van de Laar MA, Huisman AM, Vonkeman HE, Houben HH, Kadir SW, Kostense PJ, *et al*: Eradication of Helicobacter pylori does not reduce the incidence of gastroduodenal ulcers in patients on long-term NSAID treatment: double-blind, randomized, placebo-controlled trial. *Helicobacter* 2007, **12**:477–485.

22. Fu S, Ramanujam KS, Wong A, Fantry GT, Drachenberg CB, James SP, Meltzer SJ, Wilson KT: Increased expression and cellular localization of inducible nitric oxide synthase and cyclooxygenase 2 in Helicobacter pylori gastritis. *Gastroenterology* 1999, **116**:1319–1329.

23. Tatsuguchi A, Sakamoto C, Wada K, Akamatsu T, Tsukui T, Miyake K, Futagami S, Kishida T, Fukuda Y, Yamanaka N, *et al*: Localisation of cyclooxygenase 1 and cyclooxygenase 2 in Helicobacter pylori related gastritis and gastric ulcer tissues in humans. *Gut* 2000, **46**:782–789.

24. Wambura C, Aoyama N, Shirasaka D, Sakai T, Ikemura T, Sakashita M, Maekawa S, Kuroda K, Inoue T, Ebara S, *et al*: Effect of Helicobacter pylori-induced cyclooxygenase-2 on gastric epithelial cell kinetics: implication for gastric carcinogenesis. *Helicobacter* 2002, **7**:129–138.

25. Wambura C, Aoyama N, Shirasaka D, Kuroda K, Maekawa S, Ebara S, Watanabe Y, Tamura T, Kasuga M: Influence of gastritis on cyclooxygenase-2 expression before and after eradication of Helicobacter pylori infection. *Eur J Gastroenterol Hepatol* 2004, **16**:969–979.

26. Meyer F, Ramanujam KS, Gobert AP, James SP, Wilson KT: Cutting edge: cyclooxygenase-2 activation suppresses Th1 polarization in response to Helicobacter pylori. *J Immunol* 2003, **171**:3913–3917.

27. Kim TI, Lee YC, Lee KH, Han JH, Chon CY, Moon YM, Kang JK, Park IS: Effects of nonsteroidal anti-inflammatory drugs on Helicobacter pylori-infected gastric mucosae of mice: apoptosis, cell proliferation, and inflammatory activity. *Infect Immun* 2001, **69**:5056–5063.

28. Cutler AF, Prasad VM, Santogade P: Four-year trends in Helicobacter pylori IgG serology following successful eradication. *Am J Med* 1998, **105**:18–20.

29. de Leest HT, Steen KS, Lems WF, Bijlsma JW, Van de Laar MA, Huisman AM, Vonkeman HE, Houben HH, Kadir SW, Kostense PJ, *et al*: Eradication of Helicobacter pylori does not reduce the incidence of gastroduodenal ulcers in patients on long-term NSAID treatment: double-blind, randomized, placebo-controlled trial. *Helicobacter* 2007, **12**:477–485.

30. Meijer BC, Thijs JC, Kleibeuker JH, van Zwet AA, Berrelkamp RJ: Evaluation of eight enzyme immunoassays for detection of immunoglobulin G against Helicobacter pylori. *J Clin Microbiol* 1997, **35**:292–294.

31. van de Wouw BA, de Boer WA, Jansz AR, Roymans RT, Staals AP: Comparison of three commercially available enzyme-linked immunosorbent assays and biopsy-dependent diagnosis for detecting Helicobacter pylori infection. *J Clin Microbiol* 1996, **34**:94–97.

32. Kisa O, Albay A, Mas MR, Celasun B, Doganci L: The evaluation of diagnostic methods for the detection of Helicobacter pylori in gastric biopsy specimens. *Diagn Microbiol Infect Dis* 2002, **43**:251–255.

33. Malfertheiner P, Megraud F, O'Morain CA, Atherton J, Axon AT, Bazzoli F, Gensini GF, Gisbert JP, Graham DY, Rokkas T, *et al*: Management of Helicobacter pylori infection–the Maastricht IV/ Florence Consensus Report. *Gut* 2012, **61**:646–664.

34. Technical annex: tests used to assess Helicobacter pylori infection: Working Party of the European Helicobacter pylori Study Group. *Gut* 1997, **41**(Suppl 2):S10–S18.

35. Lindsetmo RO, Johnsen R, Eide TJ, Gutteberg T, Husum HH, Revhaug A: Accuracy of Helicobacter pylori serology in two peptic ulcer populations and in healthy controls. *World J Gastroenterol* 2008, **14**:5039–5045.

36. Kokkola A, Rautelin H, Puolakkainen P, Sipponen P, Farkkila M, Haapiainen R, Kosunen TU: Diagnosis of Helicobacter pylori infection in patients with atrophic gastritis: comparison of histology, 13C-urea breath test, and serology. *Scand J Gastroenterol* 2000, **35**:138–141.

37. Marchildon P, Balaban DH, Sue M, Charles C, Doobay R, Passaretti N, Peacock J, Marshall BJ, Peura DA: Usefulness of serological IgG antibody determinations for confirming eradication of Helicobacter pylori infection. *Am J Gastroenterol* 1999, **94**:2105–2108.

38. Gu Q, Xia HH, Wang WH, Wang JD, Wong WM, Chan AO, Yuen MF, Lam SK, Cheung HK, Liu XG, *et al*: Effect of cyclo-oxygenase inhibitors on Helicobacter pylori susceptibility to metronidazole and clarithromycin. *Aliment Pharmacol Ther* 2004, **20**:675–681.

39. Park SH, Park DI, Kim SH, Kim HJ, Cho YK, Sung IK, Sohn CI, Jeon WK, Kim BI, Keum DK: *Effect of high-dose aspirin on Helicobacter pylori eradication Dig Dis Sci* 2005, **50**:626–629.

40. Wang WH, Wong WM, Dailidiene D, Berg DE, Gu Q, Lai KC, Lam SK, Wong BC: Aspirin inhibits the growth of Helicobacter pylori and enhances its susceptibility to antimicrobial agents. *Gut* 2003, **52**:490–495.

19

Evaluation of a new fluorescence quantitative PCR test for diagnosing *Helicobacter pylori* infection in children

Zhiying Ou[1†], Liya Xiong[1†], Ding-You Li[2*], Lanlan Geng[1], Lixia Li[1], Peiyu Chen[1], Min Yang[1], Yongmei Zeng[1], Zhenwen Zhou[1], Huimin Xia[1] and Sitang Gong[1*]

Abstract

Background: Numerous diagnostic tests are available to detect *Helicobactor pylori* (H. pylori). There has been no single test available to detect H. pylori infection reliably. We evaluated the accuracy of a new fluorescence quantitative PCR (fqPCR) for H. pylori detection in children.

Methods: Gastric biopsy specimens from 138 children with gastritis were sent for routine histology exam, rapid urease test (RUT) and fqPCR. ^{13}C-urea breath test (^{13}C-UBT) was carried out prior to endoscopic procedure. Gastric fluids and dental plaques were also collected for fqPCR analysis.

Results: 38 children (27.5%) were considered positive for H. pylori infection by gold standard (concordant positive results on 2 or more tests). The remaining 100 children (72.5%) were considered negative for H. pylori. Gastric mucosa fqPCR not only detected all 38 H. pylori positive patients but also detected 8 (8%) of the 100 gold standard-negative children or 11 (10.7%) of the 103 routine histology-negative samples. Therefore, gastric mucosa fqPCR identified 46 children (33.3%) with H. pylori infection, significantly higher than gold standard or routine histology (P<0.01). Both gastric fluid and dental plaque fqPCR only detected 32 (23.2%) and 30 (21.7%) children with H. pylori infection respectively and was significantly less sensitive than mucosa fqPCR (P<0.05) but was as sensitive as non-invasive UBT.

Conclusions: Gastric mucosa fqPCR was more sensitive than routine histology, RUT, ^{13}C-UBT alone or in combination to detect H. pylori infection in children with chronic gastritis. Either gastric fluid or dental plaque PCR is as reliable as ^{13}C-UBT for H. pylori detection.

Keywords: Fluorescence quantitative PCR, *Helicobacter pylori*, Gastric mucosa, Gastric fluids, Dental plaques, Children

Background

Helicobacter pylori (H. pylori) is one of the most common chronic bacterial infections in developing countries. The overall prevalence of H. pylori infection in southern China is 44.2% in children and 61.6% in symptomatic patients [1,2]. It is well known that a successful eradication of H. pylori dramatically reduces the rate of recurrence of gastric and duodenal ulcers in affected children. Therefore, an accurate H. pylori test is crucial for initiation of appropriate treatment.

Numerous diagnostic tests are available to detect H. pylori infection and are divided into either invasive (histology, rapid urease test (RUT) and bacterial culture) or non-invasive tests (serology, ^{13}C-urea breath test (^{13}C-UBT), and stool antigen test) [3]. However, there has been no single test available that can be used as a gold standard to detect H. pylori infection reliably and accurately [4,5]. Bacterial culture of gastric tissues has 100% specificity but sensitivity is low. Histological exam and RUT provided excellent diagnostic sensitivity and specificity of approximately 90–95% but the detection rate for H. pylori decreased in the presence of

* Correspondence: dyli@cmh.edu; sitangg@126.com
†Equal contributors
²Department of Pediatrics, University of Missouri Kansas City School of Medicine, Division of Gastroenterology, Children's Mercy Hospital, 2401 Gillham Road, Kansas City, MO 64108, USA
¹Department of Gastroenterology, Guangzhou Women and Children's Medical Center, Guangzhou Medical College, 9 Jinsui Road, Guangzhou 510623, China

bleeding peptic ulcers or gastric atrophy [6,7]. The ^{13}C-UBT is a safe, noninvasive and reliable method for diagnosing H. pylori infection in adults but is less accurate for the diagnosis of H. pylori infection in infants and young children [8]. The accuracy of non-invasive stool antigen test is excellent and comparable to that of other methods [9]. However, a wide range for sensitivity and specificity for stool antigen test was reported depending upon types of commercial test being used, cut-off value, treatment status and interpretation of weakly-positive results [5,9]. Therefore, it is recommended that concordant results of at least two tests are needed to define the H. pylori infection status in children [5].

PCR-based methods have been shown to be the most reliable method for H. pylori diagnosis [10-13]. We recently developed and validated a new fluorescent quantitative PCR (fqPCR) to detect H. pylori infection. The aim of this prospective study was to evaluate the accuracy of this new fqPCR test for detection of H. pylori infection in children, in comparison to commonly used tests: routine histology, RUT and ^{13}C-UBT.

Methods

Patients

From July to December 2011, 138 consecutive eligible patients undergoing routinely scheduled endoscopy at Guangzhou Women and Children's Medical Center (Guangzhou, China) were selected to participate in this study after informed consent was obtained from parents. The institutional Review Board of Guangzhou Women and Children's Medical Center approved the study protocol. We included any children who had gastrointestinal symptoms and chronic gastritis determined by histology. We excluded children who had taken antibiotics, proton pump inhibitors, H2-antagonists or gastric motility drugs within 4 weeks prior to endoscopy. We also excluded patients who had acute gastrointestinal bleeding within 1 week of endoscopy.

Endoscopic procedure

Endoscopy was performed by a trained pediatric gastroenterologist. Multiple biopsy specimens were obtained from the antrum of the stomach. Two biopsies were used for RUT, 2 for histology and 2 for fqPCR assay. During endoscopy, 1 ml of gastric fluid was collected for fqPCR. In addition, dental plaque was collected from each patient for DNA extraction and fqPCR prior to endoscopic procedure.

Routine histologic evaluation

According to standard protocol, antral specimens were fixed in a 10% buffered formalin solution, embedded in paraffin and stained with hematoxylin and eosin and Giemsa for histology and the presence of H. pylori

bacteria was determined by two experienced pathologists, who were blinded to all other test results.

[13]C-UBT

[13]C-UBT was performed according to a standard protocol included in the diagnosis kit (YouErTe Inc, Beijing, China). After fasting for at least 4 hours, a baseline breath sample was collected. Another breath sample was collected 30 min after oral administration of 75 mg of ^{13}C-urea dissolved in 50 ml of water. All the breath samples were analyzed using a single gas isotope ratio mass spectrometer (Yanghe Meidcal Inc., Beijing, China). According to the manufacture's recommendation, the test was considered positive if the 30 min delta value over baseline value (DOB) exceeded 4.0, which is consistent with the cut-off value used by others [14,15].

RUT

H. pylori chemical reaction test paper (Kedi Science Developmental Inc., Zhuhai, China) has been used routinely in our hospital with comparable sensitivity and specificity to conventional RUT (CLO-test). Antral biopsy specimens were put in the middle of the test paper at room temperature. According to the manufacture's recommendation, a color change to red within three minutes was considered positive.

fqPCR

Bacterial genomic DNA was extracted by using boiling lysis. The dental plaque sample was rinsed in 500 µl of 0.9% NaCl and centrifuged (Eppendorf 5148) at 10,000 x g for 5 min. 50 µl DNA extraction buffer was added into the precipitate. Gastric fluid was centrifuged at 10,000 x g for 5 min, and 50 µl DNA extraction buffer was added into the precipitate. One gastric biopsy specimen was homogenized after adding 50 µl DNA extraction buffer.

Each sample was incubated at 100°C for 10 min in 50 µl DNA extraction buffer containing 50 mM NaOH, 10 mM Tris–HCl (pH 8.0), 1% Triton X-100, 1% NP-40, and 0.5 mM EDTA (pH 8.0). After centrifuged at 15,000 x g for 5 min, 5 microliters of the supernatant was amplified by PCR in 50 µl of 1×PCR buffer containing 200 µM of each deoxynucleoside triphosphate (dNTP), 2 U of Taq DNA polymerase, 0.12 µM of TaqMan probe and 0.2 µM of each primer. In order to prevent contamination, we replaced dTTP with dUTP and added 0.5 U of uracil-DNA glycosylase (UDG) to the PCR system. The amplification was performed by using Light-Cycler 480II (Roche) under the following conditions: incubation at 50°C for 3 min, followed by denaturation at 94°C for 3 min, and 40 cycles of 94°C for 10 s, 55°C for 45 s, and fluorescence collection at 55°C. A final extension was performed at 40°C for 1 min. PCR primers and probe for the target gene UreA were designed by

Primer Express 2.0. Forward primer sequence is 5'-GGC TGA ATT GAT GCA AGA AG-3; reverse primers sequence is 5'-GGT ATG CAC GGT TAC GAG TT-3' and TaqMan probe sequence is FAM-5'-TCCC ATC AGG AAA CAT CGC T-3'-TAMRA. Basic Local Alignment Search Tool (BLAST) database searches were performed for primers and probes to find any sequence similarities. No matches with any human or bacterial DNA targets were found for any of the selected primers and probes.

Gold standard for H. pylori infection status

We defined H. pylori infection status as positive if at least two different tests among histology, RUT and ^{13}C-UBT showed concordant positive results [5]. H. pylori-negative status is defined as all negative or just one positive result among all three tests, histology, RUT and ^{13}C-UBT.

Statistical analysis

Statistical analysis was carried out by using SPSS software version 16.0 (SPSS, Inc., Chicago, III). Chi-square and Fisher's exact tests were applied to our analysis. P values <0.05 was considered statistically significant.

Results
Patient characteristics

A total of 138 children (male 94, mean age of 8.3 years, range 2–14 years) were enrolled in this study. The indications for endoscopy included abdominal pain, nausea, vomiting, anorexia, iron-deficiency anemia, heartburn, hiccups, fullness, anorexia, and acid reflux. All participants had been diagnosed with chronic gastritis confirmed by histology.

H. pylori infection status according to reference standard and each individual test

As shown in Table 1, 38 children (27.5%) were positive for H. pylori infection according to the gold standard. The remaining 100 children (72.5%) were considered negative for H. pylori. Note that among those, 87 patients were negative in all three tests applied, and 13 patients were positive for just one test (histology: n=0; RUT: n=10; UBT: n=3).

Routine histology, RUT and ^{13}C-UBT were positive for H. pylori in 25.4%, 32.6% and 22.5% of 138 children, respectively. H. pylori positivity rate was significantly higher with RUT than with histology or ^{13}C-UBT (p < 0.01).

Gastric biopsy specimen fqPCR was positive for H. pylori in 46 (33.3%) children, significantly higher than gold standard (p < 0.01). However, both gastric fluid and dental plaque fqPCR only detected 32 (23.2%) and 30 (21.7%) children with H. pylori infection respectively and was significantly less sensitive than gold standard (P<0.05) but as sensitive as ^{13}C-UBT.

Comparison of different assays for H. pylori infection detection using gold standard or mucosa fqPCR as the reference

We conducted validation studies for fqPCR for H. pylori infection. We enrolled 10 H. pylori-negative and 10 H. pylori-positive control patients. Negative controls were those with normal routine histology and negative results on RUT, ^{13}C-UBT and stool H. pylori antigen test. Positive controls were tested positive not only on routine histology but also on RUT, ^{13}C-UBT and stool H. pylori antigen test. All the H. pylori-positive control samples were positive by fqPCR and all the H. pylori-negative control samples were negative for fqPCR, with 100% sensitivity and 100% specificity (data not shown).

As shown in Table 1, gastric mucosa fqPCR detected 46 children with H. pylori infection. All 38 gold standard positive children were positive for gastric mucosa fqPCR. In addition, 8 (8%) of the 100 gold standard negative children or 11 (10.7%) of the 103 routine histology-negative samples were also positive for gastric mucosa fqPCR. 87 patients with negative results in all three tests were negative for gastric mucosa fqPCR, whereas 8 of the 13 patients with just one positive test were positive for gastric mucosa fqPCR.

Based on the gold standard, the sensitivities of routine histology, RUT, ^{13}C-UBT, gastric fluid fqPCR and dental plaque fqPCR were 92.1%, 92.1%, 81.6%, 84.2% and 78.9%, respectively (Table 2). In comparison, the sensitivities of routine histology, RUT, ^{13}C-UBT, gastric fluid fqPCR and dental plaque fqPCR were significantly lower at 76.1%, 76.1%, 60.9%, 69.6% and 65.2% respectively if gastric mucosa fqPCR was used as a reference standard. Specificities were between 92% and 100% with gold standard or 89.1%

Table 1 Results of various methods and gold standard for detecting *Helicobacter pylori* infection in children with gastritis

H. pylori status	Gold standard	Routine Histology	RUT	^{13}C-UBT	Gastric mucosal fqPCR	Gastric fluid fqPCR	Dental plaque fqPCR
Positive n (%)	38 (27.5%)	35 (25.4%)	45 (32.6%)	31 (22.5%)	46 (33.3%)	32 (23.2%)	30 (21.7%)
Negative n (%)	100 (72.5%)	103 (74.6%)	93 (77.4%)	107 (77.5%)	92 (66.7%)	106 (76.8%)	108 (78.3%)

RUT: rapid urease test; ^{13}C-UBT, ^{13}C-urea breath test; fqPCR, florescent quantitative PCR.

Table 2 Comparison of various methods for diagnosing H. pylori infection in children with gastritis, using gold standard (GS) or mucosal florescent quantitative PCR (mfqPCR) as the reference

	Routine histology		RUT		¹³C-UBT		Gastric fluid PCR		Dental plaque PCR	
Standard	GS	mfqPCR	GS	mfqPCR	GS	mfqPCR	GS	mfqPCR	GS	mfqPCR
Sensitivity %	92.1	76.1	92.1	76.1	81.6	60.9	84.2	69.6	78.9	65.2
Specificity %	100.0	100.0	90.0	89.1	97.0	96.7	100.0	100.0	100.0	100.0
PPV %	100.0	100.0	77.8	77. 8	90.3	90.3	100.0	100.0	100.0	100.0
NPV %	97.1	89.3	96.8	88.2	90.1	83.2	94.3	86.8	92.6	85.2

PPV: positive predictive value; NPV: negative predictive value; RUT: rapid urease test; ¹³C-UBT, urea breath test.

and 100% with mucosa fqPCR. Routine histology and all the fqPCR assays had 100% specificity and 100% positive predictive value (PPV) with either gold standard or mucosa fqPCR. Negative predictive values (NPV) of routine histology, RUT, ¹³C-UBT, gastric fluid fqPCR and dental plaque fqPCR were at 85.2-97.1% with gold standard or 83.2 to 89.2% with mucosa fqPCR.

With mucosa fqPCR as reference, the sensitivity and specificity of gastric fluid fqPCR or dental plaque fqPCR are similar to that of ¹³C-UBT (p > 0.05).

Age distribution of H. pylori in children with gastritis

As shown in Figure 1, H. pylori infection rate determined by gold standard varied from 16.7% to 50% among different age groups in 138 children with gastritis. In contrast, H. pylori infection rate determined by mucosal fqPCR method is higher and varied from 25.9% to 56.5% among different age groups. H. pylori infection rate is the highest at 10–12 year-old children with gastritis.

Discussion

We recently developed a new fqPCR for H. pylori detection, using uracil-DNA glycosylase (UDG) [16] in the reaction system to prevent PCR product contamination and effectively eliminate the false positive results. In addition, single closed-tube assay for each sample reduces aerosol contamination. Our new PCR assay is fast and takes less than 3 hours from sample processing to final result.

In this study, we found that gastric mucosa fqPCR is more sensitive than routine histology, RUT, ¹³C-UBT or the commonly used gold standard for detecting H. pylori infection in children with gastritis. Not only did fqPCR detect H. pylori in all gold standard or routine histology positive samples, it also detected H. pylori infection in 11 of the 103 routine histology-negative patients or in 8 of the 100 gold standard-negative patients. To our best knowledge, this is the first report of a novel fqPCR-based assay to establish H. pylori infection in children.

PCR-based techniques have been shown to be more sensitive than conventional methods for H. pylori detection. Lage et al. [17] used an ureC gene amplification PCR assay in gastric biopsy specimens and found it more sensitive than histology staining and ¹³C-UBT for diagnosing H. pylori infection. Ramirez-Lazaro et al. [18] showed that real-time PCR was positive for 16 sRNA+urea+23sRNA in 35 (67%) of the 52 histology-negative biopsy specimens, being more sensitive than conventional histology or

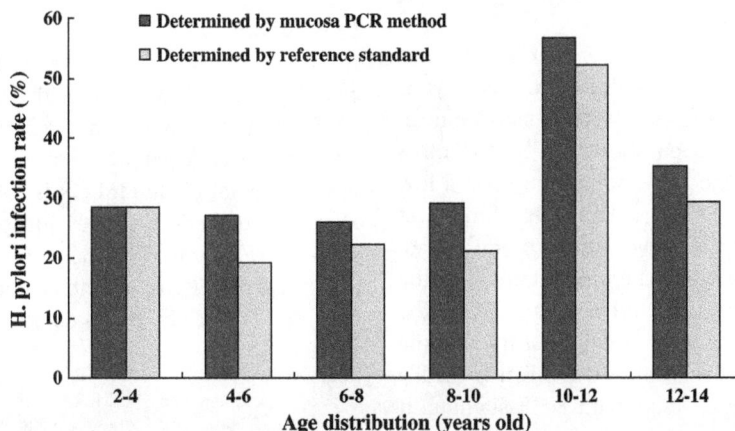

Figure 1 Age distribution of H. pylori infection rates determined by mucosal PCR method and reference standard (positive results concordant on 2 or more tests) in 138 children with gastritis.

immunohistochemistry. Most recently, Belda et al. [13] showed that a new real-time PCR system for detecting H. pylori in gastric biopsies was more sensitive than traditional diagnostic methods. In 154 symptomatic patients, the traditional gold standard detected 85 patients (55.19%) with H. pylori infection and the real-time PCR was positive for H. pylori in antral biopsies of 101 patients (65.6%).

Due to significantly high sensitivity, fqPCR detected additional H. pylori infection in 8% of gold standard negative or 10.7% of routine histology-negative gastric mucosa specimens in our study. Zsikla et al. [11] have shown that qualitative nested and quantitative PCR can detect H. pylori in about 20% of histologic-negative gastric biopsies. In patients with upper gastrointestinal bleeding, biopsy-based methods, such as RUT, histology and bacterial culture, have a low sensitivity at 45% to 70% and a high false-negative rate at 30% to 55% [6]. Weiss et al. [19] demonstrated that in gastric biopsy specimens, H. pylori was detected in 29 (52%) of cases by PCR, and only 11 (20%) by CLOtest or immunohistochemical analysis. Ramírez-Lázaro et al. [18] showed that real-time PCR detected H. pylori infection in 67% of histology-negative formalin-fixed paraffin-embedded biopsy samples obtained during peptic ulcer bleeding episodes, while immunohistochemical analysis only detected the infection in only three (6%) of the patients.

Many invasive and non-invasive tests are available to detect H. pylori in children. However, no single test is reliable enough to be the gold standard. Therefore, it is recommended to use concordant results of at least two tests to define the H. pylori infection status [5]. Using this recommended gold standard, the sensitivity and specificity of routine histology, RUT, ^{13}C-UBT in our study are excellent and consistent with other reported studies [3,4]. Since our study showed that fqPCR identified significant number of H. pylori infections that would be otherwise missed by histology and conventional assays, gastric mucosa fqPCR is superior to current gold standard for H. pylori detection.

The main limitation of this study is that we did not perform immunohistochemical staining for H. pylori infection in our biopsy samples. Immunohistochemical staining for H. pylori has been shown to be the most sensitive and specific method of staining, and has a low inter-observer variation [20-22]. However, Smith et al. [23] performed a retrospective study to investigate the usefulness of immunohistochemical stains for the diagnosis of H. pylori infection and concluded that the routine use of special stains is not necessary for the identification of H. pylori because the organism is readily identifiable in the majority of cases with H&E staining. It is possible that performing immunohistochemical stains in all our study samples might increase the sensitivity of H. pylori detection, which unlikely would change our conclusion since other studies have shown that PCR-based methods were more sensitive than immunohistochemical analysis [18,19].

Another limitation for gastric mucosa fqPCR is its invasiveness for endoscopic procedure and tissue biopsies. In clinical practice, esophagogastroduodenoscopy examination with tissue biopsy is usually performed to diagnose H. pylori infection in symptomatic children. H&E and special stains are routinely used by pathologist to identify gastritis and H. pylori organisms, in conjunction with RUT. Due to low numbers of H. pylori organisms and minimal gastric inflammation, either histology stain or RUT may not identify H. pylori infection. In this situation, PCR method would accurately diagnose H. pylori infections that would otherwise be missed.

There are reports that analysis of gastric fluids and dental plaques may be used to determine the H. pylori presence [24,25]. Using mucosal fqPCR as a reference, our study showed that gastric fluids and dental plaques fqPCR had sensitivity of 69.7% and 65.2% respectively, much less reliable than gastric mucosa fqPCR assay. However, as non-invasive assays, gastric fluids and dental plaques fqPCR was as sensitive as ^{13}C-UBT to detect H. pylori infection. Liu et al. [2] showed that the prevalence of oral H. pylori in dental plaques approximated that of gastric H. pylori in dyspeptic patients. With further studies, fqPCR in dental plaques or gastric fluid obtained from nasogastric tube can be potentially validated as an alternative non-invasive test for H. pylori detection.

Our results also showed that H. pylori infection in children with gastritis varies from 25.9% to 56.5% among different age groups, with 10 to 12 year-old age group at highest risk. However, due to small samples in each age group, the age prevalence of H. pylori infection in children needs to be confirmed by a multi-center study with a larger sample size.

Conclusion

In conclusion, our study demonstrated that gastric mucosa fqPCR was more sensitive than routine histology, RUT, ^{13}C-UBT alone or in combination to detect H. pylori infection in children with chronic gastritis. Either gastric fluid or dental plaque fqPCR is as reliable as ^{13}C-UBT for H. pylori detection. Larger prospective and multicenter studies are required to validate our finding that gastric mucosa fqPCR can potentially be established as a new gold standard for H. pylori detection.

Abbreviations

H. pylori: *Helicobacter pylori*; PCR: Polymer chain reaction; RUT: Rapid urease test; C-UBT: ^{13}C-urea breath test; fqPCR: fluorescent quantitative PCR.

Competing interests

The authors declare no competing interests associated with this manuscript.

Authors' contributions
ZO and LX: study concept and design, acquisition of data, analysis and interpretation of data and drafting of the manuscript. LG, LL, PC, MY, YZ, and ZZ: acquisition of data. DL: Critical revision of the manuscript for important intellectual content. HX and SG: study supervision. All authors read and approved the final manuscript.

Acknowledgments
This study was supported by the grant of Key Science and Technology Project of Guangzhou Bureau of Science and Information Technology (No. 2010U1-E00741), National Science foundation of China (No.30801054), Natural Science Foundation of Guangdong (S2012010009538) and Medical Health Science and Technology Foundation of Guangzhou (2008-YB-067).

References
1. Mitchell HM, Li YY, Hu PJ, Liu Q, Chen M, Du GG, Wang ZJ, Lee A, Hazell SL: Epidemiology of Helicobacter pylori in southern China: identification of early childhood as the critical period for acquisition. *J Infect Dis* 1992, **166**:149–153.
2. Liu Y, Yue H, Li A, Wang J, Jiang B, Zhang Y, Bai Y: An epidemiologic study on the correlation between oral Helicobacter pylori and gastric H. pylori. *Curr Microbiol* 2009, **58**:449–453.
3. Guarner J, Kalach N, Elitsur Y, Koletzko S: Helicobacter pylori diagnostic tests in children: review of the literature from 1999 to 2009. *Eur J Pediatr* 2010, **169**:15–25.
4. Frenck RW Jr, Fathy HM, Sherif M, Mohran Z, El Mohammedy H, Francis W, Rockabrand D, Mounir BI, Rozmajzl P, Frierson HF: Sensitivity and specificity of various tests for the diagnosis of Helicobacter pylori in Egyptian children. *Pediatrics* 2006, **118**:e1195–1202.
5. Koletzko S, Jones NL, Goodman KJ, Gold B, Rowland M, Cadranel S, Chong S, Colletti RB, Casswall T, Elitsur Y, Guarner J, Kalach N, Madrazo A, Megraud F, Oderda G: H pylori Working Groups of ESPGHAN and NASPGHAN: evidence-based guidelines from ESPGHAN and NASPGHAN for Helicobacter pylori infection in children. *J Pediatr Gastroenterol Nutr* 2011, **53**:230–243.
6. Gisbert JP, Abraira V: Accuracy of Helicobacter pylori diagnostic tests in patients with bleeding peptic ulcer: a systematic review and meta-analysis. *Am J Gastroenterol* 2006, **101**:848–863.
7. Yoo JY, Kim N, Park YS, Hwang JH, Kim JW, Jeong SH, Lee HS, Choe C, Lee DH, Jung HC, Song IS: Detection rate of Helicobacter pylori against a background of atrophic gastritis and/or intestinal metaplasia. *J Clin Gastroenterol* 2007, **41**:751–755.
8. Leal YA, Flores LL, Fuentes-Pananá EM, Cedillo-Rivera R, Torres J: 13C-urea breath test for the diagnosis of Helicobacter pylori infection in children: a systematic review and meta-analysis. *Helicobacter* 2011, **16**:327–337.
9. Choi J, Kim CH, Kim D, Chung SJ, Song JH, Kang JM, Yang JI, Park MJ, Kim YS, Yim JY, Lim SH, Kim JS, Jung HC, Song IS: Prospective evaluation of a new stool antigen test for the detection of Helicobacter pylori, in comparison with histology, rapid urease test, (13)C-urea breath test, and serology. *J Gastroenterol Hepatol* 2011, **26**:1053–1059.
10. Tiveljung A, Borch K, Jonasson J, Mårdh S, Petersson F, Monstein HJ: Identification of Helicobacter in gastric biopsies by PCR based on 16S rDNA sequences: a matter of little significance for the prediction of H. pylori-associated gastritis? *J Med Microbiol* 1998, **47**:695–704.
11. Zsikla V, Hailemariam S, Baumann M, Mund MT, Schaub N, Meier R, Cathomas G: Increased rate of Helicobacter pylori infection detected by PCR in biopsies with chronic gastritis. *Am J Surg Pathol* 2006, **30**:242–248.
12. Molnar B, Szoke D, Ruzsovics A, Tulassay Z: Significantly elevated Helicobacter pylori density and different genotype distribution in erosions as compared with normal gastric biopsy specimen detected by quantitative real-time PCR. *Eur J Gastroenterol Hepatol* 2008, **20**:305–313.
13. Belda S, Saez J, Santibáñez M, Rodríguez JC, Galiana A, Sola-Vera J, Ruiz-García M, Brotons A, López-Girona E, Girona E, Sillero C, Royo G: Quantification of Helicobacter pylori in gastric mucosa by real-time polymerase chain reaction: comparison with traditional diagnostic methods. *Diagn Microbiol Infect Dis* 2012, Epub ahead of print.
14. Kindermann A, Demmelmair H, Koletzko B, Krauss-Etschmann S, Wiebecke B, Koletzko S: Influence of age on 13C-urea breath test results in children. *J Pediatr Gastroenterol Nutr* 2000, **30**:85–91.
15. Mana F, Franken PR, Ham HR, Urbain D: Cut-off point, timing and pitfalls of the 13C-urea breath test as measured by infrared spectrometry. *Dig Liver Dis* 2001, **33**:30–35.
16. Kim GA, Lee MS, Sun Y, Lee BD, Lee JI, Lee JH, Kwon ST: Characterization of cold-active uracil-DNA glycosylase from Bacillus sp. HJ171 and its use for contamination control in PCR. *Appl Microbiol Biotechnol* 2008, **80**:785–794.
17. Lage AP, Godfroid E, Fauconnier A, Burette A, Butzler JP, Bollen A, Glupczynski Y: Diagnosis of Helicobacter pylori infection by PCR: comparison with other invasive techniques and detection of cagA gene in gastric biopsy specimens. *J Clin Microbiol* 1995, **33**:2752–2756.
18. Ramírez-Lázaro MJ, Lario S, Casalots A, Sanfeliu E, Boix L, García-Iglesias P, Sánchez-Delgado J, Montserrat A, Bella-Cueto MR, Gallach M, Sanfeliu I, Segura F, Calvet X: Real-time PCR improves Helicobacter pylori detection in patients with peptic ulcer bleeding. *PLoS One* 2011, **6**:e20009.
19. Weiss J, Tsang TK, Meng X, Zhang H, Kilner E, Wang E, Watkin W: Detection of Helicobacter pylori gastritis by PCR: correlation with inflammation scores and immunohistochemical and CLOtest findings. *Am J Clin Pathol* 2008, **129**:89–96.
20. Ashton-Key M, Diss TC, Isaacson PG: Detection of Helicobacter pylori in gastric biopsy and resection specimens. *J Clin Pathol* 1996, **49**:107–111.
21. Jonkers D, Stobberingh E, de Bruine A, Arends JW, Stockbrügger R: Evaluation of immunohistochemistry for the detection of Helicobacter pylori in gastric mucosal biopsies. *J Infect* 1997, **35**:149–514.
22. Orhan D, Kalel G, Saltik-Temizel IN, Demir H, Bulun A, Karaağaoğlu E, Cağlar M: Immunohistochemical detection of Helicobacter pylori infection in gastric biopsies of urea breath test-positive and -negative pediatric patients. *Turk J Pediatr* 2008, **50**:34–39.
23. Smith SB, Snow AN, Perry RL, Qasem SA: Helicobacter pylori: to stain or not to stain? *Am J Clin Pathol* 2012, **137**:733–738.
24. Komen NA, Bertleff MJ, van Doorn LJ, Lange JF, de Graaf PW: Helicobacter genotyping and detection in peroperative lavage fluid in patients with perforated peptic ulcer. *J Gastrointest Surg* 2008, **12**:555–560.
25. Tsami A, Petropoulou P, Kafritsa Y, Mentis YA, Roma-Giannikou E: The presence of Helicobacter pylori in dental plaque of children and their parents: is it related to their periodontal status and oral hygiene? *Eur J Paediatr Dent* 2011, **12**:225–230.

20

Association of a probiotic to a *Helicobacter pylori* eradication regimen does not increase efficacy or decreases the adverse effects of the treatment

Tomás Navarro-Rodriguez[*], Fernando Marcuz Silva, Ricardo Correa Barbuti, Rejane Mattar, Joaquim Prado Moraes-Filho, Maricê Nogueira de Oliveira, Cristina S Bogsan, Décio Chinzon and Jaime Natan Eisig

Abstract

Background: The treatment for the eradication of *Helicobacter pylori* (*H. pylori*) is complex; full effectiveness is rarely achieved and it has many adverse effects. In developing countries, increased resistance to antibiotics and its cost make eradication more difficult. Probiotics can reduce adverse effects and improve the infection treatment efficacy. If the first-line therapy fails a second-line treatment using tetracycline, furazolidone and proton-pump inhibitors has been effective and low cost in Brazil; however it implies in a lot of adverse effects. The aim of this study was to minimize the adverse effects and increase the eradication rate applying the association of a probiotic compound to second-line therapy regimen.

Methods: Patients with peptic ulcer or functional dyspepsia infected by *H. pylori* were randomized to treatment with the furazolidone, tetracycline and lansoprazole regimen, twice a day for 7 days. In a double-blind study, patients received placebo or a probiotic compound (*Lactobacillus acidophilus, Lactobacillus rhamnosus, Bifidobacterium bifidum* and *Streptococcus faecium*) in capsules, twice a day for 30 days. A symptom questionnaire was administered in day zero, after completion of antibiotic therapy, after the probiotic use and eight weeks after the end of the treatment. Upper digestive endoscopy, histological assessment, rapid urease test and breath test were performed before and eight weeks after eradication treatment.

Results: One hundred and seven patients were enrolled: 21 men with active probiotic and 19 with placebo plus 34 women with active probiotic and 33 with placebo comprising a total of 55 patients with active probiotic and 52 with placebo. Fifty-one patients had peptic ulcer and 56 were diagnosed as functional dyspepsia. The per-protocol eradication rate with active probiotic was 89.8% and with placebo, 85.1% (p = 0.49); per intention to treat, 81.8% and 79.6%, respectively (p = 0.53). The rate of adverse effects at 7 days with the active probiotic was 59.3% and 71.2% with placebo (p = 0.20). At 30 days, it was 44.9% and 60.4%, respectively (p = 0.08).

Conclusions: The use of this probiotic compound compared to placebo in the proposed regimen in Brazilian patients with peptic ulcer or functional dyspepsia showed no significant difference in efficacy or adverse effects.

Keywords: *Helicobacter pylori* eradication, Probiotic, Tetracycline, Furazolidone, Peptic ulcer, Functional dyspepsia, Treatment efficacy, Adverse effects

* Correspondence: tomasnavarro@uol.com.br
Serviço de Gastroenterologia Clínica do Hospital das Clínicas da Faculdade de Medicina da Universidade de São Paulo, Av. Dr. Enéas de Carvalho Aguiar, 255 – Cerqueira Cezar, São Paulo, SP, Brasil

Background

The *Helicobacter pylori* (*H. pylori*) eradication is a very useful tool in preventing the recurrence of peptic ulcer, in the prevention of gastric cancer and in the treatment of Malt lymphoma and gastritis [1-4]. However, the regimens used to *H. pylori* eradication are complex and require the combination of at least two antibiotics with acid suppressors that must be administered for several days [5,6]. Therefore they can lead to many adverse effects [7], most of them related to the medication but also alterations in intestinal bacterial flora due to antibiotic treatment can occur [8,9]. Most patients have trouble to adhere to treatment and to purchase the drugs that makes the eradication even more difficult.

Brazil is a densely inhabited developing country with a rate of *H. pylori* infection ranging from 58 to 80% of the adult population [10-17] and most of the infected population has low socioeconomic level. Due to specific characteristics (antibiotic prophylaxis for surgery and treatment of parasitic infections and or sexually transmitted diseases) the primary resistance to antibiotics used in the eradication of *H. pylori* is high (e.g., nitroimidazole derivatives) [18-23]. Thus, *H. pylori* eradication in Brazil should focus on the use of regimens with shorter duration and lower cost using highly effective antibiotics. The treatment of choice is the combination of proton pump inhibitor with clarithromycin and amoxicillin which has an efficacy of 85% [24].

The regimen that includes tetracycline, furazolidone and omeprazole for 7 days has been used as a second-line treatment, with 75% efficacy [25]; on the other hand furazolidone results in many adverse effects.

Adverse effects are a common cause of lack of adherence to treatment leading to treatment failure in eradicating *H. pylori* [6,26]. Treatment failure results in a higher risk of secondary resistance to antibiotics [27] and will require the use of new and usually less effective ones, with longer duration, higher cost and complex regimens [28].

Some adverse effects of treatment are intestinal alterations secondary to changes in the microbiota due to antibiotic use [29,30]. Probiotics would be an excellent tool in controlling bacterial overgrowth and reduce these effects [31-34]. There is also evidence that probiotics may also inhibit the growth of *H. pylori*, stimulate an immunological response and reduce the inflammatory effects of infection by bacteria [35-37] increasing the rate of *H. pylori* eradication [38-40].

This study aimed to detect the rate of eradication efficacy and of side effects in *H. pylori* treatment with the combination of a probiotic compound and the regimen lansoprazole, furazolidone and tetracycline in a prospective, randomized, double-blind, placebo-controlled study.

Methods

Patients

Developed in 2007 the treatment design had no previous data in literature for the proposed regimen: association of 7 days of treatment to *H. pylori* eradication added to 30 days of probiotic, both initiating at the same time. The sample calculation was based on a previous study [25] with a similar regimen, in which 20 mg of omeprazole was once a day intake, with tetracycline 500 mg and furazolidone 200 mg three times a day, for 7 days. By Fisher's exact test, with unilateral hypothesis, expecting an increase in the eradication rate of 70 to 90% with probiotic use, for a power of 0.80 and a significance level of 0.05, the sample size was 56 patients for each group, active or placebo. For a 34 to 15% reduction in the rate of adverse events with probiotic use, for a power of 0.80 and a significance level of 0.05, the sample size was 60 patients for each group.

Patients infected with *H. pylori* with a previous diagnosis of peptic ulcer or functional dyspepsia were invited to participate in the study.

Inclusion criteria were: more than 18 years old, no previous treatment for the infection, not having a chronic decompensated disease, no use of anti-inflammatory or antibiotic drugs within 4 weeks prior to enrollment and sign of informed consent.

Exclusion criteria were: patients who were pregnant or breastfeeding, patients over 80 years of age or with a history of gastrointestinal surgery and patients with erosive esophagitis or users of low-dose aspirin. Patients with difficulty to understand the treatment or to report disease symptoms and adverse effects were also excluded.

All patients were followed at the Gastroenterology outpatient clinic of this Hospital and had been previously diagnosed by upper digestive endoscopy. The study was approved by the ethics and research committee of the institution: Ethics Committee for Analysis of Research Projects - CAPPesq – of the Clinical Board of Clinics Hospital, Faculty of Medicine, University of São Paulo.

Diagnoses

All patients were underwent carbon-13 labeled urea breath test and underwent upper digestive endoscopy. If a patient was taking proton-pump inhibitors or H_2 blockers they discontinued it 10 days before the beginning of the study. The symptomatic use of aluminum hydroxide was allowed until the beginning of treatment. During endoscopy mucosal fragments were collected to perform histological assessment with HE and Giemsa staining and rapid urease test from the gastric antrum and gastric body. Eight weeks after treatment completion patients with peptic ulcer were submitted to the same examinations and those with functional dyspepsia underwent urea breath test for heal monitoring.

Symptom questionnaire

Before treatment, on the seventh and thirtieth day of treatment and 60 days after its completion, all patients answered a questionnaire on dyspeptic symptoms and the most common symptoms related to possible adverse effects due to treatment (Figure 1). Each symptom was quantified as absent (zero), mild (1), moderate (2) and severe (3). The questionnaire allowed the inclusion of new symptoms (considered as adverse effects) in the assessments after drug administration. We determined the number and intensity of symptoms in all patient evaluations. Previous symptoms that increased in intensity during and after treatment were also considered as adverse effects.

Treatment

The patients received tablets and capsules in adequate amount for 7 days of treatment, administered twice a day: 30 mg of lansoprazole, 500 mg of tetracycline and 200 mg of furazolidone. The probiotic compound consisting of *Lactobacillus acidophilus* (1.25×10^9 CFUs), *Lactobacillus rhamnosus* (1.25×10^9 CFUs), *Bifidobacterium bifidum* (1.25×10^9 CFUs) and *Streptococcus faecium* (1.25×10^9 CFUs) (Klaire Labs, Reno, NV, USA) was provided in a bottle with 60 capsules and instructions to be stored in the refrigerator and to be used regularly during 30 days

(7 days of treatment plus 23 days after cessation of the antibiotic). The placebo probiotic consisting of capsules of acidified milk powder (skim milk biologically acidified by commercial yogurt culture) was also provided at the same amount and with the same instructions.

All patients were taught at the sight of medication by the researcher himself and encouraged to maintain full and regular use of medication considering the benefits of eradicating *H. pylori*. They were also asked to maintain complete abstinence of alcohol, to hamper smoked foods, chocolate, cheese and eggs and not to use antidepressants to avoid interaction with Monoamine Oxidase Inhibitor-like effects of furazolidone during the treatment.

Randomization and study performance

Randomization was carried out using a list obtained by computer. Patients received their numbers in ascending order according to study enrollment. This number corresponded to the randomized regimen for use of medication with an active or placebo probiotic.

None of the patients knew about the randomization and investigators, blinded to the randomization, followed the treatment and performed all examinations independently. The need to disclose the randomization always resulted in the exclusion of the patient.

Symptom	Absent	Mild	Moderate	Severe
Epigastric pain				
Heartburn				
Pirosis				
Regurgitation				
Postprandial fullness				
Nausea				
Vomiting				
Diarrhea				
Abdominal pain				
Abnormal taste				
Flatulence				
Headache				
Dizziness				
Other (discriminate)				
Values	0	1	2	3

Figure 1 Symptom Questionnaire. Absent: without symptom; Mild: symptom doesn't interfere with normal activity; Moderate: symptom interferes with normal activity < 50% of evaluated time; Severe: Symptom interferes with normal activity > 50% of evaluated time, or daily, or determines the treatment interruption.

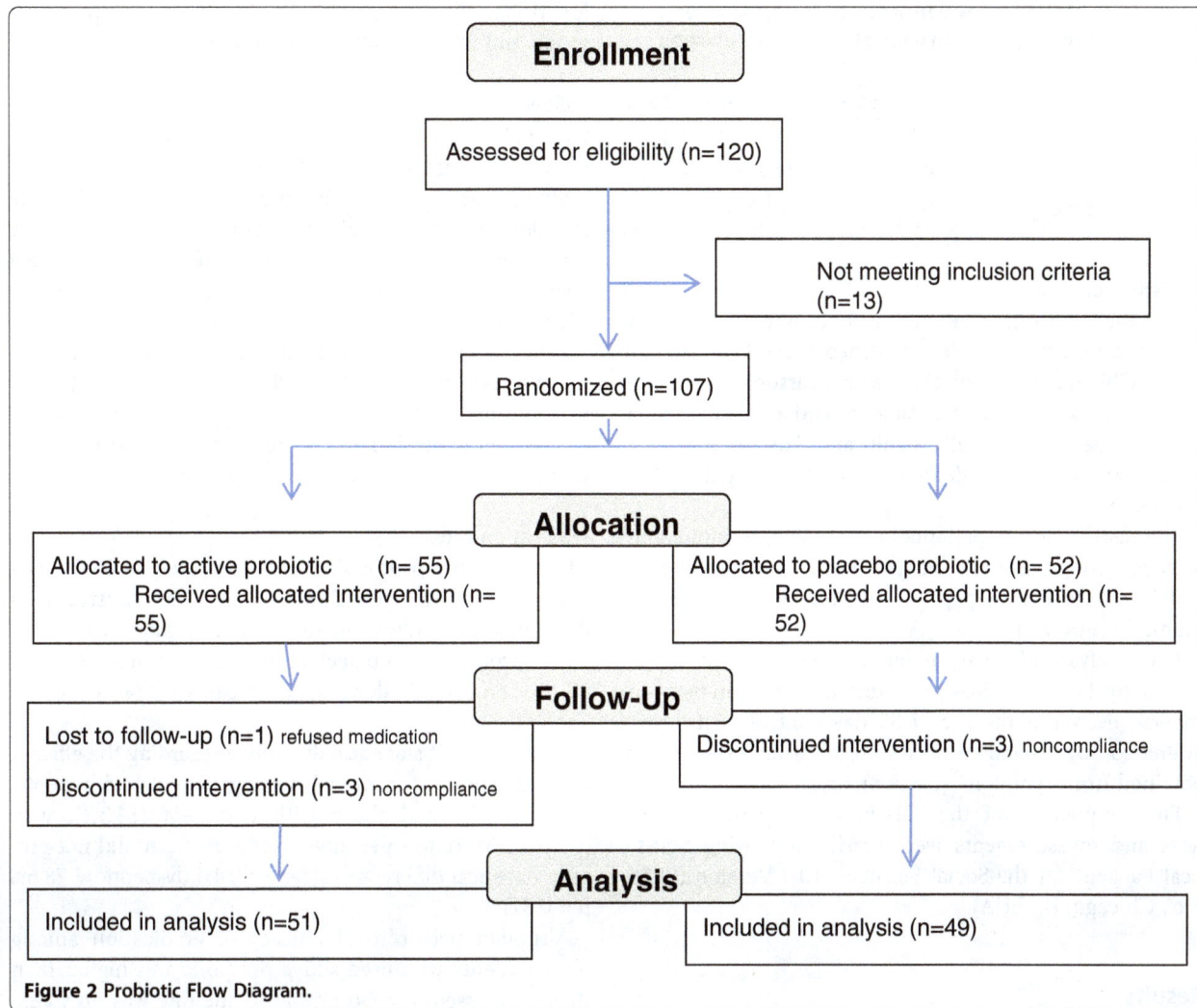

Figure 2 Probiotic Flow Diagram.

Drug use control was performed 7 and 30 days after the delivery of medication by counting the remaining tablets in the blisters and the number of probiotic capsules in the bottle. The use of at least 80% of the tablets was considered appropriate.

Patients with peptic ulcer were considered cured of infection when they had negative treatment control tests: rapid urease test, histological analysis and breath test, performed 60 days after the treatment. For patients with functional dyspepsia, they were considered cured when they had a negative urea breath test.

After treatment completion, up to control tests, patients with severe epigastric pain or heartburn symptoms were allowed to use aluminum hydroxide pills symptomatically. The use of any amount of the antacid agent characterized the intensity of the symptom as severe.

Table 1 Patient allocation in groups of active and placebo probiotic agent

		Active	Placebo	p
N		55	52	
Gender	male	21	19	
	female	34	33	0.86
Disease	peptic ulcer*	27	24	
	dyspepsia	28	28	0.76
Mean age (years)		50.4	48.4	0.78

Pearson Chi-Square.
*29 duodenal 17 gastric 5 gastric + duodenal.

Table 2 Eradication rates in groups of active and placebo probiotic

Probiotic	Active (CI 95%)	Placebo (CI 95%)	p
Per protocol	89.8% (81-99%)	85.1% (75-96%)	p = 0.49
Intention to treat	81.8% (71-92%)	76.9% (65-89%)	p = 0.53

Pearson Chi-Square.

Table 3 Eradication rates per protocol in peptic ulcer disease and dyspepsia in groups of active and placebo probiotic

	Peptic ulcer (CI 95%)	Dyspepsia (CI 95%)
Active probiotic	95.8% (87-100%)	84.0% (74-100%)
Placebo probiotic	85.7% (69-100%)	84.6% (70-99%)
Pearson Chi-Square	p = 0.23	p = 0.95

Statistical analysis

The eradication rates were analyzed per intention to treat and per protocol, with 95% confidence interval ($P<0.05$).

The Chi-square test method with Pearson's correction factor was used to compare variables and a p value < 0.05 was considered statistically significant. The homogeneity of the groups was evaluated using the nonparametric Chi-square test.

The distribution of patients in the active probiotic and placebo groups, age and gender, both for ulcer disease and for functional dyspepsia, was also evaluated by the Mann–Whitney test.

The analysis of adverse effect incidence was determined by Pearson Chi-square test and the intensity of adverse events at the 7 and 30 day control visits were evaluated by Mann–Whitney test, using the score obtained from symptom questionnaire.

The frequencies of the variables, the percentage of tests and measurements were carried out using Statistical Package for the Social Sciences, 10.0 Version (SPSS Inc., Chicago, IL, EUA).

Results

Data of included population

The flow diagram of patient enrollment in this study is shown in Figure 2.

One hundred and seven patients were included in the study, being 40 were men (37%) and 67 women (63%). The mean age was 47 years, with a median of 51 years, ranging from 21 to 74 years. Fifty-five patients (51%) were allocated in the active probiotic group and 52 (49%) in the placebo probiotic group. Fifty-one patients (48%) had peptic ulcer: duodenal 29 (57%), gastric 17 (33%) and 5 (10%) gastric and duodenal. Twenty-seven peptic ulcer patients were in the active probiotic group and 24 in the placebo group. Fifty-six patients (52%) had

functional dyspepsia, with 28 in the active probiotic group and 28 in the placebo group (Table 1).

Follow up

One patient in the active probiotic group refused the medication regimen for eradication.

Six patients did not undergo eradication control: 3 due to inappropriate use of the eradication regimen (they were concerned with the adverse effects) and three abandoned the study after the eradication regimen use. They were equally divided in the two groups.

Four patients used the eradication regimen and came for adverse effect control after seven days but then discontinued probiotic use although they returned for eradication control. Three were in the placebo probiotic group and one in the active probiotic group.

Eradication rates

The overall per protocol eradication rate was 87.5% and per intention to treat, 79.4%. There was no statistical difference in eradication rate between those who used active probiotic and placebo, both per protocol (89.8% × 85.1%) and per intention to treat (81.8% × 76.9%) Table 2.

There was not statistical difference regarding the efficacy of eradication per-protocol among patients with peptic ulcer (91.1%) and those with dyspepsia (84.3%), with p = 0.31. Moreover per-intention to treat also did not present statistical difference (ulcer = 80.4% dyspeptic = 78.6% p = 0.81).

Although per-protocol efficacy of eradication among ulcer patients who used active probiotic was higher than those who used placebo probiotic, the rate was no statistically significant (p = 0.23). Findings were similar for patients with functional dyspepsia (Table 3).

Adverse effects

At the 7-day visit 69 of 106 (65%) of patients reported side effects and at the 30-day visit, 50 of 97 patients were still reporting them (52%). Although there were differences regarding the incidence of adverse effects among patients who used active probiotic and the placebo group they did not reach statistical significance (Table 4).

The mean intensity of the adverse effects determined at 7 and 30 days was not different between groups of active probiotic and placebo (Table 5).

Table 4 Incidence of adverse effects in groups of active and placebo probiotic at 7 and 30-day visits

Visit	Active probiotic	Placebo probiotic	p
7 day	32/54 (59.3%)	37/52 (71.2%)	0.20
30 day	21/49 (44.9%)	29/48 (60.4%)	0.08

Pearson Chi-Square.

Table 5 Intensity of adverse effects in groups of active and placebo probiotic at 7 and 30 day visits

Visits	Active probiotic	Placebo probiotic	p
7 day mean/sum rank	49/2,642	58/3,028	0.11
30 day mean/sum rank	48/2,329	51/2,423	0.58

Mann–Whitney Test.

Discussion

The triple treatment regimen used in this study favored the short-term therapy (7 days), convenient dosage (twice a day) and simplicity (3 units) aimed at low cost, easy understanding and greater adherence with antibiotics which in our country show low bacterial resistance. These characteristics make treatment adherence depend more on the adverse effects that treatment complexity when compared to the classic regimen including omeprazole, clarithromycin and amoxicillin [24].

The regimen used in this study differed from a previously tested treatment [25] with furazolidone and tetracycline administered 3 × day and the proton-pump inhibitor once a day; in this regimen the drugs were equally administered twice a day for 7 days. In the first regimen the eradication effectiveness per-protocol was 75%. In this study, the per-protocol eradication efficacy was higher: 87.5% (perhaps by greater simplicity of the regimen) and this rate was similar to that obtained in our country, with a regimen that included proton-pump inhibitor, clarithromycin and amoxicillin: 88.8% (per protocol), also a short-duration regimen, preferably used as first-line eradication of H. pylori [24]. The differences between the regimens, PPI + amoxicillin + clarithromycin twice a day for 7 days or PPI once a day + Tetracycline + Furazolidone 3 times a day for 7 days were the incidence of severe adverse effects that was much lower for clarithromycin with amoxicillin (3.7%) than with furazolidone with tetracycline (15%).

This study associated a probiotic compound to the antibiotic regimen targeting a lower rate of the adverse effects. The incidence of adverse effects were higher than expected probably because of the use of a standard symptom questionnaire. Unfortunately although there was a difference in incidence and severity of adverse effects between the active probiotic and placebo groups, no statistical significance was observed.

In the literature studies have observed increase of eradication rate and decrease of adverse effects in H. pylori eradication when a probiotic is associated with the treatment of the infection [39-43]. Ojetti and coworkers [44] used a single strain of lactobacillus with 1×10^8 CFUs for 14 days also associated with a triple regimen of eradication (PPI + Levofloxacin + Amoxicillin) with 7 days in duration and obtained both increasing eradication and a reduction in adverse effects. Du and colleagues [45] also with a 7 days triple eradication regimen (PPI + Amoxicillin + Clarithomycin) also with 14 days treatment with a single strain of bacillus (3×10^7 CFUs) in patient groups approximately equal to ours also obtained eradication increased and adverse effects decreased.

Others studies achieved a decrease of adverse effects without an increase of eradication rate [34,44,46,47]. Among them, one of Manfredi at al. [46] associated a compound of the four different probiotics and prebiotics for 10 days in a sequential treatment for eradication of H. pylori and observed a reduction of adverse effects, although no increase in eradication.

On the other hand some studies didn't verified significant benefits in probiotic use [48-50]. Yoon [49] and coworkers joined a compound of 4 probiotics, for 4 weeks, to a treatment of 14 days second-line regimen for H. pylori eradication, with PPI + amoxicillin + moxifloxacin that did not increase eradication or reduce the adverse effects.

The different results are probably due to the different products used, their different concentrations, probiotic strain, dose and duration of use and also the strain of H. pylori in question, as suggested by Vitor [38] and Wilhelm [33].

Considering the fact that the use of a probiotic agent also adds more complexity to the process as it increases treatment duration, the benefit of attaining a lower incidence of adverse effects or higher eradication effectiveness with longer treatment duration is debatable, especially because the difference did not reach statistical significance, as also stated by Medeiros et al. [51].

However if probiotics can reduce the adverse effects of H. pylori eradication it could enable greater adherence to treatment and could increase the eradication rate by intention to treat.

Thus it is necessary to seek other probiotic combinations or other presentations or other dosages or other treatment duration to achieve these goals.

Conclusions

The probiotic compound used in the present study (*Lactobacillus acidophilus*, *Lactobacillus rhamnosus*, *Bifidobacterium bifidum* and *Streptococcus Faecium*), administered for 30 days associated to the H. pylori eradication regimen: Lansoprazole 30 mg, Tetracycline 500 mg and Furazolidone 200 mg administered twice a day for 7 days did not show an increase in bacterial eradication effectiveness or decrease in adverse effects of H. pylori eradication treatment in Brazilian patients with peptic ulcer and functional dyspepsia.

Competing interests
The authors declare they have no financial or non-financial competing interests.

Authors' contributions
All authors contributed to the design of the study. Acquisition of data and quality control: TNR, FMS, JNE, MNO, CSBB. Analysis and interpretation of data: TNR, FMS, JNE, MFoJP. Endoscopic examinations: RCB, DC Laboratory: RM. All authors have read and approved the final manuscript.

Acknowledgement
Drugs providing supported from *Medley Indústria Farmacêutica*, São Paulo, Brazil.

References

1. Coelho LG, Zaterka S: [Second Brazilian Consensus Conference on *Helicobacter pylori* infection]. *Arq Gastroenterol* 2005, 42:128–132.

2. Chey WD, Wong BC: American College of Gastroenterology guideline on the management of *Helicobacter pylori* infection. *Am J Gastroenterol* 2007, 102:1808–1825.

3. Malfertheiner P, Megraud F, O'Morain CA, Atherton J, Axon AT, Bazzoli F, Gensini GF, Gisbert JP, Graham DY, Rokkas T, El-Omar EM, Kuipers EJ: Management of Helicobacter pylori infection–the Maastricht IV/ Florence Consensus Report. *Gut* 2012, 61:646–664.

4. Talley NJ, Fock KM, Moayyedi P: Gastric Cancer Consensus conference recommends *Helicobacter pylori* screening and treatment in asymptomatic persons from high-risk populations to prevent gastric cancer. *Am J Gastroenterol* 2008, 103:510–514.

5. Gasparetto M, Pescarin M, Guariso G: Helicobacter pylori Eradication Therapy: Current Availabilities. *ISRN Gastroenterol* 2012, 2012:186734.

6. Cutler AF, Schubert TT: Patient factors affecting *Helicobacter pylori* eradication with triple therapy. *Am J Gastroenterol* 1993, 88:505–509.

7. Qua CS, Manikam J, Goh KL: Efficacy of 1-week proton pump inhibitor triple therapy as first-line *Helicobacter pylori* eradication regime in Asian patients: is it still effective 10 years on? *J Dig Dis* 2010, 11:244–248.

8. Periti P, Mazzei T, Mini E, Novelli A: Adverse effects of macrolide antibacterials. *Drug Saf* 1993, 9:346–364.

9. Salvo F, Polimeni G, Moretti U, Conforti A, Leone R, Leoni O, Motola D, Dusi G, Caputi AP: Adverse drug reactions related to amoxicillin alone and in association with clavulanic acid: data from spontaneous reporting in Italy. *J Antimicrob Chemother* 2007, 60:121–126.

10. Porras C, Nodora J, Sexton R, Ferreccio C, Jimenez S, Dominguez RL, Cook P, Anderson G, Morgan DR, Baker LH, Greenberg ER, Herrero R: Epidemiology of *Helicobacter pylori* infection in six Latin American countries (SWOG Trial S0701). *Cancer Causes Control* 2012. Available at http://link.springer.com/content/pdf/10.1007%2Fs10552-012-0117-5.

11. Zaterka S, Eisig JN, Chinzon D, Rothstein W: Factors related to *Helicobacter pylori* prevalence in an adult population in Brazil. *Helicobacter* 2007, 12:82–88.

12. Escobar-Pardo ML, de Godoy AP, Machado RS, Rodrigues D, Fagundes Neto U, Kawakami E: Prevalence of *Helicobacter pylori* infection and intestinal parasitosis in children of the Xingu Indian Reservation. *J Pediatr (Rio J)* 2011, 87:393–398.

13. Miranda AC, Machado RS, Silva EM, Kawakami E: Seroprevalence of *Helicobacter pylori* infection among children of low socioeconomic level in Sao Paulo. *Sao Paulo Med J* 2010, 128:187–191.

14. Dattoli VC, Veiga RV, da Cunha SS, Pontes-de-Carvalho LC, Barreto ML, Alcantara-Neves NM: Seroprevalence and potential risk factors for *Helicobacter pylori* infection in Brazilian children. *Helicobacter* 2010, 15:273–278.

15. Rodrigues MN, Queiroz DM, Rodrigues RT, Rocha AM, Braga Neto MB, Braga LL: *Helicobacter pylori* infection in adults from a poor urban community in northeastern Brazil: demographic, lifestyle and environmental factors. *Braz J Infect Dis* 2005, 9:405–410.

16. Rodrigues MN, Queiroz DM, Rodrigues RT, Rocha AM, Luz CR, Braga LL: Prevalence of *Helicobacter pylori* infection in Fortaleza, Northeastern Brazil. *Rev Saude Publica* 2005, 39:847–849.

17. Almeida Cunha RP, Alves FP, Rocha AM, Rocha GA, Camargo LM, Nogueira PO, Camargo EP, Queiroz DM: Prevalence and risk factors associated with *Helicobacter pylori* infection in native populations from Brazilian Western Amazon. *Trans R Soc Trop Med Hyg* 2003, 97:382–386.

18. Prazeres Magalhaes P, De Magalhaes Queiroz DM, Campos Barbosa DV, Aguiar Rocha G, Nogueira Mendes E, Santos A, Valle Correa PR, Camargos Rocha AM, Martins Teixeira L, Affonso de Oliveira C: *Helicobacter pylori* primary resistance to metronidazole and clarithromycin in Brazil. *Antimicrob Agents Chemother* 2002, 46:2021–2023.

19. Oleastro M, Cabral J, Ramalho PM, Lemos PS, Paixao E, Benoliel J, Santos A, Lopes AI: Primary antibiotic resistance of *Helicobacter pylori* strains isolated from Portuguese children: a prospective multicentre study over a 10 year period. *J Antimicrob Chemother* 2011, 66:2308–2311.

20. Goh KL, Navaratnam P: High *Helicobacter pylori* resistance to metronidazole but zero or low resistance to clarithromycin, levofloxacin, and other antibiotics in Malaysia. *Helicobacter* 2011, 16:241–245.

21. De Francesco V, Giorgio F, Hassan C, Manes G, Vannella L, Panella C, Ierardi E, Zullo A: Worldwide *H. pylori* antibiotic resistance: a systematic review. *J Gastrointestin Liver Dis* 2010, 19:409–414.

22. Mendonca S, Ecclissato C, Sartori MS, Godoy AP, Guerzoni RA, Degger M, Pedrazzoli J Jr: Prevalence of *Helicobacter pylori* resistance to metronidazole, clarithromycin, amoxicillin, tetracycline, and furazolidone in Brazil. *Helicobacter* 2000, 5:79–83.

23. Godoy AP, Ribeiro ML, Benvengo YH, Vitiello L, Miranda Mde C, Mendonca S, Pedrazzoli J Jr: Analysis of antimicrobial susceptibility and virulence factors in *Helicobacter pylori* clinical isolates. *BMC Gastroenterol* 2003, 3:20.

24. Felga G, Silva FM, Barbuti RC, Navarro-Rodriguez T, Zaterka S, Eisig JN: Clarithromycin-based triple therapy for *Helicobacter pylori* treatment in peptic ulcer patients. *J Infect Dev Ctries* 2010, 4:712–716.

25. Silva FM, Eisig JN, Chehter EZ, Silva JJ, Laudanna AA: Omeprazole, furazolidone, and tetracycline: an eradication treatment for resistant *H. pylori* in Brazilian patients with peptic ulcer disease. *Rev Hosp Clin Fac Med Sao Paulo* 2002, 57:205–208.

26. Glupczynski Y, Burette A: Drug therapy for *Helicobacter pylori* infection: problems and pitfalls. *Am J Gastroenterol* 1990, 85:1545–1551.

27. Peitz U, Sulliga M, Wolle K, Leodolter A, Von Arnim U, Kahl S, Stolte M, Borsch G, Labenz J, Malfertheiner P: High rate of post-therapeutic resistance after failure of macrolide-nitroimidazole triple therapy to cure *Helicobacter pylori* infection: impact of two second-line therapies in a randomized study. *Aliment Pharmacol Ther* 2002, 16:315–324.

28. Selgrad M, Malfertheiner P: Treatment of *Helicobacter pylori*. *Curr Opin Gastroenterol* 2011, 27:565–570.

29. Pérez-Cobas AE, Gosalbes MJ, Friedrichs A, Knecht H, Artacho A, Eismann K, Otto W, Rojo D, Bargiela R, von Bergen M, Neulinger SC, Däumer C, Heinsen FA, Latorre A, Barbas C, Seifert J, Dos Santos VM, Ott SJ, Ferrer M, Moya A: Gut microbiota disturbance during antibiotic therapy: a multi-omic approach. *Gut* 2012. Available at http://gut.bmj.com/content/early/2012/12/11/gutjnl-2012-303184.long.

30. Danese S, Armuzzi A, Romano A, Cremonini F, Candelli M, Franceschi F, Ojetti V, Venuti A, Pola P, Gasbarrini G, et al: Efficacy and tolerability of antibiotics in patients undergoing *H. pylori* eradication. *Hepatogastroenterology* 2001, 48:465–467.

31. Armuzzi A, Cremonini F, Bartolozzi F, Canducci F, Candelli M, Ojetti V, Cammarota G, Anti M, De Lorenzo A, Pola P, et al: The effect of oral administration of *Lactobacillus GG* on antibiotic-associated gastrointestinal side-effects during *Helicobacter pylori* eradication therapy. *Aliment Pharmacol Ther* 2001, 15:163–169.

32. Cremonini F, Di Caro S, Covino M, Armuzzi A, Gabrielli M, Santarelli L, Nista EC, Cammarota G, Gasbarrini G, Gasbarrini A: Effect of different probiotic preparations on anti-*Helicobacter pylori* therapy-related side effects: a parallel group, triple blind, placebo-controlled study. *Am J Gastroenterol* 2002, 97:2744–2749.

33. Wilhelm SM, Johnson JL, Kale-Pradhan PB: Treating bugs with bugs: the role of probiotics as adjunctive therapy for *Helicobacter pylori*. *Ann Pharmacother* 2011, 45:960–966.

34. Yasar B, Abut E, Kayadibi H, Toros B, Sezikli M, Akkan Z, Keskin O, Ovunc Kurdas O: Efficacy of probiotics in *Helicobacter pylori* eradication therapy. *Turk J Gastroenterol* 2011, 21:212–217.

35. Yang YJ, Sheu BS: Probiotics-containing yogurts suppress Helicobacter pylori load and modify immune response and intestinal microbiota in the Helicobacter pylori-infected children. *Helicobacter* 2012, 17:297–304.

36. Zhou C, Ma FZ, Deng XJ, Yuan H, Ma HS: Lactobacilli inhibit interleukin-8 production induced by *Helicobacter pylori* lipopolysaccharide-activated Toll-like receptor 4. *World J Gastroenterol* 2008, 14:5090–5095.

37. Hsieh PS, Tsai YC, Chen YC, Teh SF, Ou CM, King VA: Eradication of Helicobacter pylori infection by the probiotic strains Lactobacillus johnsonii MH-68 and L. salivarius ssp. salicinius AP-32. *Helicobacter* 2012, 17:466–477.

38. Vítor JM, Vale FF: Alternative therapies for Helicobacter pylori: probiotics and phytomedicine. *FEMS Immunol Med Microbiol* 2011, 63:153–164.

39. Canducci F, Armuzzi A, Cremonini F, Cammarota G, Bartolozzi F, Pola P, Gasbarrini G, Gasbarrini A: A lyophilized and inactivated culture of *Lactobacillus acidophilus* increases *Helicobacter pylori* eradication rates. *Aliment Pharmacol Ther* 2000, 14:1625–1629.

40. Szajewska H, Horvath A, Piwowarczyk A: Meta-analysis: the effects of

Saccharomyces boulardii supplementation on *Helicobacter pylori* eradication rates and side effects during treatment. *Aliment Pharmacol Ther* 2010, **32**:1069–1079.

41.　Zou J, Dong J, Yu X: **Meta-analysis:** *Lactobacillus* **containing quadruple therapy versus standard triple first-line therapy for** *Helicobacter pylori* **eradication.** *Helicobacter* 2009, **14**:97–107.

42.　Scaccianoce G, Zullo A, Hassan C, Gentili F, Cristofari F, Cardinale V, Gigliotti F, Piglionica D, Morini S: **Triple therapies plus different probiotics for** *Helicobacter pylori* **eradication.** *Eur Rev Med Pharmacol Sci* 2008, **12**:251–256.

43.　Wang ZH, Gao QY, Fang JY: **Meta-Analysis of the Efficacy and Safety of Lactobacillus-containing and Bifidobacterium-containing Probiotic Compound Preparation in Helicobacter pylori Eradication Therapy.** *J Clin Gastroenterol* 2013, **47**:25–32.

44.　Ojetti V, Bruno G, Ainora ME, Gigante G, Rizzo G, Roccarina D, Gasbarrini A: **Impact of Lactobacillus reuteri Supplementation on Anti-Helicobacter pylori Levofloxacin-Based Second-Line Therapy.** *Gastroenterol Res Pract* 2012, **2012**:740381.

45.　Du YQ, Su T, Fan JG, Lu YX, Zheng P, Li XH, Guo CY, Xu P, Gong YF, Li ZS: **Adjuvant probiotics improve the eradication effect of triple therapy for** *Helicobacter pylori* **infection.** *World J Gastroenterol* 2012, **18**:6302–6307.

46.　Manfredi M, Bizzarri B, Sacchero RI, Maccari S, Calabrese L, Fabbian F, De'Angelis GL: **Helicobacter pylori infection in clinical practice: probiotics and a combination of probiotics + lactoferrin improve compliance, but not eradication, in sequential therapy.** *Helicobacter* 2012, **17**:254–263.

47.　Tolone S, Pellino V, Vitaliti G, Lanzafame A, Tolone C: **Evaluation of Helicobacter Pylori eradication in pediatric patients by triple therapy plus lactoferrin and probiotics compared to triple therapy alone.** *Ital J Pediatr* 2012, **38**:63.

48.　Cats A, Kuipers EJ, Bosschaert MA, Pot RG, Vandenbroucke-Grauls CM, Kusters JG: **Effect of frequent consumption of a** *Lactobacillus casei*-**containing milk drink in** *Helicobacter pylori*-**colonized subjects.** *Aliment Pharmacol Ther* 2003, **17**:429–435.

49.　Yoon H, Kim N, Kim JY, Park SY, Park JH, Jung HC, Song IS: **Effects of multistrain probiotic-containing yogurt on second-line triple therapy for** *Helicobacter pylori* **infection.** *J Gastroenterol Hepatol* 2011, **26**:44–48.

50.　Kindermann A, Lopes AI: *Helicobacter pylori* **infection in pediatrics.** *Helicobacter* 2009, **14**(Suppl 1):52–57.

51.　Medeiros JA, Goncalves TM, Boyanova L, Pereira MI, de Carvalho JN, Pereira AM, Cabrita AM: **Evaluation of** *Helicobacter pylori* **eradication by triple therapy plus** *Lactobacillus acidophilus* **compared to triple therapy alone.** *Eur J Clin Microbiol Infect Dis* 2011, **30**:555–559.

21

Diabetes, insulin use and Helicobacter pylori eradication

Chin-Hsiao Tseng[1,2*]

Abstract

Background: Diabetic patients may have a higher risk of gastric cancer. However, whether they have a higher incidence of Helicobacter pylori (HP) eradication is not known. Furthermore, whether insulin use in patients with type 2 diabetes may be associated with a higher incidence of HP eradication has not been investigated.

Methods: This is a retrospective cohort study. The reimbursement databases from 1996 to 2005 of 1 million insurants of the National Health Insurance in Taiwan were retrieved. After excluding those aged <25 years, cases of gastric cancer, cases receiving HP eradication before 2005, patients with type 1 diabetes mellitus and those with unknown living region, the reimbursement data of a total of 601,441 insurants were analyzed. Diabetes status and insulin use in patients with type 2 diabetes before 2005 were the main exposures of interest and the first event of HP eradication in 2005 was the main outcome evaluated. HP eradication was defined as a combination use of proton pump inhibitor or H2 receptor blockers, plus clarithromycin or metronidazole, plus amoxicillin or tetracycline, with or without bismuth, in the same prescription for 7-14 days. The association between type 2 diabetes/insulin use and HP eradication was evaluated by logistic regression, considering the confounding effect of diabetes duration, comorbidities, medications and panendoscopic examination.

Results: In 2005, there were 10,051 incident cases receiving HP eradication. HP eradication was significantly increased with age, male sex, diabetes status, insulin use, use of calcium channel blocker, panendoscopic examination, hypertension, dyslipidemia, chronic obstructive pulmonary disease, stroke, nephropathy, ischemic heart disease and peripheral arterial disease. Significant differences were also seen for occupation and living region. Medications including statin, fibrate, angiotensin-converting enzyme inhibitor/angiotensin receptor blocker and oral anti-diabetic agents were not associated with HP eradication. The adjusted odds ratios for diabetes, insulin use and use of calcium channel blocker was 1.133 (1.074, 1.195), 1.414 (1.228, 1.629) and 1.147 (1.074, 1.225), respectively.

Conclusions: Type 2 diabetes and insulin use in the diabetic patients are significantly associated with a higher incidence of HP eradication. Additionally, use of calcium channel blocker also shows a significant association with HP eradication.

Keywords: Diabetes, Helicobacter pylori, Insulin, Gastric cancer, National Health Insurance, Taiwan

Background

Our population-based cohort study showed that patients with type 2 diabetes mellitus (T2DM) have a significantly higher risk of gastric cancer mortality [1]. Helicobacter pylori (HP) infection is the most important etiology for gastric cancer, and its eradication can significantly reduce gastric cancer in carriers without precancerous lesions [2].

However, the link between diabetes and HP infection has been inconsistently reported. Case-control studies suggested that patients with type 1 diabetes mellitus (T1DM) do not have a higher prevalence of HP infection [3,4] and the prevalence may decrease with longer duration of diabetes [3]. Successful HP eradication rates in patients with T1DM and T2DM are 62% and 50%, respectively, which are much lower than the recommended 80% [5-7]. Furthermore, reinfection rate is higher in patients with T1DM [8,9], and it may deteriorate metabolic control, leading to the requirement of higher insulin dosage and development of diabetic complications [8,9].

Studies regarding HP infection rate in patients with T2DM are still scarce. A hospital-based case-control study from Pakistan enrolling 74 patients with T2DM and 74

Correspondence: ccktsh@ms6.hinet.net
[1]Department of Internal Medicine, National Taiwan University Hospital, No. 7 Chung-Shan South Road, Taipei, Taiwan
[2]Department of Internal Medicine, National Taiwan University College of Medicine, Taipei, Taiwan

non-diabetic controls suggested that diabetic patients have a higher infection rate (73% vs. 51.4%) [10]. Similarly, a higher infection rate is observed in 210 patients with T2DM (vs. 210 controls) in a study from the United Arab Emirates [11]. On the other hand, a Turkish study in 141 patients with T2DM and 142 controls showed no significant difference between the two groups [12].

Based on the above observations, it is reasonable to hypothesize that diabetic patients might have a higher HP infection rate or a higher clinical activity of the infection requiring eradication therapy. It is also possible that patients with T2DM and with poor glycemic control, who require insulin therapy, may represent a group of high risk patients for HP eradication. Population-based study and incidence data evaluating these hypotheses have not been reported. Therefore, by using the population-based reimbursement databases of the National Health Insurance (NHI) in Taiwan, the present study tests these hypotheses by evaluating the incidence and odds ratios of HP eradication in patients with T2DM versus non-diabetic subjects; and in insulin users versus non-users among the patients with T2DM. The effects of diabetes duration, comorbidities, medications and the frequency of panendoscopic examination (PES) were also considered in the analyses.

Methods
Study population
This is a retrospective cohort study using the reimbursement databases of the NHI of Taiwan. According to the Ministry of Interior, >98.0% of the Taiwanese population in 2005 (22,770,383: 11,562,440 men and 11,207,943 women) were covered by the NHI [13]. A random sample of 1,000,000 insurants in 2005 was created by the National Health Research Institute. The National Health Research Institute is the only institute approved, as per local regulations, for conducting sampling of a representative sample of the whole population for the year 2005 with a predetermined sample size of 1,000,000 individuals. The reimbursement databases of these individuals were retrieved and could be provided for academic research after approval. The identification information was scrambled for the protection of the privacy of the individuals.

Figure 1 shows a flowchart for selecting cases for the study. After excluding subjects <25 years old, patients with T1DM (in Taiwan, patients with T1DM were issued a "Severe Morbidity Card" after certified diagnosis), living region unknown, cases with a diagnosis of gastric cancer and cases receiving HP eradication before 2005, the data of 601,441 subjects were analyzed.

Data retrieved from NHI databases
The reimbursement databases were available back to 1996. Identification number, sex, birth date, medications and diagnostic codes based on the *International Classification of Diseases, Ninth Revision, Clinical Modification* (ICD-9-CM) were retrieved. Diabetes was coded 250.1-250.9 and gastric cancer 151. The comorbidities (ICD-9-CM codes) included hypertension (401-405), chronic obstructive pulmonary disease (490-496, a surrogate for smoking), stroke (430-438), nephropathy (580-589), ischemic heart disease (410-414), peripheral arterial disease (250.7, 785.4, 443.81, 440-448), eye disease (250.5, 362.0, 369, 366.41, 365.44), obesity (278) and dyslipidemia (272.0-272.4).

Medications included statin, fibrate, angiotensin-converting enzyme inhibitor and/or angiotensin receptor blocker, calcium channel blocker, sulfonylurea, metformin, insulin, acarbose, pioglitazone and rosiglitazone. The NHI

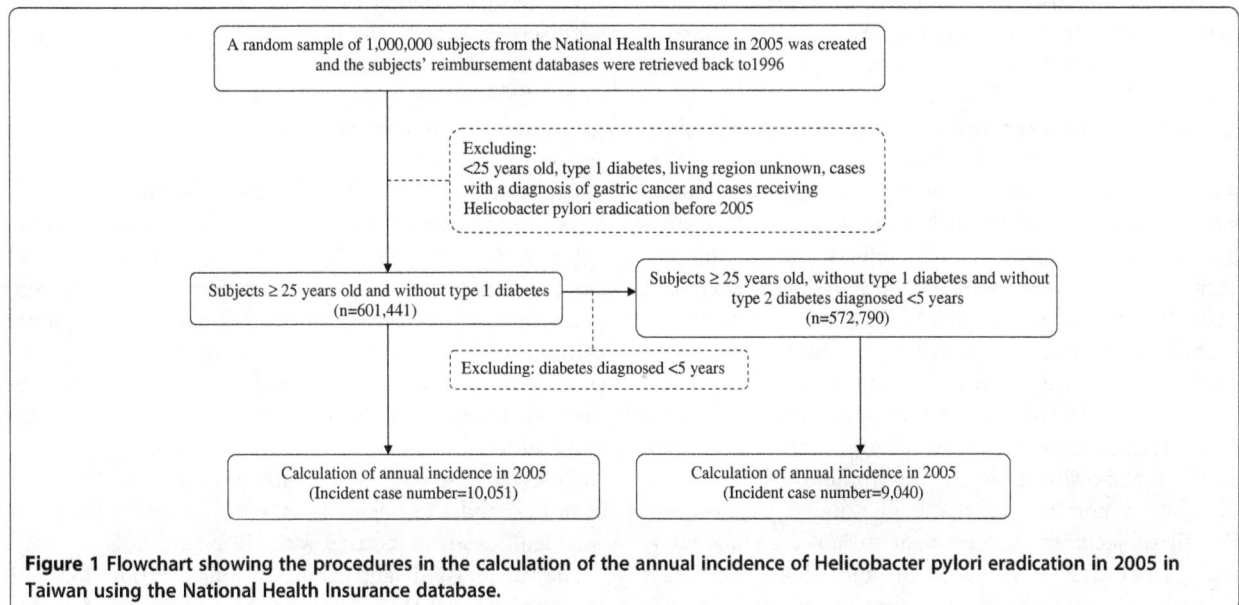

Figure 1 Flowchart showing the procedures in the calculation of the annual incidence of Helicobacter pylori eradication in 2005 in Taiwan using the National Health Insurance database.

insurants were classified according to occupation and this served as a surrogate for socioeconomic status. The living region served as a surrogate for geographical distribution of some environmental exposure. Occupation was categorized as I: civil servants, teachers, employees of governmental or private business, professionals and technicians; II: people without particular employers, self-employed or seamen, III: farmers or fishermen; and IV: low-income families supported by social welfare or veterans. Living region was categorized as Taipei, Northern, Central, Southern and Kao-Ping/Eastern.

The methods for identifying patients receiving HP eradication therapy in a previous study were followed [14]. The details for all therapeutic regimens are shown in the supplementary Table 1 of this earlier paper. In brief, HP eradication therapy was defined as a combination use of proton pump inhibitor or H2 receptor blockers, plus clarithromycin or metronidazole, plus amoxicillin or tetracycline, with or without bismuth, in the same prescription order for 7-14 days.

Statistical analyses

Diabetes status and insulin use were considered as the exposures of interest and HP eradication as the outcome in the study. To assure the correctness of temporal order of exposure and outcome, age, diabetes status, diabetes duration, use of insulin or other medications, and comorbidities were recorded as a status or diagnosis before January 1, 2005; and HP eradication was recorded as a first event occurring in the year 2005. PES done in 2005 and from 1997 to 2005 were both analyzed. The purpose to include PES done in 2005 was to assure the temporal proximity of performing PES which might be related to the conduction of HP eradication.

The baseline characteristics between diabetic and non-diabetic subjects were compared by Student's t test for continuous variables and by Chi square test for categorical variables.

Chi square test examined the differences of annual incidence of HP eradication among subgroups of age (25-44, 45-54, 55-64 and ≥65 years), sex, diabetes (for all subjects), insulin use (for diabetic patients only), occupation and living region, for all subjects and for the diabetic patients only separately, before and after excluding patients with diabetes diagnosed <5 years (Figure 1).

Logistic regression estimated the mutually-adjusted odds ratios for HP eradication in all subjects and in the diabetic patients only. For the diabetic patients only, the independent variables included age, sex, PES (1997-2005), the above-mentioned comorbidities, living region, occupation and all the above-mentioned medications. For all subjects, the independent variables included age, sex, diabetes, PES (1997-2005), the above-mentioned comorbidities, medications other than anti-diabetic

therapies (i.e., statin, fibrate, angiotensin-converting enzyme inhibitor and/or angiotensin receptor blocker, calcium channel blocker), living region and occupation.

Additional logistic models were created to examine whether the magnitude of the odds ratios for diabetes status (for all subjects), diabetes duration (for all subjects) and insulin use (for the diabetic patients only) might change by including different sets of covariates. Model I was adjusted for age and sex; model II for age, sex, occupation and living region; model III for age, sex, occupation, living region, PES (in 2005), hypertension, chronic obstructive pulmonary disease, stroke, nephropathy, ischemic heart disease, peripheral arterial disease, eye disease, obesity and dyslipidemia; model IV for age, sex, occupation, living region, PES (in 2005), hypertension, chronic obstructive pulmonary disease, stroke, nephropathy, ischemic heart disease, peripheral arterial disease, eye disease, obesity, dyslipidemia, statin, fibrate, angiotensin converting enzyme inhibitor/angiotensin receptor blocker and calcium channel blocker (model IV in diabetic patients only was additionally adjusted for oral anti-diabetic agents including sulfonylurea, metformin, acarbose, pioglitazone and rosiglitazone).

Analyses were conducted using SAS statistical software, version 9.1 (SAS Institute, Cary, NC). Data were expressed as mean (standard deviation) for continuous variables or number (%) for categorical variables. $P < 0.05$ was considered statistically significant.

Results

Table 1 compares the baseline characteristics between diabetic and non-diabetic subjects. The diabetic patients were older and female predominant, and had higher prevalence rates of comorbidities, medication use and PES (in 2005 or 1997-2005).

The annual incidences of HP eradication in different groups are shown in Table 2. HP eradication rates increased with increasing age, and were higher in men, diabetic patients and insulin users. Significant differences were also seen for occupation and living region.

The mutually-adjusted odds ratios for HP eradication are shown in Table 3. For all subjects, age, male sex, diabetes, PES (1997-2005), hypertension, chronic obstructive pulmonary disease, stroke, nephropathy, ischemic heart disease, peripheral arterial disease, dyslipidemia, calcium channel blocker, living region (northern and central) and occupation (III and IV) were significantly associated with a higher incidence. Except for dyslipidemia and living region in northern Taiwan, the significant variables for the diabetic patients only were all the same as in the model for all subjects. Furthermore, insulin use was significantly associated with HP eradication.

The unadjusted and adjusted odds ratios for HP eradication for diabetes status (for all subjects), diabetes

Table 1 Baseline characteristics of study subjects aged 25 years or older by diabetes status

Variable	Diabetes mellitus				P value
	No		Yes		
	n or mean	% or SD	*n* or mean	% or SD	
n (%)	511519	85.05	89922	14.95	
Age (years)	43.98	14.00	58.01	14.95	<0.0001
Sex (men, %)	253626	49.58	39950	44.43	<0.0001
Hypertension (%)	79292	15.50	50549	56.21	<0.0001
Chronic obstructive pulmonary disease (%)	105693	20.66	36273	40.34	<0.0001
Stroke (%)	24744	4.84	18484	20.56	<0.0001
Nephropathy (%)	24780	4.84	15971	17.76	<0.0001
Ischemic heart disease (%)	40465	7.91	28523	31.72	<0.0001
Peripheral arterial disease (%)	15732	3.08	12683	14.10	<0.0001
Eye disease (%)	1170	0.23	8763	9.75	<0.0001
Obesity (%)	4180	0.82	2410	2.68	<0.0001
Dyslipidemia (%)	51126	9.99	44973	50.01	<0.0001
Statin (%)	19608	3.83	24481	27.22	<0.0001
Fibrate (%)	16084	3.14	19053	21.19	<0.0001
Angiotensin-converting enzyme inhibitor/ Angiotensin receptor blocker (%)	6904	1.35	6638	7.38	<0.0001
Calcium channel blocker (%)	34889	6.82	18908	21.03	<0.0001
Occupation (%)					
I	282985	55.32	35103	39.04	<0.0001
II	82588	16.15	17037	18.95	
III	61580	12.04	19708	21.92	
IV	84366	16.49	18074	20.10	
Living region (%)					
Taipei	193494	37.83	31534	35.07	<0.0001
Northern	74045	14.48	11182	12.44	
Central	91087	17.81	15664	17.42	
Southern	66785	13.06	14807	16.47	
Kao-Ping/Eastern	86108	16.83	16735	18.61	
Panendoscopic examination in 2005	8211	1.61	2834	3.15	<0.0001
Panendoscopic examination in 1997-2005	37759	7.38	11762	13.08	<0.0001
Diabetic patients only					
Sulfonylurea (%)	-	-	37211	41.38	
Metformin (%)	-	-	33106	36.82	
Insulin (%)	-	-	6010	6.68	
Acarbose (%)	-	-	6968	7.75	
Pioglitazone (%)	-	-	2329	2.59	
Rosiglitazone (%)	-	-	6538	7.27	

Data are expressed as *n* (%) or mean (SD). *Occupation categories are explained in "Materials and Methods".

duration (for all subjects) and insulin use (for diabetic patients only) are shown in Table 4. Diabetes was associated with a significantly higher odds ratio of HP eradication in all models, though the odds ratio attenuated when more covariates were adjusted, especially when the comorbidities were considered (models III and IV). The odds ratios attenuated with increasing diabetes duration and with adjustment for covariates, especially when comorbidities and medications were included. The odds ratios became insignificant for diabetes duration of more than 3 years in models III and IV. Insulin use was significantly associated with a higher odds ratio though the magnitude of the odds ratios attenuated slightly after adjustment for covariates.

Table 2 Annual incidence (per 100,000) of Helicobacter pylori eradication in 2005 in Taiwan

Variable	Excluding diabetes diagnosed <5 years					
	No			Yes		
	n	Incidence	*P*	*n*	Incidence	*P*
All subjects						
Age (years)						
25-44	3250	1009.44	<0.0001	3066	974.82	<0.0001
45-54	2370	1805.69		2134	1725.63	
55-64	1687	2469.52		1462	2352.68	
≥65	2744	3433.69		2378	3281.67	
Sex						
Men	5142	1751.51	<0.0001	4612	1648.96	<0.0001
Women	4909	1594.53		4428	1510.76	
Diabetes						
No	7129	1393.69	<0.0001	7129	1393.69	<0.0001
Yes	2922	3249.48		1911	3118.93	
Occupation*						
I	4272	1343.02	<0.0001	3915	1277.81	<0.0001
II	1815	1821.83		1640	1744.48	
III	2023	2488.68		1764	2332.50	
IV	1941	1894.77		1721	1778.46	
Living region						
Taipei	3471	1542.47	<0.0001	3123	1455.34	<0.0001
Northern	1220	1431.47		1103	1349.10	
Central	1670	1564.39		1486	1461.00	
Southern	1623	1989.17		1449	1874.95	
Kao-Ping/Eastern	2067	2009.86		1879	1928.17	
Diabetic patients only						
Age (years)						
25-44	374	1999.57	<0.0001	190	1687.09	<0.0001
45-54	568	2789.51		332	2598.83	
55-64	677	3435.33		452	3339.24	
≥65	1303	4183.12		937	3953.92	
Sex						
Men	1380	3454.32	0.0020	850	3260.95	0.0818
Women	1542	3085.73		1061	3013.78	
Insulin use						
No	2619	3121.13	<0.0001	1678	2979.72	<0.0001
Yes	303	5041.60		233	4700.42	
Occupation*						
I	963	2743.36	<0.0001	606	2589.96	<0.0001
II	521	3058.05		346	3028.98	
III	778	3947.64		519	3694.74	
IV	660	3651.65		440	3547.53	
Living region						
Taipei	962	3050.68	0.0002	614	2910.64	<0.0001
Northern	330	2951.17		213	2761.57	

Table 2 Annual incidence (per 100,000) of Helicobacter pylori eradication in 2005 in Taiwan (Continued)

Central	489	3121.81	305	2870.86
Southern	548	3700.95	374	3562.92
Kao-Ping/Eastern	593	3543.47	405	3570.80

n = case number of Helicobacter pylori eradication.
*Occupation categories are explained in "Materials and Methods".
Chi-square test was used for the statistical analysis.

Discussion

This study provided for the first time a nation-wide population-based analysis with a large sample size on the association between T2DM and HP eradication. Diabetes was significantly associated with a higher incidence of HP eradication (Tables 2, 3, 4), independent of comorbidities, medications, PES, occupation and living region (Tables 3 and 4). The odds ratios attenuated with increasing diabetes duration, probably due to the increased occurrence of comorbidities, which might also affect the incidence of HP eradication (Table 4). Furthermore, use of calcium channel blockers (Table 3) and insulin use in the diabetic

Table 3 Mutually-adjusted odds ratios for Helicobacter pylori eradication in 2005 in Taiwan

Study/Variable	Interpretation	Adjusted odds ratio (95% confidence interval)	
		All subjects	Diabetic patients only
Age	Every 1-year increment	1.014 (1.012, 1.015)	1.008 (1.005, 1.011)
Sex	Men vs. Women	1.220 (1.171, 1.270)	1.155 (1.071, 1.247)
Diabetes	Yes vs. No	1.133 (1.074, 1.195)	–
Panendoscope examination (1997-2005)	Yes vs. No	8.940 (8.573, 9.321)	5.592 (5.173, 6.045)
Hypertension	Yes vs. No	1.199 (1.129, 1.273)	1.215 (1.098, 1.345)
Chronic obstructive pulmonary disease	Yes vs. No	1.257 (1.202, 1.314)	1.214 (1.121, 1.313)
Stroke	Yes vs. No	1.119 (1.051, 1.191)	1.096 (1.000, 1.201)
Nephropathy	Yes vs. No	1.268 (1.193, 1.347)	1.314 (1.203, 1.435)
Ischemic heart disease	Yes vs. No	1.246 (1.179, 1.317)	1.183 (1.086, 1.289)
Peripheral arterial disease	Yes vs. No	1.126 (1.048, 1.211)	1.133 (1.025, 1.252)
Eye disease	Yes vs. No	0.937 (0.833, 1.053)	0.898 (0.784, 1.029)
Obesity	Yes vs. No	0.971 (0.816, 1.155)	0.815 (0.627, 1.061)
Dyslipidemia	Yes vs. No	1.174 (1.110, 1.242)	1.034 (0.948, 1.127)
Statin	Yes vs. No	1.013 (0.946, 1.086)	1.015 (0.923, 1.116)
Fibrate	Yes vs. No	1.015 (0.944, 1.091)	1.007 (0.913, 1.110)
Angiotensin-converting enzyme inhibitor/ Angiotensin receptor blocker	Yes vs. No	1.011 (0.912, 1.121)	1.051 (0.913, 1.211)
Calcium channel blocker	Yes vs. No	1.147 (1.074, 1.225)	1.108 (1.004, 1.224)
Living region	Northern vs. Taipei	1.103 (1.042, 1.168)	1.082 (0.968, 1.208)
	Central vs. Taipei	1.124 (1.056, 1.195)	1.140 (1.022, 1.271)
	Southern vs. Taipei	1.027 (0.969, 1.088)	1.047 (0.941, 1.165)
	Kao-Ping/Eastern vs. Taipei	0.988 (0.924, 1.058)	0.979 (0.859, 1.116)
Occupation	II vs. I	1.022 (0.961, 1.087)	1.023 (0.910, 1.148)
	III vs. I	1.317 (1.235, 1.404)	1.286 (1.144, 1.445)
	IV vs. I	1.308 (1.235, 1.386)	1.205 (1.080, 1.345)
Sulfonylurea	Yes vs. No	-	0.978 (0.875, 1.093)
Metformin	Yes vs. No	-	0.972 (0.867, 1.091)
Insulin	Yes vs. No	-	1.414 (1.228, 1.629)
Acarbose	Yes vs. No	-	1.004 (0.863, 1.167)
Pioglitazone	Yes vs. No	-	0.999 (0.787, 1.269)
Rosiglitazone	Yes vs. No	-	0.939 (0.800, 1.101)

*Occupation categories are explained in "Materials and Methods".

Table 4 Odds ratios for Helicobacter pylori eradication for diabetes status, diabetes duration and insulin use

Diabetes-related variable	Odds ratio (95% confidence interval)				
	Unadjusted	Adjusted			
		Model I	Model II	Model III	Model IV
All subjects					
Non-diabetes	1.000	1.000	1.000	1.000	1.000
Diabetes	2.376 (2.275, 2.482)	1.644 (1.569, 1.723)	1.633 (1.558, 1.711)	1.132 (1.062, 1.208)	1.137 (1.065, 1.213)
All subjects					
Non-diabetes	1.000	1.000	1.000	1.000	1.000
Diabetes <1 year	3.596 (3.217, 4.020)	2.736 (2.444, 3.061)	2.721 (2.431, 3.045)	1.772 (1.522, 2.062)	1.772 (1.522, 2.062)
Diabetes 1-3 years	2.273 (2.062, 2.506)	1.695 (1.536, 1.871)	1.681 (1.523, 1.855)	1.293 (1.139 1.468)	1.289 (1.135, 1.463)
Diabetes 3-5 years	2.178 (1.977, 2.398)	1.587 (1.439, 1.750)	1.575 (1.428, 1.737)	1.057 (0.931, 1.200)	1.053 (0.927, 1.196)
Diabetes ≥5 years	2.303 (2.182, 2.430)	1.513 (1.428, 1.602)	1.503 (1.419, 1.592)	1.015 (0.938, 1.098)	1.022 (0.944, 1.106)
Diabetic patients only					
Non-insulin users	1.000	1.000	1.000	1.000	1.000
Insulin users	1.648 (1.459, 1.862)	1.495 (1.322, 1.690)	1.483 (1.311, 1.677)	1.319 (1.127, 1.543)	1.389 (1.178, 1.639)*

I: Adjusted for age and sex.
II: Adjusted for age, sex, occupation and living region.
III: Adjusted for age, sex, occupation, living region, panendoscopic examination (in 2005), hypertension, chronic obstructive pulmonary disease, stroke, nephropathy, ischemic heart disease, peripheral arterial disease, eye disease, obesity and dyslipidemia.
IV: Adjusted for age, sex, occupation, living region, panendoscopic examination (in 2005), hypertension, chronic obstructive pulmonary disease, stroke, nephropathy, ischemic heart disease, peripheral arterial disease, eye disease, obesity, dyslipidemia, statin, fibrate, angiotensin converting enzyme inhibitor/angiotensin receptor blocker and calcium channel blocker.
*Model IV in diabetic patients only was additionally adjusted for oral anti-diabetic agents including sulfonylurea, metformin, acarbose, pioglitazone and rosiglitazone.

patients (Tables 2, 3, 4) were also significantly associated with HP eradication.

The higher incidence of HP eradication associated with diabetes could be explained by the following possibilities: the diabetic patients might have a higher chance of being detected for HP infection, or they might have a higher HP infection rate or a higher activity of HP infection. A higher detection rate is possible because the diabetic patients were more prone to have PES (Table 1). However, this could not explain the whole picture because the higher incidence of HP eradication associated with diabetes remained significant after adjustment for PES and other covariates (Tables 3 and 4). Currently we do not have HP infection rates in Taiwanese diabetic and non-diabetic subjects. Some studies suggested that the HP infection rates are similar between non-diabetic and diabetic subjects in patients with either T1DM [3,4] or T2DM [12]. If this is the case, the higher incidence of HP eradication associated with diabetes (Tables 2, 3, 4) may implicate that HP infection in the diabetic patients is more clinically active with more severe symptoms, leading to its diagnosis and the use of medications for its eradication.

Insulin use was consistently associated with a higher incidence of HP eradication, but none of the oral anti-diabetic agents was (Tables 2, 3, 4). Insulin use may be a proxy for uncontrollable hyperglycemia with more severe disease. Therefore this observation might be explained in the following ways. HP infected patients might have deteriorated metabolic control [8,9] and

required insulin therapy; or they might have more severe diabetic conditions (e.g., diabetic gastroparesis) with gastrointestinal symptoms leading to more aggressive examination and diagnosis of HP infection.

A significantly higher rate of HP eradication was seen in subjects taking calcium channel blockers (Table 3). It is interesting that calcium channel blockers are also associated with gastroesophageal reflux disease, probably due to its relaxation effect on lower esophageal sphincter [15]. HP infection can induce pepsinogen release from chief cells (which may induce and aggravate peptic ulcer disease) via mechanisms involving calcium and calmodulin [16]. However, L-type calcium channel is not responsible for the pepsinogen release induced by HP [16]. Therefore it is unlikely that calcium channel blockers used in clinical practice would affect the peptic ulcers induced by HP. It was possible that the gastrointestinal symptoms associated with its use that led to the diagnosis of HP infection.

Recent studies suggest that HP eradication may reverse atrophic gastritis and improve intestinal metaplasia, which may contribute to the reduction of gastric cancer occurrence [17-19]. Therefore, early diagnosis of HP infection with clinical use of medications to eradicate the infection is not only important for the treatment of the clinical symptoms related to the infection, but also for the prevention of gastric cancer. One clinical implication of the present study is that patients with T2DM, especially those treated with insulin, may belong to a high risk group requiring special medical attention.

HP infection rate in a community-based study in Taiwan was 54.4%, and it showed age-dependency without sexual difference [20]. Although the present study suggested that clinical presentation of HP eradication was age-dependent (Tables 2 and 3), it also demonstrated a higher incidence of HP eradication in the male population (Tables 2 and 3). The reasons for a higher risk of HP eradication in men are still unknown. One possibility is that the activity of HP infection could be higher in men, which is correspondent to the higher risk of gastric cancer in men than in women in Taiwan [1].

Except for eye disease, obesity and dyslipidemia (in diabetic patients only) all other comorbidities were significantly associated with HP eradication (Table 3). This observation explained the attenuated odds ratios with prolonged diabetes duration (Table 4), when chronic complications might set in and interfere with the association between diabetes and HP eradication.

Some studies suggested that people living in crowded condition or with lower socioeconomic status may have a higher risk of HP infection [21-23]. In Taiwan, Taipei City is the most populated area. However, residents in relatively sparse area of Central Taiwan had significantly higher incidence of HP eradication than people living in other regions (Table 3). This suggested that living in crowded condition might not be an important predisposing factor. On the other hand, people with an occupation as farmers or fishermen (occupation III) or with low family income (occupation IV) consistently showed significantly higher odds ratios (Table 3), suggesting a possible role of socioeconomic status or its related condition of hygiene.

This study has several strengths. It is population-based with a large nationally representative sample, therefore, the study is not likely to be biased with respect to diabetes status or records of HP eradication. Because NHI is a universal and mandatory insurance with very high coverage but low co-payments, the detection rate would not tend to differ among different social classes.

Limitations included a lack of actual measurement of some recognized confounders such as personal hygiene, living condition, blood groups and genetic factors. We also did not have biochemical data including blood glucose, hemoglobin A_{1c} and lipid profiles to evaluate whether HP infection can affect metabolic control. This study evaluated the incidence of HP eradication and not the prevalence or incidence of HP infection. However, because most people infected with HP do not develop clinical disease [21], estimation of prevalence or incidence of HP infection may not have clinical relevance as the evaluation of HP eradication does. Another concern is that there might be considerable under-diagnosis and under-treatment of HP infection. However, if the misclassification of the outcome is non-differential, an underestimation of the odds ratios is expected.

Conclusions

This study shows a significantly higher incidence of HP eradication in patients with T2DM and in insulin users among the diabetic patients. The odds ratios attenuated with increasing diabetes duration, probably due to the occurrence of other comorbidities. Additionally, lower socioeconomic status and use of calcium channel blockers consistently show a higher rate of HP eradication, but the uses of oral anti-diabetic agents do not. The underlying causes for the link between T2DM and the use of medications and HP eradication are clinically important but require further investigation.

Abbreviations
HP: Helicobacter pylori; ICD-9-CM: International Classification of Diseases, Ninth Revision, Clinical Modification; NHI: National Health Insurance; PES: Panendoscopic examination; T1DM: Type 1 diabetes mellitus; T2DM: Type 2 diabetes mellitus.

Competing interests
The author declares that he has no competing interests.

Acknowledgments
The study is based in part on data from the National Health Insurance Research Database provided by the Bureau of National Health Insurance, Department of Health and managed by National Health Research Institutes (Registered number 99274). The interpretation and conclusions contained herein do not represent those of Bureau of National Health Insurance, Department of Health or National Health Research Institutes.

Author's contributions
CHT researched data and wrote manuscript.

References
1. Tseng CH: Diabetes conveys a higher risk of gastric cancer mortality despite an age-standardised decreasing trend in the general population in Taiwan. *Gut* 2011, **60**:774–779.
2. Wong BC, Lam SK, Wong WM, Chen JS, Zheng TT, Feng RE, Lai KC, Hu WH, Yuen ST, Leung SY, Fong DY, Ho J, Ching CK, Chen JS, China Gastric Cancer Study Group: **Helicobacter pylori eradication to prevent gastric cancer in a high-risk region of China: a randomized controlled trial.** *JAMA* 2004, **291**:187–194.
3. de Luis DA, de la Calle H, Roy G, de Argila CM, Valdezate S, Canton R, Boixeda D: **Helicobacter pylori infection and insulin-dependent diabetes mellitus.** *Diabetes Res Clin Pract* 1998, **39**:143–146.
4. Dore MP, Bilotta M, Malaty HM, Pacifico A, Maioli M, Graham DY, Realdi G: **Diabetes mellitus and Helicobacter pylori infection.** *Nutrition* 2000, **16**:407–410.
5. Selinger C, Robinson A: **Helicobacter pylori eradication in diabetic patients: still far off the treatment targets.** *South Med J* 2010, **103**:975–976.
6. Sargýn M, Uygur-Bayramicli O, Sargýn H, Orbay E, Yavuzer D, Yayla A: **Type 2 diabetes mellitus affects eradication rate of Helicobacter pylori.** *World J Gastroenterol* 2003, **9**:1126–1128.
7. Demir M, Gokturk HS, Ozturk NA, Serin E, Yilmaz U: **Efficacy of two different Helicobacter pylori eradication regimens in patients with type 2 diabetes and the effect of Helicobacter pylori eradication on dyspeptic symptoms in patients with diabetes: a randomized controlled study.** *Am J Med Sci* 2009, **338**:459–464.

8.   Ojetti V, Migneco A, Nista EC, Gasbarrini G, Gasbarrini A, Pitocco D, Ghirlanda
     G: H pylori re-infection in type 1 diabetes: a 5 years follow-up. *Dig Liver
     Dis* 2007, **39:**286–287.
9.   Ojetti V, Pitocco D, Bartolozzi F, Danese S, Migneco A, Lupascu A, Pola P,
     Ghirlanda G, Gasbarrini G, Gasbarrini A: **High rate of helicobacter pylori re-
     infection in patients affected by type 1 diabetes.** *Diabetes Care* 2002,
     25:1485.
10. Devrajani BR, Shah SZ, Soomro AA, Devrajani T: **Type 2 diabetes mellitus: A
     risk factor for Helicobacter pylori infection: A hospital based case-control
     study.** *Int J Diabetes Dev Ctries* 2010, **30:**22–26.
11. Bener A, Micallef R, Afifi M, Derbala M, Al-Mulla HM, Usmani MA: **Association
     between type 2 diabetes mellitus and Helicobacter pylori infection.** *Turk J
     Gastroenterol* 2007, **18:**225–229.
12. Demir M, Gokturk HS, Ozturk NA, Kulaksizoglu M, Serin E, Yilmaz U:
     **Helicobacter pylori prevalence in diabetes mellitus patients with
     dyspeptic symptoms and its relationship to glycemic control and late
     complications.** *Dig Dis Sci* 2008, **53:**2646–2649.
13. Department of Health, Taiwan: http://www.doh.gov.tw/CHT2006/DM/
     DM2_2.aspx?now_fod_list_no=10383&class_no=440&level_no=4
     (accessed March 21, 2012).
14. Wu CY, Kuo KN, Wu MS, Chen YJ, Wang CB, Lin JT: **Early Helicobacter pylori
     eradication decreases risk of gastric cancer in patients with peptic ulcer
     disease.** *Gastroenterology* 2009, **137:**1641–1648. e1-2.
15. Friedenberg FK, Hanlon A, Vanar V, Nehemia D, Mekapati J, Nelson DB,
     Richter JE: **Trends in gastroesophageal reflux disease as measured by the
     National Ambulatory Medical Care Survey.** *Dig Dis Sci* 2010, **55:**1911–1917.
16. Beil W, Wagner S, Piller M, Heim HK, Sewing KF: **Stimulation of pepsinogen
     release from chief cells by Helicobacter pylori: evidence for a role of
     calcium and calmodulin.** *Microb Pathog* 1998, **25:**181–187.
17. Kang JM, Kim N, Shin CM, Lee HS, Lee DH, Jung HC, Song IS: **Predictive
     factors for improvement of atrophic gastritis and intestinal metaplasia
     after helicobacter pylori eradication: a three-year follow-up study in
     Korea.** *Helicobacter* 2012, **17:**86–95.
18. Kodama M, Murakami K, Okimoto T, Abe T, Nakagawa Y, Mizukami K, Uchida
     M, Inoue K, Fujioka T: **Helicobacter pylori eradication improves gastric
     atrophy and intestinal metaplasia in long-term observation.** *Digestion*
     2012, **85:**126–130.
19. Kodama M, Murakami K, Okimoto T, Sato R, Uchida M, Abe T, Shiota S,
     Nakagawa Y, Mizukami K, Fujioka T: **Ten-year prospective follow-up of
     histological changes at five points on the gastric mucosa as
     recommended by the updated Sydney system after Helicobacter pylori
     eradication.** *J Gastroenterol* 2012, **47:**394–403.
20. Lin JT, Wang JT, Wang TH, Wu MS, Lee TK, Chen CJ: **Helicobacter pylori
     infection in a randomly selected population, healthy volunteers, and
     patients with gastric ulcer and gastric adenocarcinoma. A seroprevalence
     study in Taiwan.** *Scand J Gastroenterol* 1993, **28:**1067–1072.
21. Gale EA: **A missing link in the hygiene hypothesis?** *Diabetologia* 2002,
     45:588–594.
22. Aguemon BD, Struelens MJ, Massougbodji A, Ouendo EM: **Prevalence and
     risk-factors for Helicobacter pylori infection in urban and rural Beninese
     populations.** *Clin Microbiol Infect* 2005, **11:**611–617.
23. Hoang TT, Bengtsson C, Phung DC, Sörberg M, Granström M:
     **Seroprevalence of Helicobacter pylori infection in urban and rural
     Vietnam.** *Clin Diagn Lab Immunol* 2005, **12:**81–85.

22

Down-regulation of HSP70 sensitizes gastric epithelial cells to apoptosis and growth retardation triggered by *H. pylori*

Weili Liu[1], Yan Chen[2], Gaofeng Lu[3], Leimin Sun[1] and Jianmin Si[1*]

Abstract

Background: *H. pylori* infection significantly attenuated the expression of HSP70 in gastric mucosal cells. However, the role of HSP70 cancellation in *H. pylori*-associated cell damages is largely unclear.

Methods: Small interfering RNA (siRNA) was used to down-regulate HSP70 in gastric epithelial cell lines AGS. The transfected cells were then incubated with *H. pylori* and the functions of HSP70 suppression were observed by viability assay, cell cycle analyses and TUNEL assay. HSP70 target apoptotic proteins were further identified by Western blot.

Results: The inhibition of HSP70 has further increased the effect of growth arrest and apoptosis activation triggered by *H. pylori* in gastric epithelial cells. The anti-proliferation function of HSP70 depletion was at least by up-regulating p21 and cell cycle modulation with S-phase accumulation. An increase of apoptosis-inducing factor (AIF) and cytosolic cytochrome C contributes to the activation of apoptosis following down-regulation of intracellular HSP70. Extracellular HSP70 increased cellular resistance to apoptosis by suppression the release of AIF and cytochrome c from mitochondria, as well as inhibition of p21 expression.

Conclusions: The inhibition of HSP70 aggravated gastric cellular damages induced by *H. pylori*. Induction of HSP70 could be a potential therapeutic target for protection gastric mucosa from *H. pylori*-associated injury.

Background

In recent years, heat shock proteins (HSP) have been implicated to be an additional factor utilized for the gastric defence mechanisms at the intracellular level [1]. HSP70 is generally considered to be a major molecular chaperone to accelerate the cellular recovery from different stimuli by cope with unfolded or denatured proteins [2], through which HSP70 might achieve efficient mucosal defence for ulcer or inflammation healing [3,4].

Helicobacter pylori (*H. pylori*) infection leads to significant inflammations in the gastric mucosa, which is closely associated with development of atrophic gastritis, peptic ulcer, gastric cancer, and mucosa-associated lymphoid tissue (MALT) lymphoma. Animal studies have demonstrated that *H. pylori* infection damages gastric mucosa by either disrupting the balance in cell apoptosis and proliferation, or decreasing migration of epithelial cells within the gastric mucosa [1,5,6]. Recent studies have found that *H. pylori* decreases the synthesis of HSP70 in gastric epithelial cells by the inactivation of heat shock factor- 1 [7-11], however, whether the inhibition of HSP70 would be the prominent event leading to the persistent damages from *H. pylori* in gastric epithelial cells remains unclear.

H. pylori produces ammonia in gastric mucosa with its high urease activity. Our previous animal studies have introduced ammonia solution to simulate the conditions of *H. pylori* infection, and succeeded in inducing atrophic gastritis in rats [12]. Further studies demonstrated that induction of HSP70 expression is beneficial for preventing gastric atrophy and maintaining mucosal functions in gastric cells [12]. Since the induction of HSP70 is suggested to constitute a novel therapeutic approach for the prevention or treatment of *H. pylori*-associated conditions, it's conceivable that deregulation of HSP70 might be a prominent cause of *H. pylori*-associated damages. Therefore, we

* Correspondence: sijm@zju.edu.cn
[1]Gastroenterology laboratory, Clinical Research Institute, Sir Run Run Shaw Hospital, School of Medicine, Zhejiang University, 310016 Hangzhou, People's Republic of China

investigated the correlation of HSP70 inhibition with the mucosal damages induced by *H. pylori* in this study.

Methods

Cell culture and transfection

Human gastric epithelial cell line AGS (CRL-1739, ATCC, USA) were maintained in RPMI1640 medium supplemented with 10% fetal bovine serum (FBS) without antibiotics at 37°C in a humidified atmosphere of 5% CO_2 and 95% air.

Small interfering RNAs (siRNAs) were designed against the mRNA sequences targeting HSP70 (Genebank: NM_005345.5), $siRNA_1$: 5'-CTTTCCAGGTGATCAA CGA-3', $siRNA_2$: 5'-AGGACGAGTTTGAGCACAA-3'[13], $siRNA_3$: 5'-GACTTTGCATTTCCTAGTA-3'. We used RNAi-Ready vector, which contains a neomycin resistance gene and GFP for selection of stable transfectants. In the preliminary experiments, we employed three constructs that target three distinct regions of the HSP70 gene to deplete HSP70 expression, and found $siRNA_2$ was better than the others for the short-term inhibition of HSP70. Therefore, $siRNA_2$ was selected for the following stable transfection. AGS cells were transfected with the HSP70 siRNA constructs by use of lipofectamine according to the manufacturer's protocol. The total amount of plasmids was adjusted by using the empty vector plasmid in each assay. Briefly, 1×10^5 cells were plated in RPMI1640 containing 10% FBS in 6-well plates 24 h before transfection. Then transfection was performed with serum-free RPMI1640 containing 2 µg plasmid constructs and 6 µl lipofectamine. After 5 h, fresh RPMI1640 containing 10% FBS was added until 2 ml of final volume. The selection with 0.4 mg/ml neomycin was started 48 h after transfection. GFP was used as a control for transfection or selection efficiency. A control sample transfected with empty vector plasmid was included. Neomycin-resistant cell pools and single cell clone were generated, in which HSP70 expression was confirmed by immunoblot analysis and real-time PCR.

Bacterial strain and coculture conditions

H. pylori expressing CagA and VacA (ATCC 700392) were grown on Columbia agar medium with 5% of fresh sheep blood under microaerobic conditions (5%O_2, 10%CO_2, 8% N_2) at 37°C. Before the experiment, bacteria were harvested and suspended in RPMI 1640 medium (including 10% FBS but no antimicrobial agents). The bacteria were densitometrically counted according to the McFarland scale and suitable dilution was prepared for the cell culture (bacteria/cell ratio at 200:1 for most tests).

Real-time PCR

The RNA was harvested from cell culture with RNeasy columns (QIAGEN). Single stranded cDNA synthesis

was made with the TaqMan RT Kit (QIAGEN) using oligo-$(dT)_{16}$ primers. The cDNA originating from the transfected cells were used as template for the following PCR reaction and the housekeeping gene glyceraldehyde-3-phosphate dehydrogenase (GAPDH) was served as an internal control. Primers were designed as follows (Genebank: NM_005345.5): HSP70-for, 5'-AACACCGTGTTT-GACGCGAA-3'; HSP70-rev, 5'-GGTCAGCACCATGGA CGAGA-3'; HSP70-probe, 5'-FAM-CCAGGTGAT-CAACGACGGAGACAAGCCC-TAMRA-3'. The negative control contained the reaction mixture but no DNA. The reactions were performed with a real-time PCR machine (BIOER, Japan) with a Taq activation at 95°C for 5 min followed by 35 cycles of three segments consisting of 30 sec at 95°C, 30 sec at 55°C, and 30 sec at 72°C. The level of HSP70 mRNA was evaluated relative to that of GAPDH mRNA.

Growth curve and cell proliferation Assay

Cell growth curve or proliferation assessment was quantified using a tetrazolium salt colorimetric assay with 3-[4,5-dimethylthiazol-2-yl]-2,5-diphenyltetrazolium bromide (MTT, final concentration of 0.5 mg/ml, Sigma-Aldrich, St. Louis, MO, USA). Briefly, the cells stably transfected with HSP70 siRNA or the empty vector were cultured in a 96-well plate for 1~6 days. In the proliferation assay, these cells were incubated with live *H. pylori* for 0, 24, 48 or 72 hours. The absorbance of samples was measured at 492 nm in the microplate reader.

Cell apoptosis assays

Cells suspension (2×10^4) was added to each well of 48-well plates and was incubated with *H. pylori* (1:200) for 24 h. We analyzed apoptosis with the use of the terminal deoyecelotibyl transferase mediated dUTP-biotin nick end labeling assay (TUNEL) kit (Cell Death Detection kit, Roche, Germany) according to the instructions provided by the manufacturer. Quantitation of apoptotic cells was accomplished by counting the number of apoptotic bodies sighted in the microscopic fields. Labeling indices were calculated as the mean number of labeled cells (from five random fields of vision) divided by total counted cells (500 cells).

Cell cycle analysis

Cells were seeded (2×10^5) on 6-well plates and were synchronized through serum starvation for 48 hours. Then the cells were incubated with *H. pylori* at 200:1 of bacterium to cell ratio in RPMI1640 containing 10% FBS for 0, 6, 12 or 24 hours. The treated cells were collected and fixed in 70% ethanol. Cell pellets were resuspended in 500 µl of propidium iodide buffer (10 mM Tris-Cl at PH 7.5, 50 µg/ml propidium iodide, 0.1% Triton X-100, 0.1% sodium citrate and 2 mg/ml RNase) and incubated in the dark at 4°C overnight. Stained cells were analyzed by the Beckman Coulter EPICS XL flow cytometer using the CellQuest software. At least 1×10^4 cells have been tested in each test.

Immunoblotting analyses

Total proteins were isolated from the transfected cells and the concentration was measured by Bio-Rad Protein Assay. Mitochondrial or cytosolic protein was extracted in according to the protocol of Mitochondria/cytosol Fractionation Kit (BioVision). All procedures were performed at 4°C. The expressions of HSP70 (anti-HSP70, Sigma-Aldrich, St. Louis, MO, USA), Bax, caspase-3, caspase-6, caspase-7, cytochrome c, p21, PCNA (antibodies, Cell Signaling Technology, Danvers, MA, USA) and AIF (anti-AIF, Santa Cruz Biotechnology, Santa Cruz, CA) were assessed by immunoblotting with corresponding antibodies. The blotted membrane was visualized by chemiluminescent substrate (EZ-ECL, Kibbutz Beit Haemek Israel). The immunoblotting for β-actin (Santa Cruz Biotechnology, Santa Cruz, CA) was used as a loading control.

Statistical analysis

Any significance in differences between two data sets was determined by the Student's *t*-test. *P* values < 0.05 were considered significant in all analyses.

Results

H. pylori infection suppressed HSP70 expression in gastric cell line AGS cells

We first examined the influence of *H. pylori* on HSP70 expression in AGS cells. Basal HSP70 expression was found relatively high in the gastric epithelial cells, but *H. pylori* infection induced a significant suppression of HSP70. The inhibitory effect of *H. pylori* on HSP70 expression was improved with the extended incubation time from 0 h up to 48 h. The signal for HSP70 protein was detectable in AGS cells incubated in the medium containing *H. pylori* at 200:1 or 500:1 of bacterium to cell ratio, and the suppression of HSP70 in response to bacterium appeared to be concentration-dependent manner (Figure 1. A). We also explore the effect of the live bacteria on the viability of AGS cells over different periods of time. Concomitant with HSP70 inhibition by *H. pylori*, incubation of *H. pylori* with AGS cell line caused a significant decrease in cell viability. Coincidentally, the inhibitory effect of *H. pylori* on AGS cell growth was improved with the increased concentration of the bacterium and extended incubation period (Figure 1. B).

Generation of gastric cells AGS with reduced level of HSP70

To further investigate the role of HSP70 depletion in *H. pylori*-associated mucosal damage, we established AGS cell lines with down-regulated HSP70 by siRNAs (Figure 2A). Suppression of HSP70 mRNA and protein in the stable transfected cell line was confirmed, which showed approximately 50% decrease in HSP70 expression as compared to vector transfected control cells (Figure 2B&2C). The reduction of HSP70 slowed down the growth of AGS cells with the morphological senescence characterized by large and membrane blebbing (Figure 2D).

Effect of HSP70 depletion on proliferation of gastric epithelial cells with H. pylori infection

H. pylori inhibited cell growth accompanying suppression of HSP70 expression in AGS cells. We thus examined whether the suppressive effect of *H. pylori* on cell proliferation may result from the down-regulated HSP70. As the cells were cocultured with *H. pylori*, a much lower level of HSP70 expression was demonstrated in AGS/siRNA^{HSP70} cells comparing with AGS/siRNA^{control} cells (Figure 3A). Viable cells were significantly reduced to 64.5% or 28.6% in AGS/siRNA^{HSP70} cells (vs. 78.5% or 46.4% in AGS/siRNA^{control} cells, P < 0.05) following incubation with *H. pylori* for 48 h or 72 h respectively (Figure 3B).

HSP70 depletion causes cell cycle arrest in S phase in gastric cells with H. pylori infection

To determine if HSP70 depletion mediated growth inhibition was the result of its cell cycle modulation, we investigated the effect of HSP70 inhibition on cell cycle distribution in *H. pylori*-infected AGS cells. Our results revealed a significant increase in the number of cells in the S phase in AGS/siRNA^{HSP70} as compared with its control at different time interval (Figure 3C).

To elucidate the molecular basis by which HSP70 modulates cell cycle in gastric epithelial cell, p21 and PCNA, the well-known genes involved in the cell cycle regulation, were analyzed. Immunoblotting analysis confirmed that p21 protein but not PCNA was expressed at higher levels in the AGS/siRNA^{HSP70} cells compared with control vector transfected cells (Figure 3D).

HSP70 depletion induced apoptosis and pro-apoptotic proteins in gastric cells with H. pylori infection

Both *H. pylori* and HSP70 have been reported to be involved in the regulation of apoptosis. To determine whether apoptosis induced in the gastric epithelium exposed to live *H. pylori* might occur due to the elimination of HSP70 expression, TUNEL staining was performed to validate the alteration of *H. pylori*-associated-apoptosis might be induced by HSP70 depletion in AGS cells. TUNEL-positive cells were much more in AGS/siRNA^{HSP70} cells than those in the vector control cells (5.36% ± 1.22% vs 1.46% ± 0.56%, *P*< 0.01; Figure 4A).

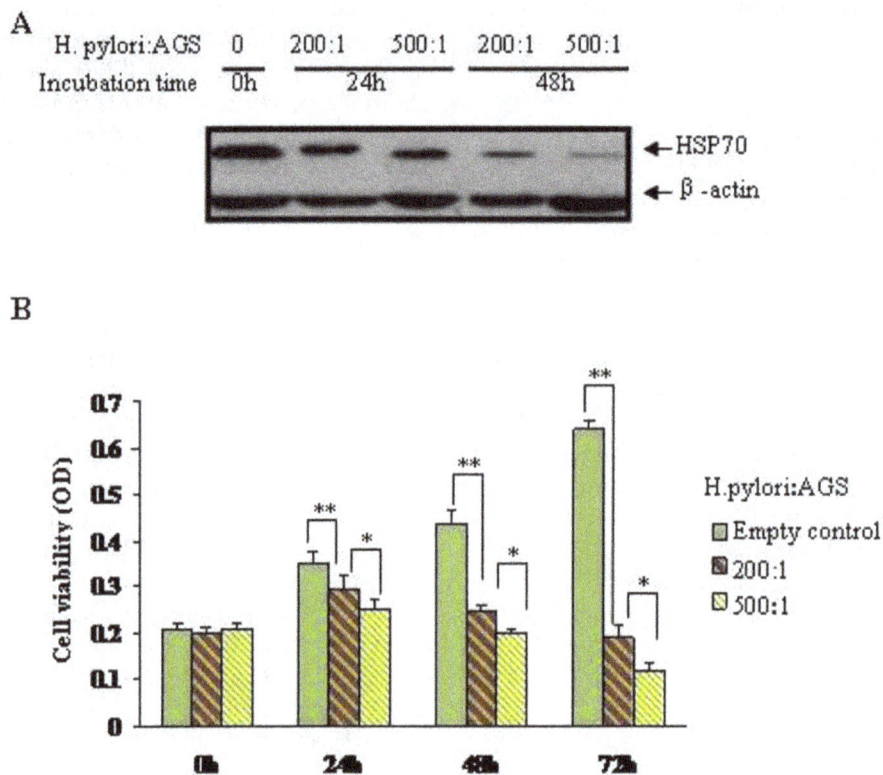

Figure 1 Effects of *H. pylori* on AGS cells. (A) AGS cells were treated with *H. pylori* at the ratio of 200:1(bacterium to cells) or 500:1 for 0, 24 or 48 hours, respectively. Suppression of HSP70 in AGS by *H. pylori* infection was evidenced by immunoblotting. (B) *H. pylori* infection significantly inhibited cell proliferation in gastric epithelial cell line in a dose- and time-dependent manner. Data are mean ± SD, *P <0.05, **P <0.01.

Identification of apoptotic genes modulated by HSP70 in AGS cells with H. pylori infection

To elucidate the molecular basis by which HSP70-suppression involved in gastric cells apoptosis, proapoptotic genes expression profile in HSP70-siRNA stably transfected AGS were analyzed by immunoblotting. The apoptosis-inducing effect by HSP70 depletion was mediated by regulating important pro-apoptotic genes including AIF and cytochrome C, as evidenced by an accumulation of AIF and the release of cytochrome c from mitochondria (Figure 4B). No considerable changes for apoptotic proteins in the down stream of the caspase-dependent apoptotic pathways, including caspase-3, caspase-6 and caspase-7 have been observed.

Extracellular HSP70 compensated for the effect of endogenous HSP70 depletion on apoptosis and proliferation

To test whether exogenously applied HSP70 might compensate for the loss of endogenous HSP70, extracellular HSP70 (50 ng/ml) were exposed to AGS/siRNA[HSP70] cells with *H. pylori* infection for 48 hours. The exogenous HSP70 inhibited cytochrome c release from

mitochondria to cytosol and AIF accumulation, as well as the expression of p21 (Figure 4C&4D).

Discussion

HSP70 protects gastric mucosal cells against intrinsic and extrinsic stimuli, and maintains the proper structure and function of the gastric mucosa [14,15], suggesting induction of HSP70 might be useful for medical treatment of diseases with mucosal damage. Tsukimi Y et al. found HSP70 may facilitate the healing of acetic acid-induced gastric ulcers in rats [16]. Our previous study has demonstrated that up-regulation of HSP70 expression by Geranylgeranylacetone (GGA) interrupts the progression of atrophic gastritis in rats, as evidenced by the improvement of inflammation and glandular restoration in gastric mucosa [12]. HSP70 could protect gastric mucosa from *H. pylori*-associated gastrointestinal diseases [17]. *H. pylori* infection destroyed gastric mucosa barrier function through inducing a significant reduction of HSP70 expression in gastric epithelial cells, which was supposed to disturb gastric adaptation and facilitate H pylori to avoid host immunity [10]. We demonstrate here that suppression of HSP70 increased the sensitivity of gastric cells to *H. pylori* infection with the inhibition

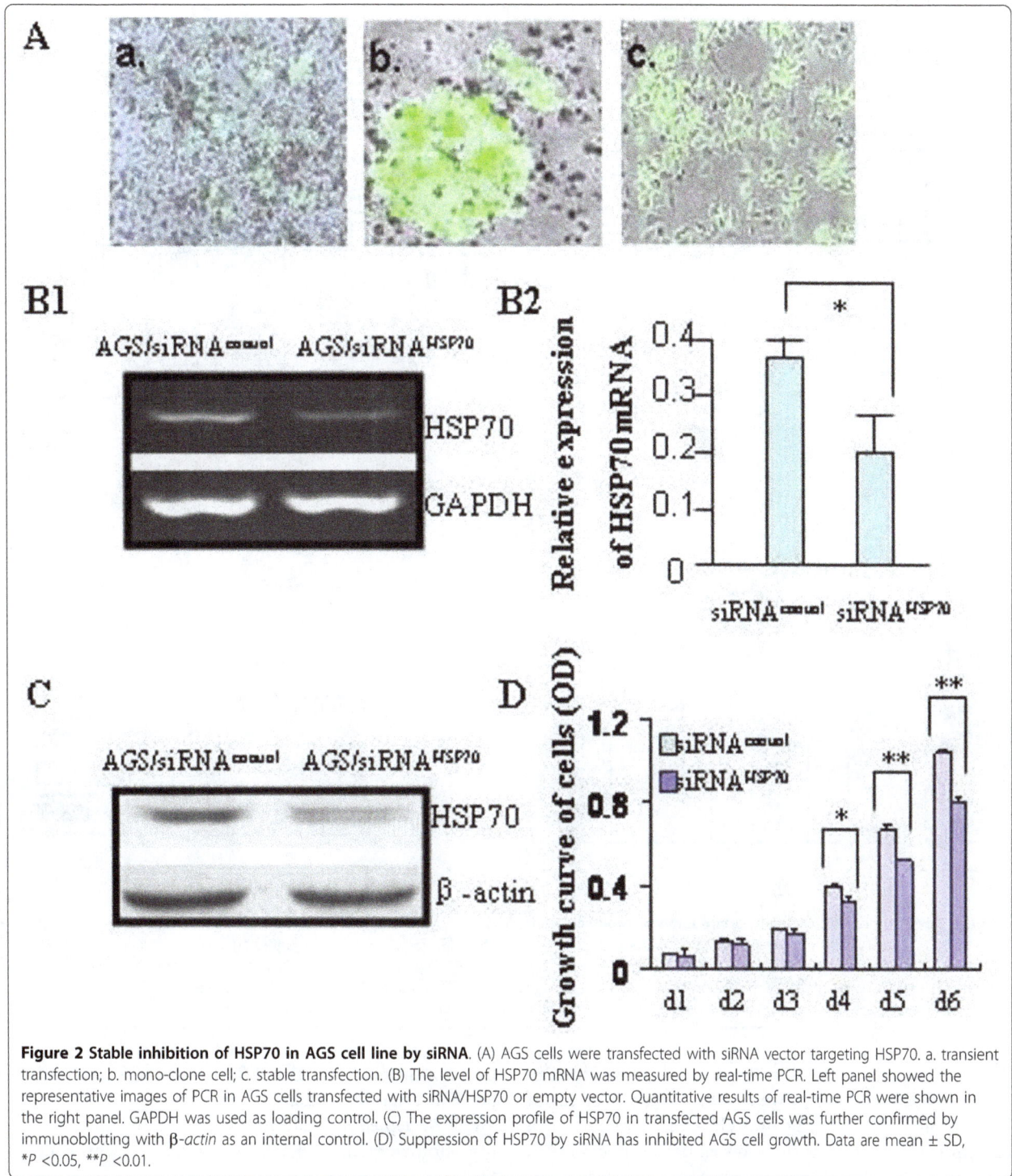

Figure 2 Stable inhibition of HSP70 in AGS cell line by siRNA. (A) AGS cells were transfected with siRNA vector targeting HSP70. a. transient transfection; b. mono-clone cell; c. stable transfection. (B) The level of HSP70 mRNA was measured by real-time PCR. Left panel showed the representative images of PCR in AGS cells transfected with siRNA/HSP70 or empty vector. Quantitative results of real-time PCR were shown in the right panel. GAPDH was used as loading control. (C) The expression profile of HSP70 in transfected AGS cells was further confirmed by immunoblotting with β-*actin* as an internal control. (D) Suppression of HSP70 by siRNA has inhibited AGS cell growth. Data are mean ± SD, *P <0.05, **P <0.01.

of cellular growth and cell cycle progression, as well as induction of apoptosis.

H. pylori infection damages gastric mucosa by disturbing equilibrium between apoptosis and proliferation. HSPs could reverse these inferiorities in mucosal healing. Inhibition of endogenous HSP70 slowed cellular multiplication, and enhanced the effect of *H. pylori* on cell viability. The

anti-proliferation role of *H. pylori* was more evident following the further depletion of HSP70 expression. HSP70 involving in cell growth could be a cell cycle event. Rohde M et al. reported that Hela cells transfected with siRNA against HSP70 revealed an arrest in G2/M phase of cell cycle [18], which resulted in growth retardation with features of cell senescence. Our previous study have found

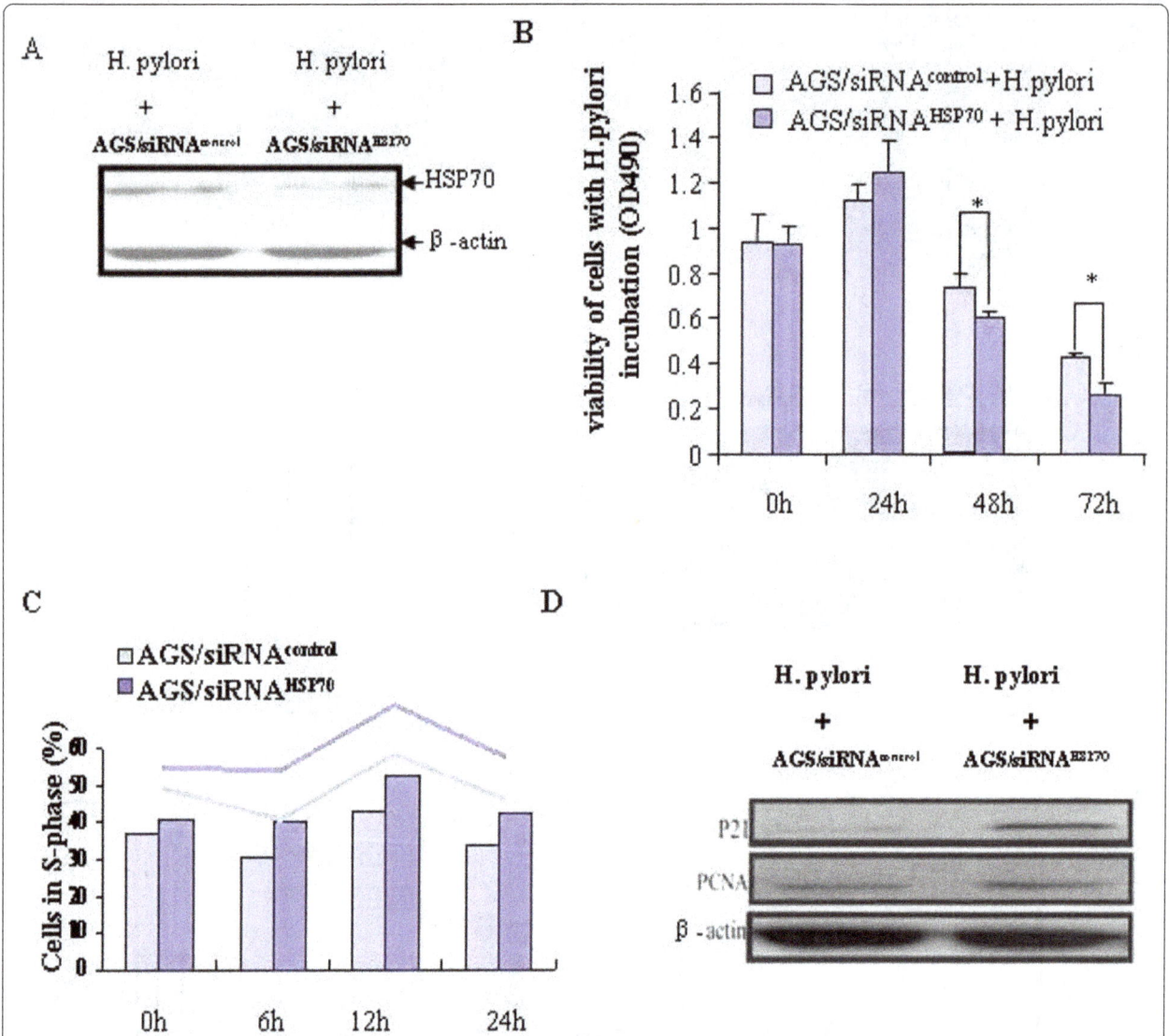

Figure 3 HSP70 depletion enhanced inhibition of proliferation in AGS cells with *H. pylori* infection. (A) Aberrant expression of HSP70 in transfected AGS cells with *H. pylori* infection was evidenced by immunoblotting. (B) HSP70 suppression further aggravated inhibitory role of *H. pylori* in cell viability in AGS cells. Data are mean ± SD, *P <0.05. (C)The effect of HSP70 depletion on proliferation was further confirmed by flow cytometre, which showed more accumulation of HSP70 siRNA transfected cells in S-phase as compared with the control vector transfected cells. (D) Protein expression of p21 and PCNA was evaluated by immunoblotting. β-*actin* was used as an internal control.

that down-regulation of HSP70 induced S-phase arrest in AGS cells. Furthermore, we investigated the effect of HSP70 on the cell cycle of AGS cells infected with *H. pylori*, and the results showed that depletion of HSP70 induced AGS cells accumulating in S-phase independent of *H. pylori* infection. Our observation that HSP70-depletion induced S-phase arrest and p21 over-expression is in agreement with the previous report that transduction of the p21 gene resulted in S-phase arrest [19,20]. The p21 protein can inhibit DNA synthesis by interacting with PCNA [21], and plays a regulatory role in S phase DNA replication and DNA damage repair [22]. Growth arrest by

p21 can promote cellular differentiation, and therefore prevents cell proliferation [23].

HSP70 depletion could make AGS more susceptible to the cytotoxicity of *H. pylori* by interference with apoptotic programs. *H. pylori* is known to cause apoptosis of gastric epithelial cells by targeting mitochondria [24,25]. Mitochondria respond to multiple death stimuli. It has been demonstrated that pro-apoptotic Bcl-2 family proteins such as Bax could induce mitochondrial membrane permeabilization and cause the release of mitochondria-mediated apoptosis signaling molecules including cytochrome c and AIF [26]. Cytochrome c triggers the

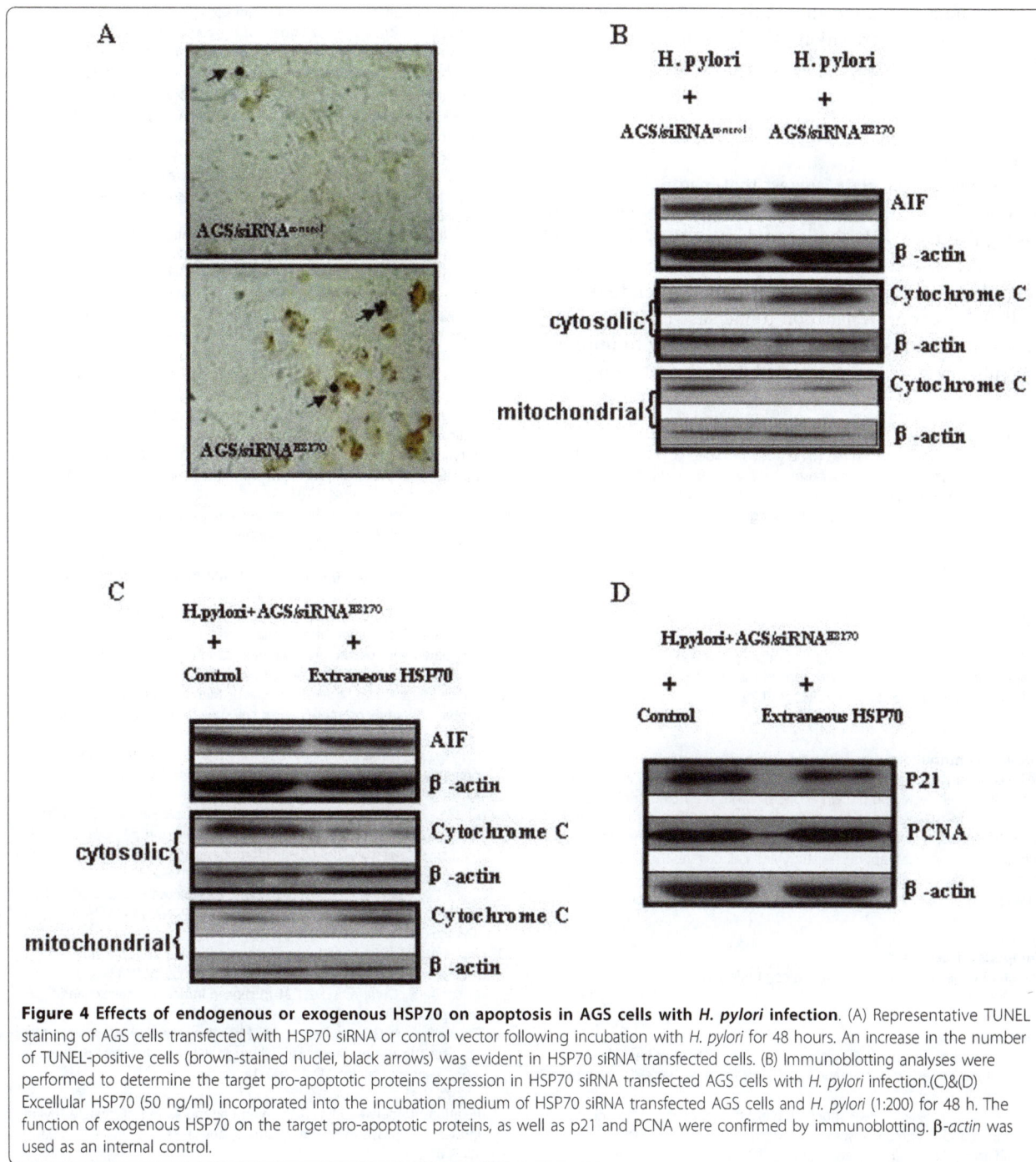

Figure 4 Effects of endogenous or exogenous HSP70 on apoptosis in AGS cells with *H. pylori* infection. (A) Representative TUNEL staining of AGS cells transfected with HSP70 siRNA or control vector following incubation with *H. pylori* for 48 hours. An increase in the number of TUNEL-positive cells (brown-stained nuclei, black arrows) was evident in HSP70 siRNA transfected cells. (B) Immunoblotting analyses were performed to determine the target pro-apoptotic proteins expression in HSP70 siRNA transfected AGS cells with *H. pylori* infection.(C)&(D) Excellular HSP70 (50 ng/ml) incorporated into the incubation medium of HSP70 siRNA transfected AGS cells and *H. pylori* (1:200) for 48 h. The function of exogenous HSP70 on the target pro-apoptotic proteins, as well as p21 and PCNA were confirmed by immunoblotting. β-*actin* was used as an internal control.

caspase-dependent cascade [27], but AIF executes cell death in the absence of caspase [28-30]. *H. pylori* has been reported to trigger apoptosis in AGS cells via release of cytochrome c and AIF from mitochondria [31]. Our study demonstrated that down-regulation of HSP70 induced the further release of cytochrome c and AIF in the AGS with *H. pylori* infection, consistent with the hypothesis that HSP70 suppression could sensitize the gastric epithelial cells to the damage from *H. pylori*.

Furthermore, we evaluated the role of extracellular HSP70 in *H. pylori*-infected AGS cells, and demonstrated that extracellular HSP70 protein could partial compensate for the decreased intracellular HSP70 by reducing release of cytochrome c and AIF, which could block apoptosis in gastric cells with *H. pylori* infection. Consistently, extracellular HSP70 could also modulate the proliferation of AGS cells by inhibiting expression of p21. The exogenous HSP70 might cross the cellular plasma membrane and reduce apoptosis with the decrease of toxicity protein aggregation [32]. Exogenous HSP70 was suggested to be a trophic factor supporting cell survival [33].

Conclusions

In conclusion, our data suggest that insufficient expression of HSP70 would render gastric epithelial cells more susceptible to *H. pylori*-induced damage than they would be if HSP70 were more abundant. The extracellular HSP70 may compensate for the deficit of endogenous HSP70 depletion. Designation to increase HSP70 protein may serve as a potential therapeutic strategy to improve the outcome of *H. pylori*-infected patients.

Acknowledgements
We thank Prof. Dai Ning who has generously provided *H. pylori* strain (ATCC 700392) to us. This study was supported by a grant from the National Natural Science Foundation of China (Grant No. J20111996), a joint grant from the Education Department of Zhe Jiang Province, China (Y200803495).

Author details
[1]Gastroenterology laboratory, Clinical Research Institute, Sir Run Run Shaw Hospital, School of Medicine, Zhejiang University, 310016 Hangzhou, People's Republic of China. [2]Department of Gastroenterology, Second Affiliated Hospital, School of Medicine, Zhejiang University, Hangzhou, People's Republic of China. [3]Department of thoracic surgery, Zhejiang Hospital, Hangzhou, People's Republic of China.

Authors' contributions
LWL acquired the majority of data (involving assay design, cell culture, cell transfection, cell cycle and protein analysis), wrote the manuscript and contributed to the design and concept of the study. CY & LGF performed cell culture, apoptosis and viability assay. LGF performed Western blot. SLM contributed to the concept of the study and cell culture. SJM conceived the studies, oversaw the experimental work and established all the collaborations. All authors read and approved the final manuscript.

Competing interests
The authors declare that they have no competing interests.

References
1. Choi SR, Lee SA, Kim YJ, Ok CY, Lee HJ, Hahm KB: **Role of heat shock proteins in gastric inflammation and ulcer healing.** *J Physiol Pharmacol* 2009, **60**(Suppl 7):5-17.
2. Basu S, Srivastava PK: **Heat shock proteins: the fountainhead of innate and adaptive immune responses.** *Cell Stress Chaperones* 2000, **5**:443-51.
3. Ishihara T, Suemasu S, Asano T, Tanaka KI, Mizushima T: **Stimulation of gastric ulcer healing by heat shock protein 70.** *Biochem Pharmacol* 2011.
4. Asai M, Kawashima D, Katagiri K, Takeuchi R, Tohnai G, Ohtsuka K: **Protective effect of a molecular chaperone inducer, paeoniflorin, on the HCl- and ethanol-triggered gastric mucosal injury.** *Life Sci* 2011, **88**:350-7.
5. Nardone G, Staibano S, Rocco A, Mezza E, D'armiento FP, Insabato L, *et al*: **Effect of helicobacter pylori infection and its eradication on cell proliferation, DNA status, and oncogene expression in patients with chronic gastritis.** *Gut* 1999, **44**:789-99.
6. Fan XG, Kelleher D, Fan XJ, *et al*: **Helicobacter pylori increases proliferation of gastric epithelial cells.** *Gut* 1996, **38**:19-22.
7. Klaamas K, Kurtenkov O, von Mensdorff-Pouilly S, Shjapnikova L, Miljukhina L, Brjalin V, *et al*: **Impact of Helicobacter pylori infection on the humoral immune response to MUC1 peptide in patients with chronic gastric diseases and gastric cancer.** *Immunol Invest* 2007, **36**(4):371-86.
8. Konturek JW, Fischer H, Konturek PC, Huber V, Boknik P, Luess H, *et al*: **Heat shock protein 70 (hsp70) in gastric adaptation to aspirin in Helicobacter pylori infection.** *J Physiol Pharmacol* 2001, **52**:153-64.
9. Pierzchalski P, Krawiec A, Ptak-Belowska A, Baranska A, Konturek SJ, Pawlik WW: **The mechanism of heat-shock protein 70 gene expression abolition in gastric epithelium caused by Helicobacter pylori infection.** *Helicobacter* 2006, **11**(2):96-104.
10. Huff JL Hansen LM, Solnick JV: **Gastric transcription profile of Helicobacter pylori infection in the rhesus macaque.** *Infect Immun* 2004, **72**:5216-26.
11. Axsen WS, Styer CM, Solnick JV: **Inhibition of heat shock protein expression by helicobacter pylori.** *Microb Pathog* 2009, **47**:231-6.
12. Liu WL, Chen SJ, Chen Y, Sun LM, Zhang W, Zeng YM, *et al*: **Protective effects of heat shock protein70 induced by geranyl-geranylacetone in atrophic gastritis in rats.** *Acta Pharmacologica Sinica* 2007, **28**:1001-6.
13. Gabai VL, Budagova KR, Sherman MY: **Increased expression of the major heat shock protein Hsp72 in human prostate carcinoma cells is dispensable for their viability but confers resistance to a variety of anticancer agents.** *Oncogene* 2005, **24**:3328-38.
14. Suemasu S, Tanaka K, Namba T, Ishihara T, Katsu T, Fujimoto M, *et al*: **A role for HSP70 in protecting against indomethacin-induced gastric lesions.** *J Biol Chem* 2009, , **284**: 19705-15.
15. Rokutan K: **Role of heat shock proteins in gastric mucosal protection.** *J Gastroenterol Hepatol* 2000, **15**(Suppl):12-9.
16. Tsukimi Y, Nakai H, Itoh S, Amagase K, Okabe S: **Involvement of heat shock proteins in the healing of acetic acid-induced gastric ulcers in rats.** *J Physiol Pharmacol* 2001, **52**:391-406.
17. Tomomitsu T, Tomoyuki S, Tomiyasu A, Masakatsu N, Daisuke Y, Masaaki O, *et al*: **The BB genotype of heat-shock protein (HSP) 70-2 gene is associated with gastric pre-malignant condition in H. pylori-infected older patients.** *Anticancer Research* 2009, **29**:3453-58, 16-20.
18. Rohde M, Daugaard M, Jensen MH, *et al*: **Members of the heat -shock protein 70 family promote cancer cell growth by distinct mechanism.** *Genes & Development* 2005, **19**:570-82.
19. Ogryzko VV, Wong P, Howard BH: **WAF1 retards S-phase progression primarily by inhibition of cyclin-dependent kinases.** *Mol Cell Biol* 1997, **17**:4877-4882.
20. Zhu Hongbo, Zhang Lidong, Wu Shuhong, Teraishi Fuminori, Davis JJohn, Jacob Dietmar, *et al*: **Induction of S-phase arrest and p21 overexpression by a small molecule 2[[3-(2,3-dichlorophenoxy)propyl] amino] ethanol in correlation with activation of ERK.** *Oncogene* 2004, **23**:4984-92.
21. Chen J, Jackson PK, Kirschner MW, Dutta A: **Separate domains of p21 involved in the inhibition of Cdk kinase and PCNA.** *Nature* 1995, **374**:386-388.
22. Gartel AL, Radhakrishnan SK, Lost in transcription: **p21 repression, mechanisms, and consequences.** *Cancer Res* 2005, **65**(10):3980-5.
23. Abbas Tarek, Dutta Anindya: **P21 in cancer: intricate networks and multiple activities.** *Nat Rev Cancer* 2009, **9**(6):400-14.
24. Zhang H, Fang DC, Lan CH, Luo YH: **Helicobacter pylori infection induces apoptosis in gastric cancer cells through the mitochondrial pathway.** *J Gastroenterol Hepatol* 2007, **22**:1051-6.
25. Chiozzi V, Mazzini G, Oldani A, Sciullo A, Ventura U, Romano M, *et al*: **Relationship between Vac A toxin and ammonia in Helicobacter pylori-induced apoptosis in human gastric epithelial cells.** *J Physiol Pharmacol* 2009, **60**:23-30.
26. Yang J, Liu XS, Bhalla K, Kim CN, Ibrada AM, Cai JY, *et al*: **Prevention of apoptosis by Bcl-2:release of cytochrome c from mitochondria blocked.** *Science* 1997, **275**:1129-32.
27. Garland JM, Rudin C: **Cytochrome c Induces Caspase-Dependent Apoptosis in Intact Hematopoietic cells and overrides apoptosis suppression mediated by bcl-2, growth factor signaling, MAP-Kinase-Kinase, and malignant change.** *Blood* 1998, **92**:1235-46.
28. Joza N, Susin SA, Daugas E, Stanford WL, Cho SK, Li CY, *et al*: **Essential role of the mitochondrial apoptosis-inducing factor in programmed cell death.** *Nature* 2001, **410**:549-54.

29. Susjin SA, Daugas E, Ravagnan L, Samejima K, Zamzami N, Loeffler M, *et al*: **Two distinct pathways leading to nuclear apoptosis.** *J Exp Med* 2000, **192**:571-80.

30. Cregan SP, Dawson VL, Slack RS: **Role of AIF in caspase-dependent and caspase-independent cell death.** *Oncogene* 2004, **23**:2785-96.

31. Ashkorab H, Dashwood RH, Dashwood MM, Zaidi SI, Hewitt SM, Green WR, *et al*: *H. pylori*-**induced apoptosis in human gastric cancer cells mediated via the release of apoptosis-inducing factor from mitochondria.** *Helicobacter* 2008, **13**:506-17.

32. Novoselova TV, Margulis BA, Novoselov SS, *et al*: **Treatment with extracellular HSP70/HSC70 protein polyglutamine toxicity and aggregation.** *J Neurochem* 2005, **94**:597-606.

33. Robinson MB, Tidwell JL, Gould T, *et al*: **Extracellular heat shock protein 70: a critical component for motoneuron survival.** *J Neurosci* 2005, **25**:9735-45.

23

Applicability of a short/rapid ^{13}C-urea breath test for *Helicobacter pylori*

Hemda Schmilovitz-Weiss[1*], Vered Sehayek-Shabat[1], Rami Eliakim[2], Eitan Skapa[3], Yona Avni[4] and Haim Shirin[3]

Abstract

Background: Carbon labeled urea breath tests usually entail a two point sampling with a 20 to 30-minute gap. Our aim was to evaluate the duration of time needed for diagnosing *Helicobacter pylori* by the BreathID® System.

Methods: This is a retrospective multicenter chart review study. Test location, date, delta over baseline, and duration of the entire test were recorded. Consecutively ^{13}C urea breath tests results were extracted from the files over a nine year period.

Results: Of the 12,791 tests results, 35.1% were positively diagnosed and only 0.1% were inconclusive. A statistically significant difference in prevalence among the countries was found: Germany showing the lowest, 13.3%, and Israel the highest, 44.1%. Significant differences were found in time to diagnosis: a positive diagnosis had the shortest and an inconclusive result had the longest. Overall test duration averaged 15.1 minutes in Germany versus approximately 13 minutes in other countries. Diagnosis was achieved after approximately 9 minutes in Israel, Italy and Switzerland, but after 10 on average in the others. The mean delta over baseline value for a negative diagnosis was 1.03 ± 0.86, (range, 0.9 - 5), versus 20.2 ± 18.9, (range, 5.1 - 159.4) for a positive one.

Conclusions: The BreathID® System used in diagnosing *Helicobacter pylori* can safely shorten test duration on average of 10-13 minutes without any loss of sensitivity or specificity and with no test lasting more than 21 minutes.

Keywords: BreathID®, breath test, *Helicobacter pylori*, test duration

Background

Among the non-endoscopic procedures used in diagnosing *Helicobacter pylori* (*H. pylori*), serology remains the most accepted. It is a widely available, inexpensive test with a high negative predictive value. However, the variable specificity, especially if the prevalence of *H. pylori* is low, and its relatively poor positive predictive value, limit the use of the test. Carbon labeled urea breath tests (UBT), which have a high sensitivity and specificity, are commonly used as a noninvasive method in detecting an active *Helicobacter pylori* (*H. pylori*) infection. UBT are the preferred method used in epidemiological studies, screening dyspeptic patients and assessing

* Correspondence: hemdaw1@netvision.net.il
[1]Gastroenterology Unit, Hasharon Hospital, Rabin Medical Center, Petach Tikva, Tel-Aviv University, Tel Aviv, Israel

eradication or recurrence of the infection [1]. These tests usually entail a two point sampling with a 20 to 30-minute gap, and necessitate a mass spectrometry for analysis. Upon modifying the sampling method, immediate results can be achieved.

One such option includes real time continuous sampling ^{13}C molecular correlation spectroscopy (MCS™) technology. The BreathID® device (Exalenz, Israel) has been validated and cleared by the FDA and has also been previously used on children and adults [2,3]. This office-based system offers several advantages over the conventional mass spectrometry-based UBT, including an immediate test result, a standardized test drink (citric acid) and, most importantly for children, a sampling method that does not require active cooperation.

For many years, test shortening procedures have been routinely practiced including the use of various ^{13}C-urea concentrations, and different citric acid test drinks. The new molecular correlation spectrometry technology enables continuous sampling of the expired breath of the patients, which in turn, enables the device to terminate the test immediately after a conclusive positive or negative result of *H. pylori* had been identified [2].

The use of a citric acid-based test drink has been shown to enhance hydrolysis of the urea and produce a more rapid rise in expired $^{13}CO_2$ [4]. The BreathID™-system combined with a citric acid drink and continuous breath sampling significantly reduces the amount of time needed for a final result compared to isotope ratio mass spectrometer. However, these test-shortening modifications have not been widely accepted by the medical community. There are limited data [5] validating these tests but they have been in use in several gastroenterology departments for many years.

The current investigation retrospectively examined over 12,000 BreathID™ test results from several randomly selected gastroenterology departments. The goal of this retrospective evaluation was to assess, on average, the minimal time required to achieve accurate, definite UBT results using the BreathID™ system.

Methods
Urea Breath Tests
The effect of the breath test sampling method in detecting *H. pylori* was examined using continuous real time methodology (i.e., the BreathID® system). The BreathID™ system is comprised of the following components: a) a kit containing 75 mg of ^{13}C-urea (a 99% ^{13}C-enriched urea tablet); b) a packet of granulated Citrica (a 4.5 gram packet containing 4 g of citric acid, 0.149 mg of aspartame, orange aroma, FD&C yellow #6); c) an IDcircuit-sampling device; and d) a BreathID® device. All patients received 75 mg of ^{13}C-urea with a 4.5 gram citric acid based powder (Citrica). The IDcircuit, a continuous nasal breath sampling device, transported the breath sample from the patient to the BreathID™ and did not require active cooperation.

Based on molecular correlation spectrometry, the BreathID® continuously measured $^{13}CO_2$ and $^{12}CO_2$ concentrations from the patient's breath, thus establishing the $^{13}CO_2/^{12}CO_2$ ratio, displayed vs. time on the screen. The results were obtained within 10-15 minutes and printed on a thermal printer.

Determining the positive or negative results from the BreathID™ was based on a device algorithm. If, after 5 minutes, the delta over baseline (DOB) of the $^{13}CO_2/^{12}CO_2$ ratio was greater than 6 at more than two time points, the patient was considered positive. If, after 5 minutes, the DOB was below 3 at more than two time points, the patient was considered negative. If, after 20 minutes, neither of the two criteria was fulfilled, then the nominal 5 DOB threshold was considered in order to distinguish positive from negative patients, unless the previous three points were within ± 1 DOB of the 5 DOB threshold. In this case, the results were defined as inconclusive.

The study protocol was approved by the Institutional Review Board of the Rabin Medical Center. Informed consent was not taken from all patients since this is retrospective study with data taken from different centers not all needing informed consent. The study was supported by Exalenz, Ltd.

Study Subjects and Protocol
A total of 12,751 consecutively selected ^{13}C urea breath tests performed between 2001 and 2009 were extracted from the files of fifteen gastrointestinal units in Israel, The Netherlands, Switzerland, Germany and Italy, representing approximately 50% of the tests performed during the 9-year period. Some patients underwent a second UBT test after *H. pylori* eradication. For subjects who had more than one test result, pre and post treatment, all of the identified tests were used. There was no obvious selection bias, as all tests were collected from these centers. ^{13}C-UBT in the gastroenterology clinical laboratories was used in subjects with gastrointestinal symptoms, such as dyspepsia, peptic ulcers and gastric malignancy. UBT was given to patients after a three-hour fast.

Exclusion criteria included: a) administration of antibiotics and/or bismuth preparations within four weeks prior to date of entry to the study; b) administration of proton pump inhibitors within 2 weeks prior to date of entry to the study; and c) pregnant or breast-feeding women. The challenges were separated into positive (DOB > 5 within 20 minutes) and negative test results (DOB < 5 within 20 minutes). Test date, country, device number, DOB, final result time (time at which the test result was obtained) and duration of the entire test were recorded. In addition, we specifically searched for the number of individuals who had an inconclusive result after 20 minutes (within 1 DOB of the threshold, as described above).

Statistical Analyses
Continuous variables are summarized by mean, standard deviation (SD), minimum, median and maximum and are compared by a t-test (two groups) or ANOVA (3 groups or more). Categorical variables are summarized by a count and percentage and compared by a chi-squared test. Since so few tests were inconclusive, subjects with inconclusive results were excluded from the analyses. In addition, there were 27 test subjects for whom duration of examination was incorrectly recorded due to a software bug. Therefore, these cases were also excluded from analyses of test duration.

Results

Prevalence of H. pylori

The diagnosis distribution was evaluated in all sites within each country. Italy - 7, Israel - 5 and Germany, The Netherlands and Switzerland, with only one site each. All sites had one device per site except for Switzerland, with two.

Study data are presented in Table 1. Out of 12,751 tests performed (Table 1), only 0.1% of the test results were inconclusive. Analysis of the *H. pylori* prevalence by country revealed a statistically significant difference in prevalence among the countries evaluated in the study. Germany had the lowest prevalence with 13.3% and Israel the highest with 44.1% (Table 2).

Duration of the Testing Procedure

The duration of the test procedure from initiation until completion (overall test duration) and the amount of time required until the device was able to provide a diagnosis (test duration until diagnosis) was compared. We found significant differences in both overall duration and time to diagnosis obtained among the three possible outcomes: positive, negative and inconclusive: a positive diagnosis had the shortest duration and an inconclusive result had the longest duration (Table 1). Significant differences in both overall duration and time to diagnosis between the countries were also found.

Overall, test duration was 15.1 minutes in Germany versus approximately 13 minutes in other countries. This may have been due to the low prevalence of *H. pylori* in Germany (Table 2) which lead to a longer test duration (Table 3). Diagnosis was obtained after approximately 9 minutes in Israel, Italy and Switzerland, but after 10 minutes in The Netherlands and Germany. Significant differences in both overall duration and time to diagnosis among the sites were also demonstrated, where the shortest mean overall test duration was 12.7 minutes in Italy versus approximately 15 minutes in Israel and Germany. Diagnosis was obtained after approximately 9 minutes in three Israeli sites, one Italian site and a little over 10 minutes on average in The Netherlands, Germany and two Italian sites. Similar results were obtained between devices within their respective countries, which may validate the differences as country- related and not device- related.

No significant differences were found in overall test duration between tests performed in the morning (until 4 pm) versus tests performed in the afternoon/evening (4 pm or later).

Delta Over Baseline Values (DOB)

Diagnosis, given by the BreathID™ device, was derived by evaluating the DOB value. The mean DOB value for a negative diagnosis was 1.03 (± 0.86) with a range of 0.9 to 5, whereas the positive cases had a mean DOB of 20.2 (± 18.9) and a range of 5.1 through 159.4. Greater variability was seen in DOB means between countries for positively diagnosed subjects than for negative subjects, although this difference was not statistically significant (Table 1).

Discussion

The optimal ^{13}C-UBT conditions for diagnosing *H. pylori* infection are still being perfected. Attempts to improve the ^{13}C-UBT have focused on decreasing the amount of substrate used and reducing the duration of the test. Urita et al. recently reported an ultra short ten second endoscopic UBT using 20 mg of ^{13}C-urea sprayed onto the gastric mucosa. The maximum sensitivity and specificity of intragastric samples were 83.7% and 100% with a cut-off point of 8 per thousand. However, their clinical cohort cannot be compared with ours because of the use of an invasive endoscopic method [6].

No consensus was demonstrated in the evaluation of different ^{13}C-UBT protocols regarding the dosage of the ^{13}C-urea, the time and interval of the breath sample collection or the test meal chosen to delay gastric emptying. Each clinical center used its own test protocol,

Table 1 Distribution of test duration and DOB by diagnosis.

Outcome	N (%)	Distribution	by test	duration	(n = 12,724)*
		Mean ± SD (Minutes)	Minimum (Minutes)	Median (Minutes)	Maximum (Minutes)
Inconclusive	8 (0.1)	18.04 ± 1.76	14.68	18.09	20.35
Negative	8254 (64.8)	10.03 ± 2.24	5.43	10.05	20.58
Positive	4462 (35.1)	8.93 ± 2.55	5.42	8.02	20.90
Outcome	N (%)	Distribution	of DOB by	diagnosis	(n = 12751)
		Mean ± SD	Minimum	Median	Maximum
Inconclusive	8 (0.1)	5.50 ± 0.24	5.20	5.55	5.80
Negative	8268 (64.8)	1.03 ± 0.86	-0.90	1.00	5.00
Positive	4475 (35.1)	20.20 ± 18.89	5.10	13.20	159.4

*(There were 27 tests without duration results, only DOB results (as mentioned in the paper).

Table 2 *H. pylori* prevalence by country

Country	Diagnosis				All
	Negative		Positive		
	N	%	N	%	
Germany	169	86.7	26	13.3	195
Netherland	1671	76.0	529	24.0	2200
Israel	3322	55.9	2619	44.1	5941
Italy	2701	70.1	1154	29.9	3855
Switzerland	405	73.4	147	26.6	552
P value*			< 0.0001		

*Between countries

making comparison of results almost impossible. Although Dominguez-Munoz et al. reported identical sensitivity and 100% specificity of ^{13}C-UBT for three different test meals (0.1 N citric acid solution, semiliquid fatty meal and semiliquid meal), the delta peak values of $^{13}CO_2$ were much higher when a citric acid solution was used as the test drink [7]. Moreover, Graham et al. using 1, 2 and 4 g of citric acid reported that the increase in urease activity was dose dependent [8].

In general, acidic gastric milieu may improve the accuracy of the UBT, probably by increasing the entrance of urea into *H. pylori* and the activity of its cytoplasmic urease, the cornerstone of the urea breath test [9-12]. Acidic gastric juices may also neutralize the ammonia, which may cause bacterial damage by itself and reduce urease activity [13].

A higher acidic gastric environment (pH approximately 2.0) induced by citric acid has been found by several investigators to increase the exhaled CO_2 isotopes (^{13}C or ^{14}C) levels in a dose dependent manner [4,7,8]. To maintain a low gastric pH, we used high dose citric acid, which also delays gastric emptying [14]. However, others have hypothesized that these two factors appear unlikely to be the critical determinants in the increased access of urea to the urease enzyme *in vivo* [15-17].

Hamlet et al. more than a decade ago, examined the efficacy and duration of ^{14}C-UBT using similar methods [18,19]. They reported that by supplying ^{14}C-urea as a

rapid -release tablet along with citric acid, it is possible to shorten the duration of the UBT to 10 minutes with excellent accuracy, even during acid suppression therapy. The tablet-based UBT proved to be accurate during omeprazole treatment, correctly identifying all of the 10 *H. pylori*-infected patients [19].

Chey et al. and our group also demonstrated that intragastric acidification by citrate administration before and during the UBT decreased the false negative results in patients receiving PPI treatment [20-22]. The decreased false negative results induced by PPIs are probably related to the use of citric acid as a test drink. Thus, the data reported by Hamlet et al. are consistent with our data.

An acknowledged weakness of our study was the absence of a gold standard to evaluate the performance of the BreathID® system. However, the device was approved by the FDA in 2001, making it a comparable test to endoscopy in diagnosing *H. pylori*. (The validation trial can be reviewed at link: http://www.accessdata. fda.gov/cdrh_docs/pdf/k011668.pdf).

Since our data is based on raw data from the devices, demographic data is unavailable. The impact of this office- based, fully automated breath collection system, showing immediate results, is that it is activated by a single button, with no need of entering other patient data. Nevertheless, the patient's name/ID can be added to the printout.

Conclusions

The BreathID® test used in our research, performed with a continuous breath test sampling device, collected data from 5 countries over a period of 9 years. Our analysis of 12,791 randomly chosen BreathID™ tests using a high dose citric acid as a test drink and continuous sampling of the expired breath indicated that completion of the UBT required 10-13 minutes on average. Only 8 subjects (0.1%) from the total population had inconclusive results and needed further time to reach a conclusive result. Our results are in agreement with an earlier report using the same technique on a smaller group of examinees [5]. Although this study is

Table 3 Distribution by country of total test duration and test duration until diagnosis

Test duration by country	Test duration (min)						Test duration until diagnosis (min)					
	N	Mean	SD	Minimum	Median	Maximum	N	Mean	SD	Minimum	Median	Maximum
Country												
Germany	195	15.10	4.18	10.43	14.48	32.77	195	10.24	2.43	6.68	10.25	20.18
Netherland	2198	13.36	2.97	6.63	12.95	41.40	2198	10.46	2.58	5.42	10.26	20.48
Israel	5918	13.13	3.18	8.18	12.05	47.12	5918	9.23	2.20	5.62	8.25	20.48
Italy	3853	12.97	3.25	8.17	11.68	55.37	3853	9.78	2.47	5.62	8.65	20.90
Switzerland	552	13.80	4.01	8.53	12.94	33.28	552	9.59	2.47	6.12	8.83	20.38
P value		< 0.0001						< 0.0001				

retrospective and *post hoc* in design, our results provide validation of the usefulness of BreathID® as a short and rapid method in diagnosing *H. pylori*.

Acknowledgements
Funding
The study was supported by Exalenz Ltd.

Author details
[1]Gastroenterology Unit, Hasharon Hospital, Rabin Medical Center, Petach Tikva, Tel-Aviv University, Tel Aviv, Israel. [2]Department of Gastroenterology, Rambam Medical Center, Technion, Haifa, Israel. [3]Gastroenterology Unit, Assaf Harofeh Medical Center, Tel Aviv, Tel-Aviv University, Tel Aviv, Israel. [4]Gastroenterology Unit, Wolfson Medical Center, Holon, Tel-Aviv University, Tel Aviv, Israel.

Authors' contributions
HS-W participated in the design of the study, drafted the manuscript and conceived the study. VS-S collected, analyzed and interpreted the data. RE collected, analyzed and interpreted the data. ES collected, analyzed and interpreted the data. YA collected, analyzed and interpreted the data. HS participated in the design of the study, drafted the manuscript and conceived the study.
All authors read and approved the final manuscript.

Competing interests
The authors declare that they have no competing interests.

References
1. Savarino V, Vigneri S, Celle G: The C urea breath test in the diagnosis of *Helicobacter pylori* infection. *Gut* 1999, 45(Suppl):I18-22.
2. Shirin H, Kenet G, Shevah O, Wardi Y, Birkenfeld S, Shahmurov M, Bruck R, Niv Y, Moss SF, Avni Y: Evaluation of a novel continuous real time ^{13}C urea breath analyzer for *Helicobacter pylori*. *Aliment Pharmacol Ther* 2001, 15:389-394.
3. Levine A, Shevah O, Miloh T, Wine E, Niv Y, Bujanover Y, Avni Y, Shirin H: Validation of a novel real time ^{13}C urea breath test for rapid evaluation of *Helicobacter pylori* in children and adolescents. *J Pediatr* 2004, 145:112-114.
4. Pathak CM, Bhasin DK, Nada R, Bhattacharya A, Khanduja KL: Changes in gastric enviroment with test meals affect the performance of ^{14}C urea breath test. *J Gastroenterol Hepatol* 2005, 20:1260-1265.
5. Israeli E, Ilan Y, Meir SB, Buenavida C, Goldin E: A novel 13C-urea breath test device for the diagnosis of Helicobacter pylori infection: continuous online measurements allow for faster test results with high accuracy. *J Clin Gastroenterol* 2003, 37:139-141.
6. Urita Y, Hike K, Torii N, Kikuchi Y, Watanbe T, Kurakata H, Sugimoto M, Miki K: Ten-second endoscopic breath test using a 20-mg dose of ^{13}C-urea to detect *Helicobacter pylori* infection. *Hepatogastroenterology* 2007, 54:951-954.
7. Dominguez-Munoz JE, Leodolter A, Sauerbruch T, Malfertheiner P: A citric acid solution in an optimal test drink in the ^{13}C-urea breath test for the diagnosis of *Helicobacter pylori* infection. *Gut* 1997, 40:459-462.
8. Graham DY, Runke D, Anderson SY, Malaty HM, Klein PD: Citric acid as the test meal for the ^{13}C-urea breath test. *Am J Gastroenterol* 1999, 94:1214-1217.
9. Rektorschek M, Weeks D, Sachs G, Melchers K: Influence of pH on metabolism and urease activity of *Helicobacter pylori*. *Gastroenterology* 1998, 115:628-641.
10. Scott DR, Weeks D, Hong C, Postius S, Melchers K, Sachs G: The role of internal urease in acid resistance of *Helicobacter pylori*. *Gastroenterology* 1998, 114:58-70.
11. Meyer-Rosberg K, Scott DR, Rex D, Melchers K, Sachs G: The effect of environmental pH on the proton motive force of *Helicobacter pylori*. *Gastroenterology* 1996, 111:886-900.
12. Weeks DL, Eskandari S, Scott DR, Sachs G: A H+ -Gated urea channel: The link between *Helicobacter pylori* urease and gastric colonization. *Science* 2000, 287:482-485.
13. Weil J, Bell GD, Powell K, Morden A, Harrison G, Gant PW, Jones PH, Trowell JE: Omeprazole and *Helicobacter pylori*: temporary suppression rather than true eradication. *Aliment Pharmacol Ther* 1991, 5:309-313.
14. Leodolter A, Dominguez-Munoz JE, Von Arnim U, Malfertheiner P: Citric acid or orange juice for the ^{13}C-urea breath test: the impact of pH and gastric emptying. *Aliment Pharmacol Ther* 1999, 13:1057-1062.
15. Shiotani A, Saeed A, Yamaoka Y, Osato MS, Klein PD, Graham DY: Citric acid-enhanced *Helicobacter pylori* urease activity in vivo is unrelated to gastric emptying. *Aliment Pharmacol Ther* 2001, 15:1763-1767.
16. Agha A, Opekun AR, Abudayyeh S, Graham DY: Effect of different organic acids (citric, malic and ascorbic) on intragastric urease activity. *Aliment Pharmacol Ther* 2005, 21:1145-1148.
17. Oztürk E, Yeşilova Z, Ilgan S, Ozgüven M, Dağalp K: Performance of acidified ^{14}C-urea capsule breath test during pantoprazole and ranitidine treatment. *J Gastroenterol Hepatol* 2009, 24:1248-1251.
18. Hamlet AK, Erlandsson KIM, Olbe L, Backman VEM, Svennerholm A-M, Pettersson AB: A simple, rapid, and highly reliable capsule-based ^{14}C urea breath test for diagnosis of *Helicobacter pylori* infection. *Scand J Gastroenterol* 1995, 30:1058-1063.
19. Hamlet A, Stage L, Lönroth H, Cahlin C, Nyström C, Pettersson A: A novel tablet-based ^{13}C urea breath test for Helicobacter pylori with enhanced performance during acid suppression therapy. *Scand J Gastroenterol* 1999, 34:367-374.
20. Chey WD, Chathadi KV, Montague J, Ahmed F, Murthy U: Intragastric acidification reduces the occurrence of false-negative urea breath test results in patients taking a proton pump inhibitor. *Am J Gastroenterol* 2001, 96:1028-1032.
21. Shirin H, Frenkel D, Shevah O, Levine A, Bruck R, Moss SF, Niv Y, Avni Y: Effect of proton pump inhibitors on the continuous real time ^{13}C-urea breath test. *Am J Gastroenterol* 2003, 98:46-50.
22. Levine A, Shevah O, Shabat-Sehayek V, Aeed H, Boaz M, Moss SF, Niv Y, Avni Y, Shirin H: Masking of ^{13}C urea breath test by proton pump inhibitors is dependent on type medication: comparison between omeprazole, pantoprazole, lansoprazole and esomeprazole. *Aliment Pharmacol Ther* 2004, 20:117-122.

24

Association between *Helicobacter pylori cagA*-related genes and clinical outcomes in Colombia and Japan

Masahide Watada[1,2], Seiji Shiota[1,2], Osamu Matsunari[1,2], Rumiko Suzuki[1], Kazunari Murakami[2], Toshio Fujioka[2] and Yoshio Yamaoka[1,3*]

Abstract

Background: Specific genotypes of several virulence factors of *Helicobacter pylori* (eg, *cagA*-positive, *vacA* s1, *oipA* "on" and *babA*-positive) have been reported to be predictors of severe clinical outcomes. Importantly, the presence of these genotypes correlates with each other. We hypothesized that novel virulence genes correlate with the presence of *cagA*. Therefore, we aimed to find novel candidate virulence genes that correlate with *cagA* and examined the association of these genes with clinical outcomes in Colombian and Japanese populations.

Methods: *cagA*-associated genes were selected based on previous *H. pylori* genome microarray data. A total of 343 strains (174 from Colombia and 169 from Japan) were examined for the status of *cagA*, *vacA*, and candidate genes by polymerase chain reaction and dot blot.

Results: Microarray data showed that 9 genes were significantly correlated with the presence of *cagA*. Among the 9 genes, the functions of 4 were known, and we selected these 4 genes as candidate genes (*hp0967*, *jhp0045*, *jhp0046*, and *jhp0951*). The prevalences of *cagA*, *vacA* s1/m1 genotype, and *hp0967* were significantly higher in Japan than Colombia, whereas those of *jhp0045* and *jhp0046* were more prevalent in Colombia than Japan. The prevalences of *jhp0045* and *jhp0046* in *cagA*-positive cases of gastric cancer were significantly higher than those from gastritis in Colombia (P = 0.015 and 0.047, respectively). In contrast, the prevalence of 4 candidate genes was independent of clinical outcomes in Japan.

Conclusions: *jhp0045* and *jhp0046* might be novel markers for predicting gastric cancer in *cagA*-positive cases in Colombia, but not in Japan.

Background

Helicobacter pylori (*H. pylori*) infection is now accepted as the major cause of chronic gastritis. In addition, several epidemiological studies have shown that *H. pylori* infection is linked to severe gastritis-associated diseases, including peptic ulcer and gastric cancer (GC) [1]. In 1994, the International Agency for Research on Cancer categorized *H. pylori* infection as a group I carcinogen [2]. Although GC is one of the most common cancers, only a minority of individuals with *H. pylori* infection ever develop it. The prevalence of GC is approximately 3% in *H. pylori*-positive patients [3].

In addition to environmental factors (eg, diet) and host factors, virulence factors of *H. pylori*, such as *cagA*, *vacA*, *oipA*, *babA*, *hopQ*, and *homA/B*, have been demonstrated to be predictors of gastric atrophy, intestinal metaplasia, and severe clinical outcomes [4-10]. The most studied virulence factor of *H. pylori* is *cagA*, which is located at the end of an approximately 40-kb cluster of genes called *cag* pathogenicity island (PAI). *cag* PAI encodes a type-IV secretion system and transfers CagA protein into host cells [11]. CagA protein is believed to have oncogenic potential [12,13], and *cagA*-positive strains are reported to be associated with severe clinical outcomes [14].

* Correspondence: yyamaoka@oita-u.ac.jp
[1]Department of Environmental and Preventive Medicine, Oita University Faculty of Medicine, 1-1 Idaigaoka, Hasama-machi, Yufu-City, Oita 879-5593, Japan

However, these factors are not enough to distinguish markers for severe outcomes (eg, GC) in Japan because most *H. pylori* strains isolated in Japan possess these virulence factors. Likewise, our previous report showed that these genes were not virulence markers for GC in Colombia [10]. Importantly, the presence of these genotypes correlate with each other; the *cagA*-positive strain usually possesses the *vacA* s1/m1 genotype, and it is further closely linked to the presence of *babA* and *oipA* "on" status [14]. Therefore, we hypothesized that novel virulence genes correlate with the presence of *cagA*. Although *cagA* is not a distinguishing marker for severe outcomes in Japan and Colombia, the importance of *cagA* has been shown in both in vitro and in vivo experiments [14]. For example, our study showed that histological scores were significantly higher in *cagA*-positive subjects than *cagA*-negative ones, even in Japan [15]. Therefore, subjects infected with *cagA*-positive *H. pylori* can be considered as a higher risk population than those with *cagA*-negative strains, even in Japan and Colombia. However, only a minority of individuals with *cagA*-positive *H. pylori* infection develop severe outcomes in both countries. This suggests that other virulence factors in *cagA*-positive strains are necessary to develop severe outcomes.

Previous whole *H. pylori* genome microarray data revealed that several genes were associated with the presence of *cagA* and/or clinical outcomes. For example, Romo-González et al. examined 42 *H. pylori* strains and found that several genes were associated with gastroduodenal diseases [16]. In addition, Salama et al. used the microarray of 15 *H. pylori* strains and identified several genes that correlated with the presence of *cag* PAI [17], although they did not examine the association between these genes and clinical outcomes. However, these microarray data are not sufficient as conclusive evidence of the association due to the small sample size. Previously, we also performed whole *H. pylori* genome microarray and examined 1,531 genes, including *cagA*, in 56 *H. pylori* strains isolated from several countries [18].

In this study, we aimed to find novel candidate virulence genes that correlate with the presence of *cagA*, and we examined the association of these genes with clinical outcomes in Colombian and Japanese populations.

Methods
Microarray experiments

Initially, candidate genes were selected from previous studies by Salama et al. [17] and Romo-González et al. [16]. Microarray data from 56 strains in our previous report was then used for the examination of the association of candidate virulence genes with the presence of *cagA* [18].

Patients

H. pylori strains were obtained from the gastric mucosa of *H. pylori*-infected patients who underwent endoscopy at Oita University Faculty of Medicine, Oita, Japan, and Universidad Nacional de Colombia, Bogota, Colombia. Presentations included gastritis, duodenal ulcer (DU), gastric ulcer (GU), and GC. DU, GU, and GC were identified by endoscopy, and GC was further confirmed by histopathology. Gastritis was defined as *H. pylori* gastritis in the absence of peptic ulcers or gastric malignancy. Patients with a history of partial gastric resection were excluded. Patients who received *H. pylori* eradication therapy or treatment with antibiotics, bismuth-containing compounds, H2-receptor blockers, or proton pump inhibitors within 4 weeks prior to the study were also excluded. Informed consent was obtained from all participants, and the protocol was approved by the ethics committees of Oita University and Universidad Nacional de Colombia.

H. pylori genotyping

Antral biopsy specimens were obtained for the isolation of *H. pylori* using standard culture methods, as previously described [19]. Chromosomal DNA was extracted from confluent plate cultures expanded from a single colony using a commercially available kit (QIAGEN Inc., Valencia, CA, USA). Two *H. pylori* strains with full-sequenced genomes, 26695 (ATCC 700392) and J99 (ATCC 700824) deposited in the GenBank, were used as control strains. The *cagA* status was determined by polymerase chain reaction (PCR) using primer pair 5'-ACC CTA GTC GGT AAT GGG-3' and 5'-GCT TTA GCT TCT GAY ACY GC-3' (Y = C+T), as described previously [20]. The *vacA* genotyping (s1, s2, m1, and m2) was performed by PCR, as described previously [21,22]. Primers for the signal region yielded a fragment of 259 bp for s1 variants and one of 286 bp for s2 variants. Primers for the middle region yielded a fragment of 570 bp for m1 variants and one of 645 bp for m2 variants.

Two primer sets for each candidate gene were designed with software Primer 3 (version. 0.4.0) based on the published sequences of *H. pylori* (Table 1). Amplification of *H. pylori* genomic DNA sequences was carried out in a total volume of 25 μL containing 2.5 μL of PCR buffer, 0.2 mM of each deoxynucleotide, 0.625 U of Blend Taq DNA polymerase (Blend Taq, Toyobo Co., Ltd., Osaka, Japan), 0.2 μM of each primer, and more than 10 ng of *H. pylori* DNA. Each reaction mixture was amplified as follows: initial denaturation at 94°C for 5 min, which was followed by 30 cycles of denaturation at 94°C for 30 s, annealing at the indicated temperature in Table 1 for 30 s, extension at 72°C for 1 min, and then final extension at 72°C for 5 min. The

Table 1 Primer sequences

Primer Name	Primer Sequence (5'-3') Forward	Primer Sequence (5'-3') Reverse	AT (°C)	Product size
hp0967-1	CATGGCTTTAAATGGCAACA	CCGGCATTAAATCGTTGTTT	58	169
hp0967-2	TAGCGTGTATTTTGGCGATG	GATAGCCGGCATTAAATCGT	59	151
jhp0045-1	TGGCAAAAGAGTCCAAGACA	CGTTGCAATAAAAACGCAGA	59	180
jhp0045-2	AAAACAACGCCTGGTATTGC	GATTGCACTTTATGCGTGTGA	60	158
jhp0046-1	AAGCAAGCGATAATGTCATGG	AATTGAGCGTTTTGGTGTCC	59	154
jhp0046-2	AGCAAGCGATAATGTCATGG	AATTGAGCGTTTTGGTGTCC	58	153
jhp0951-1	CAAAGCGTGAATGATTTGGA	AGATTGCGCAAGGATTTGAG	56	194
jhp0951-2	ATGCGTGGCTAAGCGATACT	GACCCAACGCTCTTGAAGTT	57	243

AT; annealing temperature

amplified fragment was detected by 2.0% agarose gel electrophoresis using an ultraviolet transilluminator.

Dot blot

For each sample, 500 ng of total DNA was added to 100 μL of TE buffer and mixed with 100 μL of a denaturing buffer (0.5 M NaOH; 1.5 M NaCl). The denatured DNA was transferred to a Hybond-N$^+$ membrane (GE Health-Care, Piscataway, NJ, USA) by means of a Bio-Dot Microfiltration Apparatus (Bio-Rad Laboratories, Inc., Hercules, CA, USA). DNA of J99 and human DNA were also transferred to the membrane and used as positive and negative controls, respectively. The membranes were hybridized at 42°C overnight in plastic bags containing ECL Gold hybridization buffer supplemented with 5% (wt/vol) blocking agent and 0.5 M NaCl. The membranes were washed 3 times in primary washing buffer (0.5× SSC [1× SSC is 0.15 M NaCl plus 0.015 M sodium citrate] [pH 7.0], 0.4% sodium dodecyl sulfate) at room temperature for 15 min and 3 times in secondary washing buffer (2× SSC) at room temperature for 15 min. Finally, the membranes were exposed to Hyperfilm ECL film (GE HealthCare). Gene status was considered positive when at least one of the PCR reactions was positive. When gene status was considered negative by PCR, we further confirmed the results using dot-blot analyses. If PCR results yielded negative results but the dot blot showed a positive blot, we considered the samples positive.

DNA sequencing

DNA sequencing for the full length of jhp0045 (1,032 bp) was performed with several primer pairs located at jhp0044 and jhp0046. Likewise, DNA sequencing for the full length of jhp0046 (783 bp) was performed with several primer pairs located at jhp0045 and jhp0047. PCR products were purified with Centri-sep Columns (Applied Biosystems by Life Technologies, Tokyo, Japan), and the amplified fragments were sequenced with Hi-Di Formamide (Applied Biosystems by Life Technologies) using an ABI Prism 310 Genetic Analyzer (Applied

Biosystems by Life Technologies, Carlsbad, CA, USA) in accordance with the manufacturer's instructions.

Statistical analysis

Variables such as gender, mean age, and the presence of each candidate gene and cagA were evaluated. The univariate association between each genotype and the clinical outcomes were quantified by the chi-square test. A multivariate logistic regression model was used to calculate the odds ratios (OR) of the clinical outcomes by including age, sex, and H. pylori genotypes. All determinants with P values of < 0.10 were entered together in the full model of logistic regression, and the model was reduced by excluding variables with P values of > 0.10. ORs and 95% confidence intervals (CIs) were used to estimate the risk. Spearman rank coefficients (r) were also determined to evaluate the association between the different genotypes of the strains. A P value of less than 0.05 was accepted as statistically significant. The SPSS statistical software package version 18.0 (IBM Corporation, Armonk, NY, USA) was used for all statistical analyses.

Results
Selection of candidate genes

Twelve genes that were strongly associated with cagA status in the report by Salama et al. [17] were selected. In addition, 26 genes that were associated with severe gastric diseases in the report by Romo-González et al. [16] were selected. Because hp1426 was reported in both reports, a total of 37 genes were selected as candidate genes, as shown in additional file 1.

Among the 37 genes, the status of 9 genes (hp0186, hp0713, hp0967, hp1409, hp1410, jhp0045, jhp0046, jhp0950, and jhp0951) were significantly correlated with the cagA status in our microarray data [18] (P = 0.026, 0.026, 0.014, 0.048, 0.030, 0.033, 0.033, 0.017, and 0.005 for each above gene, respectively). Among the 9 genes, 4 genes (hp0967, jhp0045, jhp0046, and jhp0951) were selected in our analyses because the functions of these genes are known. The presence of 3 genes (hp0967, jhp0045, and jhp0046) was inversely correlated with the presence of *cagA*, but that of *jhp0951* was positively correlated with the presence of *cagA*. We examined the presence of these candidate genes in 28 full sequenced strains deposited in Genbank. The *hp0967*, *jhp0045*, *jhp0046*, and *jhp0951* were found in 18, 7, 7, and 13 strains, respectively.

Prevalence of candidate genes in Japan and Colombia

The distribution of the status of *cagA*, *vacA*, *hp0967*, *jhp0045*, *jhp0046*, and *jhp0951* in the two countries is shown in Table 2. Three samples from Colombia showed the positive for both *vacA* m1 and m2 genotypes, which suggest the mixed infection, were excluded in the final analysis. Finally, a total of 343 patients were included in this study: 174 from Colombia (68 with gastritis, 43 with DU, and 63 with GC) and 169 from Japan (49 with gastritis, 50 with DU, 50 with GU, and 20 with GC). The results from PCR and dot blot matched well: there were no cases with negative results by PCR and only positive results by dot blot. There were significant differences in the status of *cagA*, *hp0967*, *jhp0045*, and *jhp0046* between strains isolated from Japanese and Colombian populations. The prevalence of *cagA* was 100% in Japan, whereas it was 65.5% in Colombia (P < 0.0001). Higher prevalences of *vacA* s1 and m1 genotypes were found in Japan than Colombia (100 vs. 76.8%, P < 0.001; 100 vs. 62.7%, < 0.001, respectively). The prevalence of *hp0967* was significantly higher in Japan than Colombia (62.1 vs. 48.0%, P = 0.013). However, the prevalences of *jhp0045* and *jhp0046* were more prevalent in Colombia than Japan (23.7 vs. 8.9%, P < 0.0001; 28.2 vs. 8.9%, P < 0.0001, respectively). There was no difference in the prevalence of *jhp0951* between the 2 countries.

The association between candidate genes and clinical outcomes in Colombia

The prevalence of each gene was examined according to clinical outcomes. The prevalence of the *vacA* m1 genotype was significantly higher in strains from patients with GC than those with gastritis (75.0 vs. 55.1%, P = 0.014) (Table 2). Although it is accepted that *cagA* is an important virulence factor, the prevalence of *cagA* was not different between the strains from patients with DU, GC, and gastritis in Colombia (61.4, 70.3, and 63.8%, P > 0.05), which was in agreement with our previous study [23]. Therefore, we hypothesized that the presence/absence of novel factors that accompany the presence of *cagA* leads to severe clinical outcomes in the Colombian population. Based on this hypothesis, the prevalences of these 4 candidate genes were examined in the *cagA*-positive cases. In *cagA*-positive cases, *vacA* status was not associated with clinical outcomes. Interestingly, the prevalence of *jhp0045* in *cagA*-positive cases from GC was significantly higher than that of gastritis (30.4 vs. 11.4%, P = 0.023) (Table 3). The prevalence of *jhp0046* in *cagA*-positive cases from GC also tended to be higher than that of gastritis (34.8 vs. 18.2%, P = 0.06), although this did not reach statistical significance. However, there were no associations of these candidates between gastritis and DU. Table 4 shows the association determined by a multivariate analysis between clinical outcomes and the presence of *jhp0045* or *jhp0046* in *cagA*-positive cases in the Colombian population. After adjustment for age and gender, *jhp0045* was an independent factor for discriminating GC from gastritis in *cagA*-positive cases (adjusted OR = 3.24; 95% CI = 1.00-10.42; Table 4). Likewise, *jhp0046* was an independent factor for discriminating GC from gastritis in *cagA*-positive cases (adjusted OR = 3.16; 95% CI = 1.05-9.47). On the other hand, the prevalences of *hp0967* and *jhp0951* in *cagA*-positive cases were not associated with clinical outcomes.

The association between candidate genes and clinical outcomes in Japan

All samples from Japan showed *cagA*-positive and *vacA* s1m1. The prevalences of the 4 candidate genes in

Table 2 Relationship between each gene and clinical outcomes in Colombia

n	Total 174		gastritis 68		DU 43		P	GC 63		P
mean age	53.4 ± 16.4		52.0 ± 16.5		48.4 ± 15.9		0.50	58.1 ± 15.5		0.01
male	90	(50.8%)	28	(40.6%)	22	(50.0%)	0.30	40	(62.5%)	0.01
cagA	116	(65.5%)	44	(63.8%)	27	(61.4%)	0.83	45	(70.3%)	0.41
vacA s1	136	(76.8%)	50	(72.5%)	33	(75.0%)	0.70	54	(84.4%)	0.08
vacA m1	111	(62.7%)	38	(55.1%)	26	(59.1%)	0.63	48	(75.0%)	0.01
hp0967	85	(48.0%)	33	(47.8%)	20	(45.5%)	0.83	32	(50.0%)	0.79
jhp0045	42	(23.7%)	14	(20.3%)	13	(29.5%)	0.24	15	(23.4%)	0.65
jhp0046	50	(28.2%)	18	(26.1%)	15	(34.1%)	0.34	17	(26.6%)	0.94
jhp0951	102	(57.6%)	40	(58.0%)	26	(59.1%)	0.86	36	(56.3%)	0.84

DU, duodenal ulcer; GC, gastric cancer
*P value was compared with gastritis

Table 3 Relationship between each gene and clinical outcomes in *cagA*-positive cases in Colombia

n	Gastritis 44		DU 27		P	GC 45		P
mean age	51.0 ± 15.3		47.2 ± 14.3		0.51	57.6 ± 14.3		0.02
male	19	(43.2%)	13	(46.4%)	0.68	31	(67.4%)	0.02
vacA s1	42	(95.5%)	24	(85.7%)	0.27	42	(91.3%)	0.51
vacA m1	33	(75.0%)	19	(67.9%)	0.66	36	(78.3%)	0.37
hp0967	24	(54.5%)	12	(42.9%)	0.40	27	(58.7%)	0.60
jhp0045	5	(11.4%)	7	(25.0%)	0.10	14	(30.4%)	0.02
jhp0046	8	(18.2%)	7	(25.0%)	0.43	16	(34.8%)	0.06
jhp0951	25	(56.8%)	19	(67.9%)	0.25	27	(58.7%)	0.76

DU, duodenal ulcer; GC, gastric cancer
*P value was compared with gastritis

cagA-positive cases were independent of clinical outcomes (Table 5).

Sequence analysis of *jhp0045* and *jhp0046* in Colombia and Japan

In order to clarify whether the sequence variants in *jhp0045* and *jhp0046* contributed to the different outcomes in Colombia and Japan, sequences of these 2 genes were compared using 8 randomly selected strains. For *jhp0045*, one-point mutation in the Japanese strains was found at 643-bp position of J99 (A643G). Therefore, the amino acid was changed from Ile to Val. The sequence of *jhp0045* from the Colombian strains matched with J99. On the other hand, there was no difference in the sequence of *jhp0046* between the strains from the 2 countries.

Nucleotide sequence accession numbers

The nucleotide sequences of *jhp0045* and *jhp0046* for 8 strains (Japanese strains: 01-401, 04-156, 05-262, and 07-238; Colombian strains: Colombia 64, Colombia 114, Colombia 174, and Colombia 229) have been deposited in the GenBank database under accession no. AB647162 to AB647169 for *jhp0045* and AB647170 to AB647176 for *jhp0046*, respectively.

Table 4 Multivariate analyses of the risk for GC by age, gender, and *jhp0045* or *jhp0046* status in *cagA*-positive cases in Colombia

	Adjusted OR	95% CI	P
Age (per 1 year)	1.02	0.99-1.05	0.10
Gender (male)	3.19	1.29-7.89	0.01
jhp0045	3.24	1.00-10.42	0.04
Age (per 1 year)	1.02	0.99-1.05	0.11
Gender (male)	3.15	1.27-7.80	0.01
jhp0046	3.16	1.05-9.47	0.03

CI, confidence interval; GC, gastric cancer; OR, odds ratio

Discussion

Our study revealed that *jhp0045* and *jhp0046* were independent discriminating factors for GC from gastritis in *cagA*-positive cases in Colombia. This suggests that *jhp0045* and *jhp0046* play a role in high-risk subjects, such as *cagA*-positive *H. pylori*-infected cases.

Several genes of *H. pylori* were reported as virulence factors, and these include *cagA, vacA, oipA, babA, hopQ*, and *homA/B* [4-10]. Importantly, most virulence factors correlated with each other; *cagA*-positive strains also possess the *vacA* s1/m1 genotype, and this is closely linked to the presence of the *babA* and *oipA* "on" status [14]. Therefore, we hypothesized that undefined novel virulence genes could exist in genes correlated with *cagA* status. Although previous microarray data showed that several genes correlated with *cagA* status, the sample number in these microarray reports was not enough to be conclusive (eg, [15] strains in the report by Salama *et al.* [17]). Among the 37 genes we selected, 9 genes were significantly correlated with the presence of *cagA*. In the present study, we focused on 4 genes whose functions have been revealed. *hp0967* is considered a virulence-associated protein D, and *jhp0951*, which encodes an integrase of the XerCD family, has been reported to be related to modifications in the response to low pH and iron limitations [16,24]. The putative functions of *jhp0045* and *jhp0046* have been described as type-II DNA methyltransferase and type-II restriction enzymes, respectively [17,25].

Among these 4 genes, *jhp0045* and *jhp0046* were significantly associated with severe clinical outcomes in *cagA*-positive cases in Colombia. Although *hp0967* has been reported to be negatively associated with DU [16], there was no association in this study. The *jhp0951* has been positively associated with DU [16]; however, an association was not found in this study. These findings suggest that these microarray data are not conclusive. A larger group of subjects is necessary to clarify the association.

Table 5 Prevalence of each gene and relationship between each gene and clinical outcomes in Japan

	Total		gastritis		DU		P	GU		P	GC		P
n	169		49		50			50			20		
mean age	60.0 ± 12.8		59.3 ± 12.8		56.0 ± 13.6		0.19	62.9 ± 12.1		0.25	64.3 ± 9.4		0.13
male	91	(53.8%)	24	(49.0%)	29	(58.0%)	0.36	27	(54.0%)	0.61	11	(55.0%)	0.65
cagA	169	(100.0%)	49	(100.0%)	50	(100.0%)	-	50	(100.0%)	-	20	(100.0%)	-
vacA s1	169	(100.0%)	49	(100.0%)	50	(100.0%)	-	50	(100.0%)	-	20	(100.0%)	-
vacA m1	169	(100.0%)	49	(100.0%)	50	(100.0%)	-	50	(100.0%)	-	20	(100.0%)	-
hp0967	105	(62.1%)	30	(61.2%)	31	(62.0%)	0.93	34	(68.0%)	0.48	10	(50.0%)	0.39
jhp0045	15	(8.9%)	2	(4.1%)	6	(12.0%)	0.14	5	(10.0%)	0.22	2	(10.0%)	0.32
jhp0046	15	(8.9%)	2	(4.1%)	6	(12.0%)	0.14	5	(10.0%)	0.22	2	(10.0%)	0.32
jhp0951	108	(63.9%)	31	(63.3%)	30	(60.0%)	0.73	35	(70.0%)	0.47	12	(60.0%)	0.80

DU, duodenal ulcer; GU, gastric ulcer; GC, gastric cancer

The mechanisms of the development of GC in those patients infected with *jhp0045* or *jhp0046* are unclear, although the putative functions of *jhp0045* and *jhp0046* have been described as a type-II DNA methyltransferase and a type-II restriction enzyme, respectively [17,25]. In this study, most strains possessing *jhp0045* had *jhp0046*. This suggests that these 2 genes may work together. This combination of a restriction enzyme and a methyltransferase is known as a restriction-modification (R-M) system [26]. It has been reported that *H. pylori* possess an extraordinary number of genes with homology to R-M genes in other bacterial species [25,27,28]. However, not all R-M systems have that function. Kong *et al.* reported that, among the 16 completely tested Type II R-M systems in J99, only 4 were fully functional in that they contained both active endonucleases and methylases [29]. The *jhp0045* and *jhp0046* were included in these functional ones. Because several R-M systems are correlated with pathogenicity [26], strains possessing *jhp0045* and *jhp0046* may be considered as truly virulent strains. Interestingly, recent reports showed that *H. pylori* strains possessing *cagA* from Colombia can be divide into 2 groups by 7 housekeeping genes [30]. This grouping was related with severe histological scores and the prevalence of GC. The *jhp0045* and *jhp0046* may be a discriminating factor for this grouping. Further study is necessary in order to examine the relationship between *jhp0045* and *jhp0046* and the grouping by 7 housekeeping genes.

Only 1 change of an amino acid resulted from a point mutation of *jhp0045* in Japanese strains compared with Colombian strains and J99. It is not clear whether this difference contributed to the different results between the 2 countries. Variants of virulence factors in different areas may result in different clinical outcomes. For example, *cagA* can be divided into 2 types (East-Asian-type *cagA* and Western-type *cagA*) according to differences in the 3' region [6,20,21]. Some reports have shown that individuals infected with East-Asian-type

cagA strains have an increased risk of peptic ulcer or GC compared to those infected with Western-type *cagA* strains [31,32]. Further studies to clarify the mechanisms or functions according to the different amino acid sequences are necessary to explain this.

Our study had several limitations. First, not only the *H. pylori* virulence factors, but also environmental factors (eg, diet) and host factors have been demonstrated to be predictors of severe clinical outcomes [33]. Especially, inflammatory cytokine gene polymorphisms (*IL-1* gene cluster, *TNF-α*, *IL-10*, and *IL-8*) have been reported to be correlated with gastric cancer [34-39]. Further study will be necessary in order to elucidate the role of our candidate genes of *H. pylori*. Second, we did not examine known virulence factors other than *cagA* and *vacA* of *H. pylori*. It is possible that our candidate genes might correlate with other known virulence factors, even in *cagA*-positive cases. It is better to examine host factors and other known virulence factors in order to clarify the role of our candidate genes in future studies. Finally, we examined the status of the genes by only positivity or negativity. The levels of gene expression can be affected by clinical outcomes. In addition, gene expression is not always correlated with protein expression patterns. For example, the expression of the blood group antigen-binding adhesin (BabA) protein is not always correlated with *babA* gene expression [40]. Further analysis using real-time PCR or immunoblotting techniques is necessary to clarify the significance of our candidate genes.

Conclusions

The *jhp0045* and *jhp0046* were associated with GC in *cagA*-positive cases in Colombia but not in Japan. In Colombia, the status of *jhp0045* and *jhp0046* may predict the future development of GC for patients with gastritis. A prospective study is necessary to confirm this. Moreover, the study of the distribution of these genes in other populations would be interesting in order to further elucidate the associations found in the present study and the possible virulence role of these factors in *H. pylori* infection.

Acknowledgements
This report is based on work supported in part by grants from the National Institutes of Health (DK62813), grants-in-aid for Scientific Research from the Ministry of Education, Culture, Sports, Science, and Technology (MEXT) of Japan (22390085, 22659087 and 30583778), and Special Coordination Funds for Promoting Science and Technology from MEXT of Japan. The authors would like to thank Ms. Kudo, Ms. Matsuda, and Ms. Takahashi for their excellent technical assistance.
Financial support: None

Author details
[1]Department of Environmental and Preventive Medicine, Oita University Faculty of Medicine, 1-1 Idaigaoka, Hasama-machi, Yufu-City, Oita 879-5593, Japan. [2]Department of General Medicine, Oita University Faculty of Medicine, 1-1 Idaigaoka, Hasama-machi, Yufu-City, Oita 879-5593, Japan. [3]Department of Medicine-Gastroenterology, Baylor College of Medicine and Michael E. DeBakey Veterans Affairs Medical Center, 2002 Holcombe Blvd., Houston, Texas 77030 USA.

Authors' contributions
Conceived and designed the experiments: MW SS YY. Performed experiments: MW OM. Analyzed the data: MW SS RS YY. Contributed reagents/materials/analysis tools: MW OM SS YY KM TF. Wrote the paper: MW SS YY. All authors read and approved the final manuscript.

Competing interests
The authors declare that they have no competing interests.

References
1. Suerbaum S, Michetti P: **Helicobacter pylori infection.** *N Engl J Med* 2002, **347**(15):1175-1186.
2. **Schistosomes, liver flukes and Helicobacter pylori.** IARC Working Group on the Evaluation of Carcinogenic Risks to Humans. Lyon, 7-14 June 1994. *IARC Monogr Eval Carcinog Risks Hum* 1994, **61**:1-241.
3. Uemura N, Okamoto S, Yamamoto S, Matsumura N, Yamaguchi S, Yamakido M, Taniyama K, Sasaki N, Schlemper R: **Helicobacter pylori infection and the development of gastric cancer.** *N Engl J Med* 2001, **345**(11):784-789.
4. Jung SW, Sugimoto M, Graham DY, Yamaoka Y: **homB status of Helicobacter pylori as a novel marker to distinguish gastric cancer from duodenal ulcer.** *J Clin Microbiol* 2009, **47**(10):3241-3245.
5. Lu H, Hsu PI, Graham DY, Yamaoka Y: **Duodenal ulcer promoting gene of Helicobacter pylori.** *Gastroenterology* 2005, **128**(4):833-848.
6. Yamaoka Y, Kodama T, Kashima K, Graham DY, Sepulveda AR: **Variants of the 3' region of the cagA gene in Helicobacter pylori isolates from patients with different H. pylori-associated diseases.** *J Clin Microbiol* 1998, **36**(8):2258-2263.
7. Yamaoka Y, Kwon DH, Graham DY: **A M(r) 34,000 proinflammatory outer membrane protein (oipA) of Helicobacter pylori.** *Proc Natl Acad Sci USA* 2000, **97**(13):7533-7538.
8. Sugimoto M, Zali MR, Yamaoka Y: **The association of vacA genotypes and Helicobacter pylori-related gastroduodenal diseases in the Middle East.** *Eur J Clin Microbiol Infect Dis* 2009, **28**(10):1227-1236.
9. Ohno T, Sugimoto M, Nagashima A, Ogiwara H, Vilaichone RK, Mahachai V, Graham DY, Yamaoka Y: **Relationship between Helicobacter pylori hopQ genotype and clinical outcome in Asian and Western populations.** *J Gastroenterol Hepatol* 2009, **24**(3):462-468.
10. Yamaoka Y, Kikuchi S, el-Zimaity HM, Gutierrez O, Osato MS, Graham DY: **Importance of Helicobacter pylori oipA in clinical presentation, gastric inflammation, and mucosal interleukin 8 production.** *Gastroenterology* 2002, **123**(2):414-424.
11. Backert S, Selbach M: **Role of type IV secretion in Helicobacter pylori pathogenesis.** *Cell Microbiol* 2008, **10**(8):1573-1581.
12. Hatakeyama M: **Oncogenic mechanisms of the Helicobacter pylori CagA protein.** *Nat Rev Cancer* 2004, **4**(9):688-694.
13. Hatakeyama M: **Helicobacter pylori CagA – a bacterial intruder conspiring gastric carcinogenesis.** *Int J Cancer* 2006, **119**(6):1217-1223.
14. Yamaoka Y: **Mechanisms of disease: Helicobacter pylori virulence factors.** *Nat Rev Gastroenterol Hepatol* 2010, **7**(11):629-641.
15. Yamaoka Y, Kita M, Kodama T, Sawai N, Kashima K, Imanishi J: **Induction of various cytokines and development of severe mucosal inflammation by cagA gene positive Helicobacter pylori strains.** *Gut* 1997, **41**(4):442-451.
16. Romo-González C, Salama NR, Burgeño-Ferreira J, Ponce-Castañeda V, Lazcano-Ponce E, Camorlinga-Ponce M, Torres J: **Differences in genome content among Helicobacter pylori isolates from patients with gastritis, duodenal ulcer, or gastric cancer reveal novel disease-associated genes.** *Infect Immun* 2009, **77**(5):2201-2211.
17. Salama N, Guillemin K, McDaniel TK, Sherlock G, Tompkins L, Falkow S: **A whole-genome microarray reveals genetic diversity among Helicobacter pylori strains.** *Proc Natl Acad Sci USA* 2000, **97**(26):14668-14673.
18. Gressmann H, Linz B, Ghai R, Pleissner KP, Schlapbach R, Yamaoka Y, Kraft C, Suerbaum S, Meyer TF, Achtman M: **Gain and loss of multiple genes during the evolution of Helicobacter pylori.** *PLoS Genet* 2005, **1**(4):e43.
19. Yamaoka Y, Kodama T, Kita M, Imanishi J, Kashima K, Graham D: **Relationship of vacA genotypes of Helicobacter pylori to cagA status, cytotoxin production, and clinical outcome.** *Helicobacter* 1998, **3**(4):241-253.
20. Yamaoka Y, Osato M, Sepulveda A, Gutierrez O, Figura N, Kim J, Kodama T, Kashima K, Graham D: **Molecular epidemiology of Helicobacter pylori: separation of H. pylori from East Asian and non-Asian countries.** *Epidemiol Infect* 2000, **124**(1):91-96.
21. Yamaoka Y, El-Zimaity H, Gutierrez O, Figura N, Kim J, Kodama T, Kashima K, Graham D, Kim J: **Relationship between the cagA 3' repeat region of Helicobacter pylori, gastric histology, and susceptibility to low pH.** *Gastroenterology* 1999, **117**(2):342-349.
22. van Doorn L, Figueiredo C, Sanna R, Plaisier A, Schneeberger P, de Boer W, Quint W: **Clinical relevance of the cagA, vacA, and iceA status of Helicobacter pylori.** *Gastroenterology* 1998, **115**(1):58-66.
23. Yamaoka Y, Kodama T, Gutierrez O, Kim JG, Kashima K, Graham DY: **Relationship between Helicobacter pylori iceA, cagA, and vacA status and clinical outcome: studies in four different countries.** *J Clin Microbiol* 1999, **37**(7):2274-2279.
24. Gancz H, Censini S, Merrell DS: **Iron and pH homeostasis intersect at the level of Fur regulation in the gastric pathogen Helicobacter pylori.** *Infect Immun* 2006, **74**(1):602-614.
25. Alm RA, Ling LS, Moir DT, King BL, Brown ED, Doig PC, Smith DR, Noonan B, Guild BC, deJonge BL, et al: **Genomic-sequence comparison of two unrelated isolates of the human gastric pathogen Helicobacter pylori.** *Nature* 1999, **397**(6715):176-180.
26. Ando T, Ishiguro K, Watanabe O, Miyake N, Kato T, Hibi S, Mimura S, Nakamura M, Miyahara R, Ohmiya N, et al: **Restriction-modification systems may be associated with Helicobacter pylori virulence.** *J Gastroenterol Hepatol* 2010, **25**(Suppl 1):S95-98.
27. Tomb JF, White O, Kerlavage AR, Clayton RA, Sutton GG, Fleischmann RD, Ketchum KA, Klenk HP, Gill S, Dougherty BA, et al: **The complete genome sequence of the gastric pathogen Helicobacter pylori.** *Nature* 1997, **388**(6642):539-547.
28. Akopyants NS, Fradkov A, Diatchenko L, Hill JE, Siebert PD, Lukyanov SA, Sverdlov ED, Berg DE: **PCR-based subtractive hybridization and differences in gene content among strains of Helicobacter pylori.** *Proc Natl Acad Sci USA* 1998, **95**(22):13108-13113.
29. Kong H, Lin LF, Porter N, Stickel S, Byrd D, Posfai J, Roberts RJ: **Functional analysis of putative restriction-modification system genes in the Helicobacter pylori J99 genome.** *Nucleic Acids Res* 2000, **28**(17):3216-3223.
30. de Sablet T, Piazuelo MB, Shaffer CL, Schneider BG, Asim M, Chaturvedi R, Bravo LE, Sicinschi LA, Delgado AG, Mera RM, et al: **Phylogeographic origin of Helicobacter pylori is a determinant of gastric cancer risk.** *Gut* 2011.
31. Vilaichone RK, Mahachai V, Tumwasorn S, Wu JY, Graham DY, Yamaoka Y: **Molecular epidemiology and outcome of Helicobacter pylori infection in Thailand: a cultural cross roads.** *Helicobacter* 2004, **9**(5):453-459.

32. Jones KR, Joo YM, Jang S, Yoo YJ, Lee HS, Chung IS, Olsen CH, Whitmire JM, Merrell DS, Cha JH: **Polymorphism in the CagA EPIYA motif impacts development of gastric cancer.** *J Clin Microbiol* 2009, **47(4)**:959-968.

33. Tsugane S, Sasazuki S: **Diet and the risk of gastric cancer: review of epidemiological evidence.** *Gastric Cancer* 2007, **10(2)**:75-83.

34. El-Omar E, Carrington M, Chow W, McColl K, Bream J, Young H, Herrera J, Lissowska J, Yuan C, Rothman N, *et al*: **Interleukin-1 polymorphisms associated with increased risk of gastric cancer.** *Nature* 2000, **404(6776)**:398-402.

35. Machado JC, Pharoah P, Sousa S, Carvalho R, Oliveira C, Figueiredo C, Amorim A, Seruca R, Caldas C, Carneiro F, *et al*: **Interleukin 1B and interleukin 1RN polymorphisms are associated with increased risk of gastric carcinoma.** *Gastroenterology* 2001, **121(4)**:823-829.

36. El-Omar EM, Rabkin CS, Gammon MD, Vaughan TL, Risch HA, Schoenberg JB, Stanford JL, Mayne ST, Goedert J, Blot WJ, *et al*: **Increased risk of noncardia gastric cancer associated with proinflammatory cytokine gene polymorphisms.** *Gastroenterology* 2003, **124(5)**:1193-1201.

37. Machado JC, Figueiredo C, Canedo P, Pharoah P, Carvalho R, Nabais S, Castro Alves C, Campos ML, Van Doorn LJ, Caldas C, *et al*: **A proinflammatory genetic profile increases the risk for chronic atrophic gastritis and gastric carcinoma.** *Gastroenterology* 2003, **125(2)**:364-371.

38. Sugimoto M, Furuta T, Shirai N, Nakamura A, Xiao F, Kajimura M, Sugimura H, Hishida A: **Different effects of polymorphisms of tumor necrosis factor-alpha and interleukin-1 beta on development of peptic ulcer and gastric cancer.** *J Gastroenterol Hepatol* 2007, **22(1)**:51-59.

39. Sugimoto M, Furuta T, Shirai N, Nakamura A, Kajimura M, Sugimura H, Hishida A: **Effects of interleukin-10 gene polymorphism on the development of gastric cancer and peptic ulcer in Japanese subjects.** *J Gastroenterol Hepatol* 2007, **22(9)**:1443-1449.

40. Yamaoka Y: **Roles of *Helicobacter pylori* BabA in gastroduodenal pathogenesis.** *World J Gastroenterol* 2008, **14(27)**:4265-4272.

Permissions

The contributors of this book come from diverse backgrounds, making this book a truly international effort. This book will bring forth new frontiers with its revolutionizing research information and detailed analysis of the nascent developments around the world.

We would like to thank all the contributing authors for lending their expertise to make the book truly unique. They have played a crucial role in the development of this book. Without their invaluable contributions this book wouldn't have been possible. They have made vital efforts to compile up to date information on the varied aspects of this subject to make this book a valuable addition to the collection of many professionals and students.

This book was conceptualized with the vision of imparting up-to-date information and advanced data in this field. To ensure the same, a matchless editorial board was set up. Every individual on the board went through rigorous rounds of assessment to prove their worth. After which they invested a large part of their time researching and compiling the most relevant data for our readers.

The editorial board has been involved in producing this book since its inception. They have spent rigorous hours researching and exploring the diverse topics which have resulted in the successful publishing of this book. They have passed on their knowledge of decades through this book. To expedite this challenging task, the publisher supported the team at every step. A small team of assistant editors was also appointed to further simplify the editing procedure and attain best results for the readers.

Apart from the editorial board, the designing team has also invested a significant amount of their time in understanding the subject and creating the most relevant covers. They scrutinized every image to scout for the most suitable representation of the subject and create an appropriate cover for the book.

The publishing team has been an ardent support to the editorial, designing and production team. Their endless efforts to recruit the best for this project, has resulted in the accomplishment of this book. They are a veteran in the field of academics and their pool of knowledge is as vast as their experience in printing. Their expertise and guidance has proved useful at every step. Their uncompromising quality standards have made this book an exceptional effort. Their encouragement from time to time has been an inspiration for everyone.

The publisher and the editorial board hope that this book will prove to be a valuable piece of knowledge for researchers, students, practitioners and scholars across the globe.

List of Contributors

Chidi V Nweneka and Andrew M Prentice
Nutrition Programme, Medical Research Council Laboratories, The Gambia, Banjul, The Gambia

Andrew M Prentice
MRC International Nutrition Group, London School of Hygiene and Tropical Medicine, Keppel Street, London, UK

Kazuhiro Watanabe, Naoyoshi Nagata, Ryo Nakashima, Etsuko Furuhata, Toshiyuki Sakurai, Naoki Akazawa, Chizu Yokoi, Masao Kobayakawa and Junichi Akiyama
Department of Gastroenterology and Hepatology, National Center for Global Health and Medicine, 1-21-1 Toyama, Shinjuku-ku, Tokyo 162-8655, Japan

Takuro Shimbo
Department of Clinical Research and Informatics, National Center for Global Health and Medicine, 1-21-1 ToyamaShinjuku-ku, Tokyo 162-8655, Japan

Masashi Mizokami
Research Center for Hepatitis and Immunology, National Center for Global Health and Medicine, Kohnodai Hospital, 1-7-1 Kohnodai, Ichikawa City, Chiba 272-8516, Japan

Naomi Uemura
Department of Gastroenterology and Hepatology, National Center for Global Health and Medicine, Kohnodai Hospital, 1-7-1 Kohnodai, Ichikawa City, Chiba 272-8516, Japan

Hassan Momtaz
Department of Microbiology, Faculty of Veterinary Medicine, ShahreKord Branch, Islamic Azad University, ShahreKord, Iran

Hossein Dabiri
Department of Medical Microbiology, Faculty of Medicine, Shahid Beheshti University of Medical Science, Tehran, Iran

Negar Souod
Young Researchers and Elite club, Central Tehran Branch, Islamic Azad University, Tehran, Iran

Mohsen Gholami
Graduated of Veterinary Medicine, Faculty of Veterinary Medicine, ShahreKord Branch, Islamic Azad University, ShahreKord, Iran

Carolina Rosal Teixeira de Souza, Aline Damasceno Seabra, Raquel Carvalho Montenegro and Rommel Rodríguez Burbano
Laboratório de Citogenética Humana, Instituto de Ciências Biológicas, Universidade Federal do Pará, Rua Augusto Corrêa, 01 – Guamá. CEP 66075-110. Caixa postal 479, Belém, PA, Brasil

Kátia Soares de Oliveira
Instituto de Ciências da Saúde, Universidade Federal do Pará, Belém, PA, Brasil

Jefferson José Sodré Ferraz
Centro Universitário do Pará, Belém, PA, Brasil

Mariana Ferreira Leal
Departamento de Ortopedia e Traumatologia, Universidade Federal de São Paulo, São Paulo, SP, Brazil

Marília Cardoso Smith and Mariana Ferreira Leal
Disciplina de Genética, Departamento de Morfologia e Genética, Universidade Federal de São Paulo, São Paulo, SP, Brasil

Paulo Pimentel Assumpção, Danielle Queiroz Calcagno and André Salim Khayat
Núcleo de Pesquisa em Oncologia, Universidade Federal do Pará, Belém, PA, Brasil

Ana Paula Negreiros Nunes Alves
Departamento de Patologia Oral, Faculdade de Odontologia, Universidade Federal do Ceará, Fortaleza, CE, Brasil

Nuno Almeida, José Manuel Romãozinho and Carlos Sofia
Gastroenterology Department, Centro Hospitalar e Universitário de Coimbra, Praceta Mota Pinto e Avenida Bissaya Barreto, 3000-075 Coimbra, Portugal

Maria Manuel Donato, Alexandra Fernandes, Carlos Calhau, José Manuel Romãozinho and Carlos Sofia
Gastroenterology Centre, Faculty of Medicine, Coimbra University, Praceta Mota Pinto e Avenida Bissaya Barreto, 3000-075 Coimbra, Portugal

Cristina Luxo and Olga Cardoso
Laboratory of Microbiology, Faculty of Pharmacy, Coimbra University, Azinhaga de Santa Comba, 3000-548 Coimbra, Portugal

Maria Augusta Cipriano and Carol Marinho
Pathology Department, Coimbra University Hospital Centre, Praceta Mota Pinto e Avenida Bissaya Barreto, 3000-075 Coimbra, Portugal

Shahidi Jamaludin, Nazri Mustaffa, Syed Hassan Syed Abdul Aziz and Yeong Yeh Lee
School of Medical Sciences, Universiti Sains Malaysia, Kubang Kerian, Kelantan, Malaysia

Nor Aizal Che Hamzah
Pasir Gudang Specialist Hospital, Pasir Gudang, Johor, Malaysia

Yanan Gong, Xianhui Peng, Lihua He, Hao Liang, Yuanhai You and Jianzhong Zhang
State Key Laboratory of Infectious Disease Prevention and Control, National Institute for Communicable Disease Control and Prevention, Chinese Center for Disease Control and Prevention, 155 Changbai Road, Changping District, Beijing 102206, China

Yanan Gong, Xianhui Peng, Lihua He, Hao Liang, Yuanhai You and Jianzhong Zhang
Collaborative Innovation Center for Diagnosis and Treatment of Infectious Diseases, Hangzhou, China

Kosuke Sakitani, Nobumi Suzuki, Ayako Yanai, Kei Sakamoto, Masao Akanuma, Yasuhiko Iwamoto and Shoji Kawazu
The Institute for Adult Diseases, Asahi Life Foundation, 2-2-6 Bakuro-cho, Nihon-Bashi, Chuo-ku, Tokyo 113-8655, Japan

Satoki Shichijo, Takako Serizawa, Kazuhiko Koike, Yutaka Yamaji and Yoshihiro Hirata
Department of Gastroenterology, Graduate School of Medicine, The University of Tokyo, Tokyo, Japan

Shin Maeda
Gastroenterology Division, Yokohama City University Graduate School of Medicine, Yokohama, Japan

Ju Yup Lee and Nayoung Kim
Department of Internal Medicine, Seoul National University Bundang Hospital, Seongnam, South Korea

Kyung Sik Park and Ju Yup Lee
Department of Internal Medicine, Keimyung University School of Medicine, Daegu, South Korea

Hyun Jin Kim
Department of Internal Medicine and Institute of Health Science, Gyeongsang National University School of Medicine, Jinju, Gyeongsangnam-do, South Korea

Seon Mee Park
Department of Internal Medicine, College of Medicine, Chungbuk National University, Cheongju, South Korea

Gwang Ho Baik
Department of Internal Medicine, Hallym University College of Medicine, Chuncheon Sacred Heart Hospital, Chuncheon, South Korea

Ki-Nam Shim
Department of Internal Medicine, Ewha Womans University School of Medicine, Seoul, South Korea

Jung Hwan Oh
Departments of Internal Medicine, College of Medicine, The Catholic University of Korea, Seoul, Republic of Korea

Suck Chei Choi
Department of Internal Medicine, Wonkwang University School of Medicine, Iksan, South Korea

Sung Eun Kim
Department of Internal Medicine, Kosin University College of Medicine, Busan, South Korea

Won Hee Kim
Digestive Disease Center, CHA Bundang Medical Center, CHA University, Seongnam, South Korea

Seon-Young Park
Department of Internal Medicine, Chonnam National University Medical School, Gwangju, South Korea

Gwang Ha Kim and Bong Eun Lee
Department of Internal Medicine, Pusan National University School of Medicine and Biomedical Research Institute, Pusan National University Hospital, Busan, South Korea

Yunju Jo
Department of Internal Medicine, Eulji General Hospital, Eulji University School of Medicine, Seoul, South Korea

Su Jin Hong
Department of Internal Medicine and Research Institute, Soonchunhyang University College of Medicine, Bucheon, South Korea

Chika Kasai, Kazushi Sugimoto, Isao Moritani, Junichiro Tanaka, Yumi Oya, Hidekazu Inoue, Masahiko Tameda, Katsuya Shiraki and Kojiro Takase
Department of Gastroenterology, Mie Prefectural General Medical Center, Yokkaichi, Japan

Masahiko Tameda and Kazushi Sugimoto
Department of Molecular and Laboratory Medicine, Mie University School of Medicine, 2-174 Edobashi, Tsu, Mie 514-8507, Japan

Yoshiyuki Takei, Masahiko Tameda and Kazushi Sugimoto
Department of Gastroenterology and Hepatology, Mie University School of Medicine, Tsu, Japan

Masaaki Ito
Department of Cardiology and Nephrology, Mie University School of Medicine, Tsu, Japan

Li-Wei Chen, Bor-Jen Hsieh, Shuo-Wei Chen and Rong-Nan Chien
Departments of Gastroenterology and Hepatology, Chang-Gung Memorial Hospital and University, 12F, No 222, Mai-Jin Road, Keelung, Taiwan

Liang-Che Chang
Departments of Pathology, Chang-Gung Memorial Hospital and University, 12F, No 222, Mai-Jin Road, Keelung, Taiwan

Chung-Ching Hua
Departments of Internal Medicine, Chang-Gung Memorial Hospital and University, 12F, No 222, Mai-Jin Road, Keelung, Taiwan

Diogo Branquinho, Nuno Almeida, Carlos Gregório, José Eduardo Pina Cabral, Adriano Casela and Luís Tomé
Gastroenterology Department, Coimbra University Hospital, Praceta Prof. Mota Pinto, 3000-075 Coimbra, Portugal

Maria Manuel Donato, Luís Tomé, Diogo Branquinho and Nuno Almeida
Gastroenterology Centre, Faculty of Medicine, Coimbra University, R. Larga, 3004-504 Coimbra, Portugal

Chao Lu, Lan Li, Chaohui Yu and Ping Xu
Department of Gastroenterology, the First Affiliated Hospital, College of Medicine, Zhejiang University, No. 79 Qingchun Road, Hangzhou 310003, China

Ye Yu
Department of Rheumatology, the First Affiliated Hospital, College of Medicine, Zhejiang University, Hangzhou 310003, China

Bo-Lin Pan, Chih-Fang Huang, Jui-Chin Chiang and Song-Seng Loke
Department of Family Medicine, Kaohsiung Chang Gung Memorial Hospital and Chang Gung University College of Medicine, 123, Dapi Road, Niaosong District, Kaohsiung 833, Taiwan

Seng-Kee Chuah
Division of Hepatogastroenterology, Department of Internal Medicine, Kaohsiung Chang Gung Memorial Hospital and Chang Gung University College of Medicine, 123, Dapi Road, Niaosong District, Kaohsiung 833, Taiwan

Patricio Gonzalez-Hormazabal, V. Gonzalo Castro and Lilian Jara
Human Genetics Program, Institute of Biomedical Sciences, School of Medicine, University of Chile, Av. Independencia 1027, 8380453 Santiago, CL, Chile

Susana Escandar, Zoltan Berger, Maher Musleh, Hector Valladares and Enrique Lanzarini
Department of Gastroenterology, University of Chile Clinical Hospital, Santiago, Chile

Maher Musleh, Hector Valladares and Enrique Lanzarini
Department of Surgery, University of Chile Clinical Hospital, Santiago, Chile

Rodrigo Buzinaro Suzuki
Department of Genotyping, Hemocenter, Marilia Medical School, Marilia, SP, Brazil

Cristiane Maria Almeida and Márcia Aparecida Sperança
Department of Molecular Biology, Marilia Medical School, Marilia, SP, Brazil

Márcia Aparecida Sperança and Rodrigo Buzinaro Suzuki
Center of Natural and Human Sciences, Universidade Federal do ABC, Rua Santa Adélia, 166 Bloco A, Torre 3, 6° andar, Sala 625, CEP 09210-170 Bairro Bangu, Santo André, SP, Brazil

Jing Jiang, Zhi-Fang Jia, Fei Kong and Suyan Tian
Division of Clinical Epidemiology, Jilin University First Hospital, Changchun, China

Mei-Shan Jin and Yin-Ping Wang
Division of Pathology, Jilin University First Hospital, Changchun, China

Xueyuan Cao and Jian Suo
Department of Gastric and Colorectal Surgery, Jilin University First Hospital, Changchun, China

Harald E Vonkeman and MAFJ van deLaar
Arthritis Center Twente, Department of Rheumatology and Clinical Immunology, Medisch Spectrum Twente Hospital and University of Twente, 7500 KA Enschede, The Netherlands

HTJI deLeest, KSS Steen, WF Lems and BAC Dijkmans
Department of Rheumatology, VU University Medical Center and Jan van Breemen Institute, Amsterdam, The Netherlands

J vanBaarlen
Laboratorium Pathologie Oost-Nederland, Enschede, The Netherlands

JWJ Bijlsma
Department of Rheumatology and Clinical Immunology, University Medical Center Utrecht, Utrecht, The Netherlands

EJ Kuipers
Department of Gastroenterology and Hepatology, Erasmus MC UniversityMedical Center, Rotterdam, The Netherlands

HHML Houben
Department of Rheumatology, Atrium Medical Center, Heerlen, The Netherlands

M Janssen
Department of Rheumatology, Rijnstate Hospital, Arnhem, The Netherlands

Ding-You Li
Department of Pediatrics, University of Missouri Kansas City School of Medicine, Division of Gastroenterology, Children's Mercy Hospital, 2401 Gillham Road, Kansas City, MO 64108, USA

Min Yang, Yongmei Zeng, Zhenwen Zhou, Huimin Xia, Sitang Gong, Zhiying Ou, Liya Xiong, Lanlan Geng, Lixia Li and Peiyu Chen
Department of Gastroenterology, Guangzhou Women and Children's Medical Center, Guangzhou Medical College, 9 Jinsui Road, Guangzhou 510623, China

Tomás Navarro-Rodriguez, Fernando Marcuz Silva, Ricardo Correa Barbuti, Rejane Mattar, Joaquim Prado Moraes-Filho, Maricê Nogueira de Oliveira, Cristina S Bogsan, Décio Chinzon and Jaime Natan Eisig
Serviço de Gastroenterologia Clínica do Hospital das Clínicas da Faculdade de Medicina da Universidade de São Paulo, Av. Dr. Enéas de Carvalho Aguiar, 255 – Cerqueira Cezar, São Paulo, SP, Brasil

Chin-Hsiao Tseng
Department of Internal Medicine, National Taiwan University Hospital, No. 7 Chung-Shan South Road, Taipei, Taiwan
Department of Internal Medicine, National Taiwan University College of Medicine, Taipei, Taiwan

Weili Liu, Leimin Sun and Jianmin Si
Gastroenterology laboratory, Clinical Research Institute, Sir Run Run Shaw Hospital, School of Medicine, Zhejiang University, 310016 Hangzhou, People's Republic of China

Yan Chen
Department of Gastroenterology, Second Affiliated Hospital, School of Medicine, Zhejiang University, Hangzhou, People's Republic of China

Gaofeng Lu
Department of thoracic surgery, Zhejiang Hospital, Hangzhou, People's Republic of China

Hemda Schmilovitz-Weiss and Vered Sehayek-Shabat
Gastroenterology Unit, Hasharon Hospital, Rabin Medical Center, Petach Tikva, Tel-Aviv University, Tel Aviv, Israel

Rami Eliakim
Department of Gastroenterology, Rambam Medical
Center, Technion, Haifa, Israel

Haim Shirin and Eitan Skapa
Gastroenterology Unit, Assaf Harofeh Medical Center,
Tel Aviv, Tel-Aviv University, Tel Aviv, Israel

Yona Avni
Gastroenterology Unit, Wolfson Medical Center,
Holon, Tel-Aviv University, Tel Aviv, Israel

**Masahide Watada, Seiji Shiota, Osamu Matsunari,
Rumiko Suzuki and Yoshio Yamaoka**
Department of Environmental and Preventive
Medicine, Oita University Faculty of Medicine, 1-1
Idaigaoka, Hasama-machi, Yufu-City, Oita 879-
5593, Japan

**Masahide Watada, Seiji Shiota, Osamu Matsunari,
Kazunari Murakami and Toshio Fujioka**
Department of General Medicine, Oita University
Faculty of Medicine, 1-1 Idaigaoka, Hasama-machi,
Yufu-City, Oita 879-5593, Japan

Yoshio Yamaoka
Department of Medicine-Gastroenterology, Baylor
College of Medicine and Michael E. DeBakey
Veterans Affairs Medical Center, 2002 Holcombe
Blvd., Houston, Texas 77030 USA

Index